Fractional Mathematical Modelling: Theory, Methods and Applications

Fractional Mathematical Modelling: Theory, Methods and Applications

Guest Editors

Faranak Rabiei
Dongwook Kim
Zeeshan Ali

MDPI

Basel • Beijing • Wuhan • Barcelona • Belgrade • Novi Sad • Cluj • Manchester

Guest Editors

Faranak Rabiei
Department of Mathematics
Texas A&M University
Kingsville
Kingsville, TX
USA

Dongwook Kim
Department of Mathematics
Texas A&M University
Kingsville
Kingsville, TX
USA

Zeeshan Ali
School of Science
Monash University
Sunway
Malaysia

Editorial Office
MDPI AG
Grosspeteranlage 5
4052 Basel, Switzerland

This is a reprint of the Special Issue, published open access by the journal *Fractal and Fractional* (ISSN 2504-3110), freely accessible at: https://www.mdpi.com/journal/fractalfract/special_issues/GY37SR31H3.

For citation purposes, cite each article independently as indicated on the article page online and as indicated below:

Lastname, A.A.; Lastname, B.B. Article Title. *Journal Name* **Year**, *Volume Number*, Page Range.

ISBN 978-3-7258-5511-7 (Hbk)
ISBN 978-3-7258-5512-4 (PDF)
https://doi.org/10.3390/books978-3-7258-5512-4

Contents

About the Editors

Faranak Rabiei

Faranak Rabiei is an Assistant Professor in the Department of Mathematics, Texas A&M University Kingsville, USA. Her research interests are in areas of numerical analysis, computational mathematics, mathematical modeling, fractional calculus, and fuzzy logic. Dr. Rabiei has published several research articles in high-ranked journals.

Dongwook Kim

Dongwook Kim is an Associate Professor in the Department of Mathematics at Texas A&M University Kingsville, USA. His research focuses on differential equations, numerical analysis, mathematical biology modeling, nonlinear stability analysis, computational mathematics, and computational neuroscience. He has authored several works on computational approaches to mathematical models, with applications in biology, engineering, and applied sciences.

Zeeshan Ali

Zeeshan Ali is a Lecturer in Mathematics in the School of Science, Monash University Malaysia. He earned his PhD in Applied Mathematics in 2023 from the School of Engineering at Monash University Malaysia. His research expertise includes mathematical modeling, mathematical biology, fractional calculus, nonlinear analysis, boundary value problems, AI-based models, and numerical analysis. He has published numerous research articles in reputable journals and has presented his work at international conferences.

Preface

This Reprint brings together a collection of recent research contributions that explore the theoretical foundations, methodological advances, and practical applications of fractional calculus. Its central focus is on fractional differential and integral equations, their analytical and numerical treatment, and their effectiveness in modeling complex systems with memory and nonlocal effects.

The scope of the Reprint extends from rigorous studies of new fractional operators and solution techniques to innovative applications in engineering, physics, materials science, biology, and medicine. The aim is to provide a comprehensive resource that highlights the versatility of fractional approaches in addressing problems that are beyond the reach of classical models.

The motivation for compiling this Reprint is to support the scientific community with a unified volume in which theoretical developments, methodological advances, and practical applications are represented side by side. It reflects the growing interest in fractional models as powerful tools that bridge pure mathematics with real-world challenges.

This Reprint is intended for mathematicians, engineers, physicists, biologists, applied scientists, and graduate students. By presenting a balanced view of mathematical rigor, computational methods, and interdisciplinary applications, it is designed to serve as both a reference and a source of inspiration for future research in fractional mathematical modelling.

Faranak Rabiei, Dongwook Kim, and Zeeshan Ali
Guest Editors

fractal and fractional

MDPI

Editorial

Fractional Mathematical Modelling: Theory, Methods and Applications

Faranak Rabiei [1,*], Dongwook Kim [1] and Zeeshan Ali [2,*]

1 Department of Mathematics, Texas A&M University Kingsville, 700 University Blvd., Kingsville, TX 78363, USA; dongwook.kim@tamuk.edu

2 School of Science, Monash University Malaysia Jalan Lagoon Selatan, Bandar Sunway 47500, Selangor, Malaysia

* Correspondence: faranak.rabiei@tamuk.edu (F.R.); zeeshan.ali@monash.edu or zeeshanmaths1@gmail.com (Z.A.)

1. Introduction

Fractional calculus shares its historical roots with classical calculus and has lately become a powerful mathematical tool for modeling complex systems. The concept dates back to 1695, when L'Hôpital posed a question to Leibniz about the possibility of a derivative of non-integer order, later developed by Liouville, Riemann, Caputo, Grünwald, Letnikov, Hadamard, and others [1–3]. These contributions have led to the establishment of multiple definitions of fractional-order operators, each with distinct advantages and limitations [4]. By extending classical calculus through fractional operators, it captures memory, hereditary effects, and nonlocal interactions [5,6]. Unlike integer-order models, fractional formulations are uniquely capable of describing processes with long-term memory and anomalous diffusion. Its wide-ranging applications in physics, engineering, biology, medicine and health sciences, finance, and the social sciences [7–10] make it an indispensable tool for analyzing complex processes. In recent years, the field has gained remarkable momentum, supported by the introduction of new operators, improvements in numerical schemes, and diverse real-world applications [11,12]. These advances have strengthened its theoretical foundations while expanding its practical relevance, positioning fractional calculus as a unifying framework that bridges mathematics with diverse applications.

Building on this broad relevance, the aim of this Reprint is to showcase recent advances in fractional calculus across theory, methodology, and applications. Out of 51 submissions received, 12 high-quality papers were accepted for publication, giving an acceptance rate of 23.5%. The selected contributions highlight new operator formulations, analytical results, numerical techniques, and interdisciplinary applications ranging from control theory and fuzzy systems to engineering devices, materials science, and biomedical systems. The rapid pace of progress in the field, particularly with the emergence of novel operator definitions, advanced numerical techniques, and diverse real-world applications, motivated the launch of this Reprint. By bringing together contributions from different perspectives, it provides a concise snapshot of current developments in fractional calculus and serves as a resource to foster further collaboration across diverse disciplines.

2. Overview of the Contributions in the Reprint

The contributions in this Reprint are grouped into three main themes, in line with the Special Issue: theoretical developments, methodological advances, and applications.

Fractal Fract. **2025**, *9*, 636 https://doi.org/10.3390/fractalfract9100636

2.1. Theoretical Developments

Theoretical developments are illustrated in two contributions. Albidah (1.) investigated two forms of the Riemann–Liouville derivative for second-order fractional differential equations, showing that the choice of lower bound yields either implicit solutions in terms of Mittag-Leffler functions or explicit solutions involving trigonometric and hyperbolic functions. Alkandari et al. (2.) developed anomalous diffusion models using regularized general fractional derivatives with Sonin kernels, linking them to continuous-time random walks and deriving explicit expressions for waiting-time densities, mean squared displacement, and conditions ensuring non-negativity and maximum principles.

2.2. Methodological Advances

Methodological advances are demonstrated in several papers. Sengül et al. (3.) employed the optimal q-Homotopy Analysis Method to study Abel-type equations, demonstrating improved convergence and accuracy over classical approaches. AlBaidani (4.) compared the homotopy perturbation transform method with a new iterative method for the time-fractional Burger-Fisher equation, showing that both approaches yield reliable and computationally efficient solutions, further validated against techniques such as Haar wavelets, OHAM, and q-HATM. Abdelfattah et al. (5.) extended the fractional differential quadrature method (FDQM) to nonlinear Riccati and Lorenz systems using generalized Caputo derivatives, demonstrating superior accuracy and convergence compared with existing methods.

2.3. Applications

Applications are explored across fuzzy systems, engineering models, materials science, and biomedical systems. Muhammad et al. (6.) analyzed fuzzy fractional two-dimensional continuous-time linear systems based on Roesser and Fornasini-Marchesini models, using granular Laplace transforms to address parameter uncertainty and validating their approach with applications in signal processing and wireless sensor networks. Al-Dosari (7.) examined Hilfer fuzzy fractional inclusions with infinite delay, proving controllability of mild solutions through nonlinear functional analytic techniques and establishing new results supported by the properties of Mittag-Leffler functions.

Engineering and materials science applications include Yu et al. (8.), who proposed a Caputo-Fabrizio-based model of a fractional-order boost converter with inductive loads, constructing both large- and small-signal models and confirming their accuracy through simulations. Xu et al. (9.) introduced a fractional-order Zener model incorporating temperature-order equivalence for viscoelastic dampers, validated experimentally and optimized using a chaotic fractional-order particle swarm algorithm. García-de-los-Ríos et al. (10.) applied fractional models to ZnO micro- and nanostructures, explaining photoconduction and nonlinear optical effects relevant for optoelectronic devices. Abdelfattah et al. (11.) applied FDQM to simulate charge dynamics in polymer solar cells, achieving high accuracy and efficiency.

In the biomedical field, Mihai et al. (12.) proposed a personalized fractional-order autotuner for the maintenance phase of anaesthesia. Using small-amplitude sine tests to non-invasively estimate patient parameters, they designed a fractional-order PID controller to regulate the Bispectral Index during Propofol infusion. Closed-loop simulations confirmed the effectiveness of this approach, highlighting its potential for clinical practice.

3. Concluding Remarks

The contributions gathered in this Reprint reflect the richness and vitality of fractional calculus research today. They bring together rigorous theoretical work, efficient numerical methods, and impactful applications spanning engineering, materials science, physics, and medicine. As guest editors, we are grateful to the authors for their contributions, the reviewers for their careful evaluations, and the editorial team of *Fractal and Fractional* for their support. We hope this collection will serve as a valuable reference for the research community and stimulate further studies at the intersection of mathematics, engineering, and applied sciences, reinforcing the role of fractional calculus as a unifying tool across disciplines.

Funding: This research received no external funding.

Conflicts of Interest: The authors declare no conflict of interest.

List of Contributions:

1. Albidah, A.B. Application of Riemann–Liouville Derivatives on Second-Order Fractional Differential Equations: The Exact Solution. *Fractal Fract.* **2023**, *7*, 843. https://doi.org/10.3390/fractalfract7120843.
2. Alkandari, M.; Loutchko, D.; Luchko, Y. Anomalous Diffusion Models Involving Regularized General Fractional Derivatives with Sonin Kernels. *Fractal Fract.* **2025**, *9*, 363. https://doi.org/10.3390/fractalfract9060363.
3. Şengül, S.; Bekiryazici, Z.; Merdan, M. Approximate Solutions of Fractional Differential Equations Using Optimal q-Homotopy Analysis Method: A Case Study of Abel Differential Equations. *Fractal Fract.* **2024**, *8*, 533. https://doi.org/10.3390/fractalfract8090533.
4. AlBaidani, M.M. Comparative Study of the Nonlinear Fractional Generalized Burger–Fisher Equations Using the Homotopy Perturbation Transform Method and New Iterative Transform Method. *Fractal Fract.* **2025**, *9*, 390. https://doi.org/10.3390/fractalfract9060390.
5. Abdelfattah, W.M.; Ragb, O.; Salah, M.; Mohamed, M. A Robust and Versatile Numerical Framework for Modeling Complex Fractional Phenomena: Applications to Riccati and Lorenz Systems. *Fractal Fract.* **2024**, *8*, 647. https://doi.org/10.3390/fractalfract8110647.
6. Muhammad, G.; Akram, M.; Alsulami, H.; Hussain, N. Granular Fuzzy Fractional Continuous-Time Linear Systems: Roesser and Fornasini–Marchesini Models. *Fractal Fract.* **2025**, *9*, 398. https://doi.org/10.3390/fractalfract9070398.
7. Al-Dosari, A.A.M. Controllability of Mild Solution to Hilfer Fuzzy Fractional Differential Inclusion with Infinite Continuous Delay. *Fractal Fract.* **2024**, *8*, 235. https://doi.org/10.3390/fractalfract8040235.
8. Yu, D.; Liao, X.; Wang, Y. Modeling and Analysis of Caputo–Fabrizio Definition-Based Fractional-Order Boost Converter with Inductive Loads. *Fractal Fract.* **2024**, *8*, 81. https://doi.org/10.3390/fractalfract8020081.
9. Xu, K.; Chen, L.; Lopes, A.M.; Wang, M.; Wu, R.; Zhu, M. Fractional-Order Zener Model with Temperature–Order Equivalence for Viscoelastic Dampers. *Fractal Fract.* **2023**, *7*, 714. https://doi.org/10.3390/fractalfract7100714.
10. Garcia-de-los-Rios, V.M.; Arano-Martínez, J.A.; Trejo-Valdez, M.; Hernández-Pichardo, M.L.; Vidales-Hurtado, M.A.; Torres-Torres, C. Fractional Photoconduction and Nonlinear Optical Behavior in ZnO Micro and Nanostructures. *Fractal Fract.* **2023**, *7*, 885. https://doi.org/10.3390/fractalfract7120885.
11. Abdelfattah, W.M.; Ragb, O.; Salah, M.; Matbuly, M.S.; Mohamed, M. Fractional Partial Differential Equation Modeling for Solar Cell Charge Dynamics. *Fractal Fract.* **2024**, *8*, 729. https://doi.org/10.3390/fractalfract8120729.
12. Mihai, M.D.; Birs, I.R.; Badau, N.E.; Hegedus, E.T.; Ynineb, A.; Muresan, C.I. Personalised Fractional-Order Autotuner for the Maintenance Phase of Anaesthesia Using Sine-Tests. *Fractal Fract.* **2025**, *9*, 317. https://doi.org/10.3390/fractalfract9050317.

References

1. Oliveira, E.C.D.; Machado, J.A.T. A Review of Definitions for Fractional Derivatives and Integral. *Math. Probl. Eng.* **2014**, *2014*, 238459 . [CrossRef]
2. Caputo, M.; Fabrizio, M. A new definition of fractional derivative without singular kernel. *Prog. Fract. Differ. Appl.* **2015**, *1*, 73–85.
3. Atangana, A.; Baleanu, D. New fractional derivatives with nonlocal and non-singular kernel: Theory and application to heat transfer model. *Therm. Sci.* **2016**, *20*, 763–769. [CrossRef]
4. Atangana, A. Fractional Operators and Their Applications. In *Fractional Operators with Constant and Variable Order with Application to Geo-Hydrology*; Academic Press: Amsterdam, The Netherlands , 2018; pp. 79–112. [CrossRef]
5. Podlubny, I. *Fractional Differential Equations: An Introduction to Fractional Derivatives, Fractional Differential Equations, to Methods of Their Solution and Some of Their Applications*; Elsevier: Amsterdam, The Netherlands, 1998; Volume 198.
6. Kilbas, A.A.; Srivastava, H.M.; Trujillo, J.J. *Theory and Applications of Fractional Differential Equations*; Elsevier: Amsterdam, The Netherlands, 2006; Volume 204.
7. Baleanu, D.; Agarwal, R.P. Fractional calculus in the sky. *Adv. Differ. Equ.* **2021**, *117*, 1–9 . [CrossRef]
8. Sun, H.; Zhang, Y.; Baleanu, D.; Chen, W.; Chen, Y.Q. A new collection of real world applications of fractional calculus in science and engineering. *Commun. Nonlinear Sci. Numer. Simul.* **2018**, *64*, 213–231. [CrossRef]
9. Madani, Y.A.; Ali, Z.; Rabih, M.; Alsulami, A.; Eljaneid, N.H.E.; Aldwoah, K.; Muflh, B. Discrete Fractional-Order Modeling of Recurrent Childhood Diseases Using the Caputo Difference Operator. *Fractal Fract.* **2025**, *9*, 55. [CrossRef]
10. Kumar, D.; Singh, J. (Eds.) *Fractional Calculus in Medical and Health Science*, 1st ed.; CRC Press: Boca Raton, FL, USA, 2020. [CrossRef]
11. Hafez, M.; Alshowaikh, F.; Voon, B.W.N.; Alkhazaleh, S.; Al-Faiz, H. Review on Recent Advances in Fractional Differentiation and its Applications. *Prog. Fract. Differ. Appl.* **2025**, *11*, 245–261. [CrossRef]
12. Volos, C. *Introductory Chapter: Fractional Calculus-From Theory to Applications*; IntechOpen: London, UK, 2025. [CrossRef]

fractal and fractional

MDPI

Article

Application of Riemann–Liouville Derivatives on Second-Order Fractional Differential Equations: The Exact Solution

Abdulrahman B. Albidah

Department of Mathematics, College of Science, Majmaah University, Al-Majmaah 11952, Saudi Arabia; a.albedah@mu.edu.sa

Abstract: This paper applies two different types of Riemann–Liouville derivatives to solve fractional differential equations of second order. Basically, the properties of the Riemann–Liouville fractional derivative depend mainly on the lower bound of the integral involved in the Riemann–Liouville fractional definition. The Riemann–Liouville fractional derivative of first type considers the lower bound as a zero while the second type applies negative infinity as a lower bound. Due to the differences in properties of the two operators, two different solutions are obtained for the present two classes of fractional differential equations under appropriate initial conditions. It is shown that the zeroth lower bound implies implicit solutions in terms of the Mittag–Leffler functions while explicit solutions are derived when negative infinity is taken as a lower bound. Such explicit solutions are obtained for the current two classes in terms of trigonometric and hyperbolic functions. Some theoretical results are introduced to facilitate the solutions procedures. Moreover, the characteristics of the obtained solutions are discussed and interpreted.

Keywords: Riemann–Liouville fractional derivative; fractional differential equations; Laplace transform; exact solution

1. Introduction

The fractional calculus (FC) is a growing field of research due to its numerous applications in several areas of sciences and engineering. The FC is a natural extension of classical calculus (CC) and has been utilized to analyze a considerable number of physical and engineering problems [1–3]. In this context, various models have been studied in the literature such as Narahari et al. [4] who applied the FC concept on the dynamics of the fractional oscillator. Propagation of ultrasonic wave in human cancelous bone was introduced by Sebaa et al. [5] via the FC approach. The physical aspect of the fractional Heisenberg equation has been addressed by Tarasov [6]. Application of the FC on the HIV infectious disease has been discussed by Ding and Yea [7]. In quantum mechanics, Wang et al. [8] investigated the time-fractional diffusion equation while other fractional models in different areas of research can be found in Refs. [9–14]. In addition, the fractional models of the projectile motion were solved by Ebaid [15] and Ebaid et al. [16] utilizing the Caputo fractional derivative (CFD) and by Ahmed et al. [17] by means of the Riemann–Liouville fractional derivative (RLFD).

In Refs. [18,19], the FC was extended to solve an astronomical model using the CFD while El-Zahar et al. [20] derived a closed form solution for the same model via applying the RLFD. Moreover, Aljohani et al. [21] obtained the exact solution of the chlorine transport model in fractional form in terms of the Mittag–Leffler function. Furthermore, the application of the RLFD on a class of engineering oscillatory problems was addressed by Ebaid and Al-Jeaid [22] for a class of first-order fractional initial value problems in which the dual solution was obtained. In addition, Seddek et al. [23] applied the RLFD to solve non-homogeneous fractional differential system containing periodic terms. Very recently, Algehyne et al. [24] presented a promise application of the FC on the concept of time dilation.

The objective of this paper is to extend the application of the RLFD to solve the following two classes:

$$ {}_{c}^{RL}D_t^{2\beta}y(t) + \omega^2 y(t) = a\cos(\Omega t), \ \frac{1}{2} < \beta \le 1, \tag{1} $$

and

$$ {}_{c}^{RL}D_t^{2\beta}y(t) - \varpi^2 y(t) = a\cos(\Omega t), \ \frac{1}{2} < \beta \le 1, \tag{2} $$

where β is none-integer order of the Riemann–Liouville derivative and a, ω, Ω, and A are constants. The two classes are to be solved under the initial conditions (ICs):

$$ {}_{c}^{RL}D_t^{2\beta-2}y(0) = A, \ {}_{c}^{RL}D_t^{2\beta-1}y(0) = B, \tag{3} $$

at two different cases for c, mainly when $c \to 0$ and $c \to -\infty$. The properties of the Riemann–Liouville derivatives ${}_{0}^{RL}D_t$ and ${}_{-\infty}^{RL}D_t$ are completely different and accordingly the nature of solutions of the present two classes are also different. The exact solution, when available, is the optimal solution for any physical/engineering model. So, the obtained exact solution reflects the importance and the main contribution of this paper. The paper is organized as follows. In Section 2, some preliminaries are introduced. In Section 3, theoretical results are derived for the particular solution of class (1). Section 4 is devoted to obtain the exact solution of class (1) while Section 5 presents the solution of class (2) in addition to the behavior of the obtained solution. The paper is concluded in Section 6.

2. Preliminaries

The Riemann–Liouville fractional integral of order α of function $f : [c, d] \to \mathbb{R}$ $(-\infty < c < d < \infty)$ is defined as [1–3]

$$ {}_{c}I_t^{\alpha}f(t) = \frac{1}{\gamma(\alpha)}\int_c^t \frac{f(\tau)}{(t-\tau)^{1-\alpha}}d\tau, \quad t > c, \ \alpha > 0. \tag{4} $$

The Riemann–Liouville fractional derivative (RLFD) of order $\alpha \in (1, 2)$ is [1–3]

$$ {}_{c}^{RL}D_t^{\alpha}f(t) = \frac{1}{\gamma(2-\alpha)}\frac{d^2}{dt^2}\left(\int_c^t \frac{f(\tau)}{(t-\tau)^{\alpha-1}}d\tau\right), \quad t > c. \tag{5} $$

For $t \in \mathbb{R}$ and $\alpha = 2\beta$ $(\frac{1}{2} < \beta \le 1)$, we have the following RLFD of the functions $e^{i\omega t}$, $\cos(\omega t)$, and $\sin(\omega t)$ as $c \to -\infty$ [22,23]:

$$ \begin{aligned} {}_{-\infty}^{RL}D_t^{2\beta}e^{i\omega t} &= (i\omega)^{2\beta}e^{i\omega t}, \\ {}_{-\infty}^{RL}D_t^{2\beta}\cos(\omega t) &= \omega^{2\beta}\cos(\omega t + \beta\pi), \\ {}_{-\infty}^{RL}D_t^{2\beta}\sin(\omega t) &= \omega^{2\beta}\sin(\omega t + \beta\pi). \end{aligned} \tag{6} $$

The Laplace transform (LT) of the RLFD (5) as $c \to 0$ is [22]

$$ \mathcal{L}\left[{}_{0}^{RL}D_t^{\alpha}y(t)\right] = s^{\alpha}Y(s) - {}_{0}^{RL}D_t^{\alpha-1}y(0) - s\,{}_{0}^{RL}D_t^{\alpha-2}y(0), \tag{7} $$

which yields

$$ \mathcal{L}\left[{}_{0}^{RL}D_t^{2\beta}y(t)\right] = s^{2\beta}Y(s) - {}_{0}^{RL}D_t^{2\beta-1}y(0) - s\,{}_{0}^{RL}D_t^{2\beta-2}y(0), \tag{8} $$

for $\alpha = 2\beta$. The Mittag–Leffler function of two parameters is defined by [1–3]

$$ E_{\delta,\gamma}(z) = \sum_{n=0}^{\infty}\frac{z^n}{\gamma(\delta n + \gamma)}, \quad (\delta > 0, \ \gamma > 0). \tag{9} $$

In particular, we have the following properties

$$E_{2,1}(-z^2) = \cos(z), \quad E_{2,1}(z^2) = \cosh(z), \quad E_{2,2}(-z^2) = \frac{\sin z}{z}, \quad E_{2,2}(z^2) = \frac{\sinh z}{z}. \quad (10)$$

The inverse LT of some expressions can be given via the Mittag–Leffler function as [2,3]

$$\mathcal{L}^{-1}\Big(\frac{s^{\delta-\gamma}}{s^\delta+\omega^2}\Big) = t^{\gamma-1}E_{\delta,\gamma}(-\omega^2 t^\alpha), \quad Re(s) > |\omega^2|^{\frac{1}{\delta}}, \quad (11)$$

which gives the equalities [16,22,23]:

$$\mathcal{L}^{-1}\Big(\frac{s^{\delta-1}}{s^\delta+1}\Big) = E_\alpha(-t^\delta), \quad (12)$$

$$\mathcal{L}^{-1}\Big(\frac{1}{s^\delta+\omega^2}\Big) = t^{\delta-1}E_{\delta,\delta}(-\omega^2 t^\delta), \qquad Re(s) > |\omega^2|^{\frac{1}{\delta}}, \quad (13)$$

$$\mathcal{L}^{-1}\Big(\frac{s^{-1}}{s^\delta+\omega^2}\Big) = t^{\delta}E_{\delta,\delta+1}(-\omega^2 t^\delta), \qquad Re(s) > |\omega^2|^{\frac{1}{\delta}}. \quad (14)$$

3. Analysis

Theorem 1. *The particular solution $y_p(t)$ of the class (1) as $c \to -\infty$ is given by*

$$y_p(t) = \lambda_1(\beta)\cos(\Omega t) + \lambda_2(\beta)\sin(\Omega t), \quad (15)$$

where $\lambda_1(\beta)$ and $\lambda_2(\beta)$ are given by

$$\lambda_1(\beta) = a\Big(\frac{\omega^2+\Omega^{2\beta}\cos(\pi\beta)}{\omega^4+\Omega^{4\beta}+2\omega^2\Omega^{2\beta}\cos(\pi\beta)}\Big), \quad \lambda_2(\beta) = a\Big(\frac{\Omega^{2\beta}\sin(\pi\beta)}{\omega^4+\Omega^{4\beta}+2\omega^2\Omega^{2\beta}\cos(\pi\beta)}\Big), \quad (16)$$

and hence,

$$y_p(t) = a\Big(\frac{\omega^2\cos(\Omega t)+\Omega^{2\beta}\cos(\Omega t-\pi\beta)}{\omega^4+\Omega^{4\beta}+2\omega^2\Omega^{2\beta}\cos(\pi\beta)}\Big). \quad (17)$$

Proof. Suppose that y_p is in the form of Equation (15), then

$$\begin{aligned} {}^{RL}_{-\infty}D_t^{2\beta} y_p &= \lambda_1(\beta)\, {}^{RL}_{-\infty}D_t^{2\beta}\cos(\Omega t) + \lambda_2(\beta)\, {}^{RL}_{-\infty}D_t^{2\beta}\sin(\Omega t), \\ &= \Omega^{2\beta}\cos(\Omega t)(\lambda_1(\beta)\cos(\pi\beta)+\lambda_2(\beta)\sin(\pi\beta)) + \\ &\quad \Omega^{2\pi\beta}\sin(\Omega t)(\lambda_2(\beta)\cos(\pi\beta)-\lambda_1(\beta)\sin(\pi\beta)), \end{aligned} \quad (18)$$

and hence

$$\begin{aligned} {}^{RL}_{-\infty}D_t^{2\beta} y_p + \omega^2 y_p &= \Big[\Big(\Omega^{2\beta}\cos(\pi\beta)+\omega^2\Big)\lambda_1(\beta) + \Omega^{2\beta}\sin(\pi\beta)\lambda_2(\beta)\Big]\cos(\Omega t) + \\ &= \Big[\Big(\Omega^{2\beta}\cos(\pi\beta)+\omega^2\Big)\lambda_2(\beta) - \Omega^{2\beta}\sin(\pi\beta)\lambda_1(\beta)\Big]\sin(\Omega t). \end{aligned} \quad (19)$$

The unknowns $\lambda_1(\beta)$ and $\lambda_2(\beta)$ can be obtained by solving the following coupled algebraic equations:

$$\begin{aligned} \Big(\Omega^{2\beta}\cos(\pi\beta)+\omega^2\Big)\lambda_1(\beta) + \Omega^{2\beta}\sin(\pi\beta)\lambda_2(\beta) &= a, \\ \Big(\Omega^{2\beta}\cos(\pi\beta)+\omega^2\Big)\lambda_2(\beta) - \Omega^{2\beta}\sin(\pi\beta)\lambda_1(\beta) &= 0, \end{aligned} \quad (20)$$

which give

$$\lambda_1(\beta) = a\Big(\frac{\omega^2+\Omega^{2\beta}\cos(\pi\beta)}{\omega^4+\Omega^{4\beta}+2\omega^2\Omega^{2\beta}\cos(\pi\beta)}\Big), \quad \lambda_2(\beta) = a\Big(\frac{\Omega^{2\beta}\sin(\pi\beta)}{\omega^4+\Omega^{4\beta}+2\omega^2\Omega^{2\beta}\cos(\pi\beta)}\Big). \quad (21)$$

Therefore, y_p takes the form:

$$y_p(t) = a\left(\frac{\omega^2\cos(\Omega t) + \Omega^{2\beta}\cos(\Omega t - \pi\beta)}{\omega^4 + \Omega^{4\beta} + 2\omega^2\Omega^{2\beta}\cos(\pi\beta)}\right), \tag{22}$$

which completes the proof. □

Lemma 1. *The particular solution $y_p(t)$ of the class (2) as $c \to -\infty$ is given by*

$$y_p(t) = a\left(\frac{-\varpi^2\cos(\Omega t) + \Omega^{2\beta}\cos(\Omega t - \pi\beta)}{\varpi^4 + \Omega^{4\beta} - 2\varpi^2\Omega^{2\beta}\cos(\pi\beta)}\right). \tag{23}$$

Proof. The proof follows immediately by replacing ω with $-i\varpi$ in Equation (17) of theorem 1, where $i = \sqrt{-1}$. □

4. Solution of the First Class: ${}_{c}^{RL}D_t^{2\beta}y(t) + \omega^2 y(t) = a\cos(\Omega t)$

In this section, two types of solutions are to be determined for the class (1) when $c \to 0$ and $c \to -\infty$, respectively. The analysis introduced in Refs. [22,23] is followed here to obtain such types of solutions.

4.1. Solution in Terms of the Mittag–Leffler Function as $c \to 0$

In this case, the first class takes the form:

$${}_{0}^{RL}D_t^{2\beta}y(t) + \omega^2 y(t) = a\cos(\Omega t), \quad \frac{1}{2} < \beta \le 1, \tag{24}$$

under the ICs:

$${}_{0}^{RL}D_t^{2\beta-2}y(0) = A, \quad {}_{0}^{RL}D_t^{2\beta-1}y(0) = B. \tag{25}$$

Applying the LT on Equation (24) yields

$$s^{2\beta}Y(s) - {}_{0}^{RL}D_t^{2\beta-1}y(0) - s\,{}_{0}^{RL}D_t^{2\beta-2}y(0) + \omega^2 Y(s) = \frac{as}{s^2+\Omega^2}. \tag{26}$$

Solving (26) for $Y(s)$ gives

$$Y(s) = \frac{As}{s^{2\beta}+\omega^2} + \frac{B}{s^{2\beta}+\omega^2} + \frac{as}{(s^{2\beta}+\omega^2)(s^2+\Omega^2)}. \tag{27}$$

Applying the inverse LT on $Y(s)$, then $y(t)$ is given by

$$y(t) = At^{2\beta-2}E_{2\beta,2\beta-1}\left(-\omega^2 t^{2\beta}\right) + Bt^{2\beta-1}E_{2\beta,2\beta}\left(-\omega^2 t^{2\beta}\right) + a\mathcal{L}^{-1}\left(\frac{1}{s^{2\beta}+\omega^2}\right) * \mathcal{L}^{-1}\left(\frac{s}{s^2+\Omega^2}\right), \tag{28}$$

where $(*)$ refers to the convolution operation, hence

$$\begin{aligned} y(t) = {} & At^{2\beta-2}E_{2\beta,2\beta-1}\left(-\omega^2 t^{2\beta}\right) + Bt^{2\beta-1}E_{2\beta,2\beta}\left(-\omega^2 t^{2\beta}\right) + \\ & a\int_0^t \tau^{2\beta-1}E_{2\beta,2\beta}\left(-\omega^2\tau^{2\beta}\right)\cos[\Omega(t-\tau)]d\tau, \end{aligned} \tag{29}$$

which can be written as

$$\begin{aligned} y(t) = {} & At^{2\beta-2}E_{2\beta,2\beta-1}\left(-\omega^2 t^{2\beta}\right) + Bt^{2\beta-1}E_{2\beta,2\beta}\left(-\omega^2 t^{2\beta}\right) + a\cos(\Omega t) \times \\ & \int_0^t \tau^{2\beta-1}E_{2\beta,2\beta}\left(-\omega^2\tau^{2\beta}\right)\cos(\Omega\tau)d\tau + a\sin(\Omega t)\int_0^t \tau^{2\beta-1}E_{2\beta,2\beta}\left(-\omega^2\tau^{2\beta}\right)\sin(\Omega\tau)d\tau. \end{aligned} \tag{30}$$

The involved integrals are difficult to compute explicitly. However, the solution in the integral form (30) reduces to the corresponding solution of the ordinary version of the class (1) as $\beta \to 1$.

Special Case as $\beta \to 1$

The solution in the integral form (30) as $\beta \to 1$ becomes

$$y(t) = AE_{2,1}\left(-\omega^2 t^2\right) + BtE_{2,2}\left(-\omega^2 t^2\right) + a\cos(\Omega t) \times \int_0^t \tau E_{2,2}\left(-\omega^2\tau^2\right)\cos(\Omega\tau)d\tau + a\sin(\Omega t)\int_0^t \tau E_{2,2}\left(-\omega^2\tau^2\right)\sin(\Omega\tau)d\tau, \quad (31)$$

i.e.,

$$y(t) = A\cos(\omega t) + \frac{B}{\omega}\sin(\omega t) + \frac{a}{\omega}\cos(\Omega t)\int_0^t \sin(\omega\tau)\cos(\Omega\tau)d\tau + \frac{a}{\omega}\sin(\Omega t)\int_0^t \sin(\omega\tau)\sin(\Omega\tau)d\tau. \quad (32)$$

Performing the integrals, we obtain

$$y(t) = A\cos(\omega t) + \frac{B}{\omega}\sin(\omega t) + a\left(\frac{\cos(\Omega t) - \cos(\omega t)}{\omega^2 - \Omega^2}\right), \quad (33)$$

which is the corresponding solution of the ordinary version $y''(t) + \omega^2 y(t) = a\cos(\Omega t)$ under the ICs $y(0) = A$ and $y'(0) = B$.

Remark 1. *It is noticed that the solution (30) is not analytic at* $t = 0 \ \forall\ \beta \in (1/2, 1)$ *for the existence of the term* $t^{2\beta-2}$. *In the next subsection, we are able to derive the analytic solution in the whole domain* $t \geq 0$.

4.2. Solution in Terms of Trigonometric Functions as $c \to -\infty$

As $c \to -\infty$, the first class is in the form:

$${}^{RL}_{-\infty}D_t^{2\beta} y(t) + \omega^2 y(t) = a\cos(\Omega t), \quad \frac{1}{2} < \beta \leq 1, \quad (34)$$

and the ICs are

$${}^{RL}_{-\infty}D_t^{2\beta-2} y(0) = A, \quad {}^{RL}_{-\infty}D_t^{2\beta-1} y(0) = B. \quad (35)$$

The solution of Equations (34) and (35) consists of the complementary solution y_c and the particular solution $y_p(t)$. However, the $y_p(t)$ is already given by Equation (17) in Theorem 1 while $y_c(t)$ can be assumed in the form [22,23]:

$$y_c(t) = c(\beta)e^{i\sigma t}, \quad (36)$$

where $c(\beta)$ and σ are unknowns and to be determined. The assumption (36) satisfies the homogeneous part of the fractional Equation (34):

$${}^{RL}_{-\infty}D_t^{2\beta} y_c(t) + \omega^2 y_c(t) = 0, \quad (37)$$

if

$$ce^{i\sigma t}\left[(i\sigma)^{2\beta} + \omega^2\right] = 0, \quad (38)$$

which implies two values of σ as

$$\sigma_1 = i\left(-\omega^2\right)^{\frac{1}{2\beta}}, \quad \sigma_2 = -i\left(-\omega^2\right)^{\frac{1}{2\beta}}, \quad (39)$$

or simply

$$\sigma_1 = \nu, \quad \sigma_2 = -\nu, \quad \nu = i\left(-\omega^2\right)^{\frac{1}{2\beta}}. \quad (40)$$

Accordingly, $y_c(t)$ becomes

$$y_c(t) = c_1(\beta)e^{ivt} + c_2(\beta)e^{-ivt}, \tag{41}$$

where $c_1(\beta)$ and $c_2(\beta)$ are unknown constants. The general solution is

$$y(t) = c_1(\beta)e^{ivt} + c_2(\beta)e^{-ivt} + y_p(t), \tag{42}$$

where $y_p(t)$ is given by Equation (17). From (42), we have

$$D_t^{2\beta-1}y(t) = c_1(\beta)(iv)^{2\beta-1}e^{ivt} + c_2(\beta)(-iv)^{2\beta-1}e^{-ivt} + D_t^{2\beta-1}y_p(t), \tag{43}$$

$$D_t^{2\beta-2}y(t) = c_1(\beta)(iv)^{2\beta-2}e^{ivt} + c_2(\beta)(-iv)^{2\beta-2}e^{-ivt} + D_t^{2\beta-2}y_p(t). \tag{44}$$

At $t = 0$, Equations (43) and (44) become

$$D_t^{2\beta-1}y(0) = (iv)^{2\beta-1}[c_1(\beta) - c_2(\beta)] + D_t^{2\beta-1}y_p(0), \tag{45}$$

$$D_t^{2\beta-2}y(0) = (iv)^{2\beta-2}[c_1(\beta) + c_2(\beta)] + D_t^{2\beta-2}y_p(0). \tag{46}$$

Applying the ICs (35), we obtain

$$c_1(\beta) = \frac{(iv)^{1-2\beta}}{2}\left[(B + ivA) - \left(D_t^{2\beta-1}y_p(0) + ivD_t^{2\beta-2}y_p(0)\right)\right], \tag{47}$$

$$c_2(\beta) = \frac{(iv)^{1-2\beta}}{2}\left[(-B + ivA) + \left(D_t^{2\beta-1}y_p(0) - ivD_t^{2\beta-2}y_p(0)\right)\right]. \tag{48}$$

To calculate $D_t^{2\beta-1}y_p(0)$ and $D_t^{2\beta-2}y_p(0)$, one can use $y_p(t)$ in Equation (15) in terms of λ_1 and λ_2 to obtain

$$D_t^{2\beta-1}y_p(0) = \Omega^{2\beta-1}[\lambda_1 \sin(\pi\beta) - \lambda_2 \cos(\pi\beta)], \tag{49}$$

$$D_t^{2\beta-2}y_p(0) = -\Omega^{2\beta-2}[\lambda_1 \cos(\pi\beta) + \lambda_2 \sin(\pi\beta)], \tag{50}$$

where λ_1 and λ_2 are given by Equation (16). Therefor, the solution takes the final form:

$$y(t) = c_1(\beta)e^{-(-\omega^2)^{\frac{1}{2\beta}}t} + c_2(\beta)e^{(-\omega^2)^{\frac{1}{2\beta}}t} + a\left[\frac{\omega^2\cos(\Omega t) + \Omega^{2\beta}\cos(\Omega t - \pi\beta)}{\omega^4 + \Omega^{4\beta} + 2\omega^2\Omega^{2\beta}\cos(\pi\beta)}\right], \tag{51}$$

where $c_1(\beta)$ and $c_2(\beta)$ are defined by Equations (47) and (48), respectively.

Remark 2. *The solution in the case $c \to -\infty$ is obtained in the explicit form (51) unlike the implicit integral form (30) when $c \to 0$. Moreover, the solution (51) is analytic in the whole domain $t \in \mathbb{R}$. In addition, the explicit form (51) is also equivalent to the corresponding solution of ordinary version of the first class as indicated in the below section.*

Special Case as $\beta \to 1$

To check, we have from (51) as $\beta \to 1$ that

$$y(t) = c_1e^{-i\omega t} + c_2e^{i\omega t} + \frac{a\cos(\Omega t)}{\omega^2 - \Omega^2}. \tag{52}$$

From (49) and (50), we have

$$\left[D_t^{2\beta-1}y_p(0)\right]_{\beta\to 1} = \Omega[\lambda_2]_{\beta\to 1} = 0, \quad \left[D_t^{2\beta-2}y_p(0)\right]_{\beta\to 1} = [\lambda_1]_{\beta\to 1} = \frac{a}{\omega^2 - \Omega^2}. \tag{53}$$

The quantities c_1 and c_2 in Equations (47) and (48) become

$$c_1 = \frac{(i\nu)^{-1}}{2}\left[(B + i\nu A) - \frac{ai\nu}{\omega^2 - \Omega^2}\right] = -\frac{B}{2i\omega} + \frac{1}{2}\left(A - \frac{a}{\omega^2 - \Omega^2}\right), \tag{54}$$

$$c_2 = \frac{(i\nu)^{-1}}{2}\left[(-B + i\nu A) - \frac{ai\nu}{\omega^2 - \Omega^2}\right] = \frac{B}{2i\omega} + \frac{1}{2}\left(A - \frac{a}{\omega^2 - \Omega^2}\right). \tag{55}$$

Substituting (54) and (55) into (52), yields

$$y(t) = \frac{B}{2i\omega}\left(e^{i\omega t} - e^{-i\omega t}\right) + \frac{1}{2}\left(A - \frac{a}{\omega^2 - \Omega^2}\right)\left(e^{i\omega t} + e^{-i\omega t}\right) + \frac{a\cos(\Omega t)}{\omega^2 - \Omega^2}, \tag{56}$$

or

$$y(t) = \frac{B}{\omega}\sin(\omega t) + \left(A - \frac{a}{\omega^2 - \Omega^2}\right)\cos(\omega t) + \frac{a\cos(\Omega t)}{\omega^2 - \Omega^2}, \tag{57}$$

which is equivalent to the solution of the ordinary version $y''(t) + \omega^2 y(t) = a\cos(\Omega t)$ under the ICs $y(0) = A$ and $y'(0) = B$.

5. Solution of the Second Class: ${}^{RL}_{c}D_t^{2\beta} y(t) - \varpi^2 y(t) = a\cos(\Omega t)$

5.1. Solution in Terms of the Mittag–Leffler Function as $c \to 0$

In this case we consider the fractional differential equation:

$${}^{RL}_{0}D_t^{2\beta} y(t) - \varpi^2 y(t) = a\cos(\Omega t), \quad \frac{1}{2} < \beta \leq 1, \tag{58}$$

under the ICs:

$${}^{RL}_{0}D_t^{2\beta-2} y(0) = A, \quad {}^{RL}_{0}D_t^{2\beta-1} y(0) = B. \tag{59}$$

Following the same analysis in Section 4.1, one can obtain the solution in the form:

$$y(t) = At^{2\beta-2}E_{2\beta,2\beta-1}\left(\varpi^2 t^{2\beta}\right) + Bt^{2\beta-1}E_{2\beta,2\beta}\left(\varpi^2 t^{2\beta}\right) + a\cos(\Omega t) \times \int_0^t \tau^{2\beta-1}E_{2\beta,2\beta}\left(\varpi^2\tau^{2\beta}\right)\cos(\Omega\tau)d\tau + a\sin(\Omega t)\int_0^t \tau^{2\beta-1}E_{2\beta,2\beta}\left(\varpi^2\tau^{2\beta}\right)\sin(\Omega\tau)d\tau. \tag{60}$$

As $\beta \to 1$, the solution in the integral form (60) reads

$$y(t) = AE_{2,1}\left(\varpi^2 t^2\right) + BtE_{2,2}\left(\varpi^2 t^2\right) + a\cos(\Omega t) \times \int_0^t \tau E_{2,2}\left(\varpi^2\tau^2\right)\cos(\Omega\tau)d\tau + a\sin(\Omega t)\int_0^t \tau E_{2,2}\left(\varpi^2\tau^2\right)\sin(\Omega\tau)d\tau, \tag{61}$$

i.e.,

$$y(t) = A\cosh(\varpi t) + \frac{B}{\varpi}\sin(\varpi t) + \frac{a}{\varpi}\cos(\Omega t)\int_0^t \sinh(\varpi\tau)\cos(\Omega\tau)d\tau + \frac{a}{\varpi}\sin(\Omega t)\int_0^t \sinh(\varpi\tau)\sin(\Omega\tau)d\tau. \tag{62}$$

Performing the integrals, we obtain

$$y(t) = A\cosh(\varpi t) + \frac{B}{\varpi}\sin(\varpi t) - a\left(\frac{\cos(\Omega t) - \cosh(\varpi t)}{\varpi^2 + \Omega^2}\right), \tag{63}$$

which is the corresponding solution of the ordinary version $y''(t) - \varpi^2 y(t) = a\cos(\Omega t)$ under the ICs $y(0) = A$ and $y'(0) = B$.

5.2. Solution in Terms of Trigonometric and Hyperbolic Functions as $c \to -\infty$

Here, we consider

$$ {}_{-\infty}^{RL}D_t^{2\beta} y(t) - \varpi^2 y(t) = a\cos(\Omega t), \quad \frac{1}{2} < \beta \le 1, \tag{64} $$

under the ICs:

$$ {}_{-\infty}^{RL}D_t^{2\beta-2} y(0) = A, \quad {}_{-\infty}^{RL}D_t^{2\beta-1} y(0) = B. \tag{65} $$

Following the same procedure of Section 4.2, we can get the solution in the form:

$$ y(t) = c_1(\beta)e^{-(\varpi^2)^{\frac{1}{2\beta}} t} + c_2(\beta)e^{(\varpi^2)^{\frac{1}{2\beta}} t} + a\left[\frac{-\varpi^2\cos(\Omega t) + \Omega^{2\beta}\cos(\Omega t - \pi\beta)}{\varpi^4 + \Omega^{4\beta} - 2\varpi^2\Omega^{2\beta}\cos(\pi\beta)}\right], \tag{66} $$

or

$$ y(t) = c_1(\beta)e^{-\varpi^{\frac{1}{\beta}} t} + c_2(\beta)e^{\varpi^{\frac{1}{\beta}} t} + a\left[\frac{-\varpi^2\cos(\Omega t) + \Omega^{2\beta}\cos(\Omega t - \pi\beta)}{\varpi^4 + \Omega^{4\beta} - 2\varpi^2\Omega^{2\beta}\cos(\pi\beta)}\right], \tag{67} $$

where $c_1(\beta)$ and $c_2(\beta)$ can be determined from Equations (47) and (48) by replacing ω with $-i\varpi$ ($i = \sqrt{-1}$), thus

$$ c_1(\beta) = -\frac{\varpi^{1/\beta-2}}{2}\left[B - {}_{-\infty}^{RL}D_t^{2\beta-1} y_p(0) - \varpi^{1/\beta}\left(A - {}_{-\infty}^{RL}D_t^{2\beta-2} y_p(0)\right)\right], \tag{68} $$

$$ c_2(\beta) = -\frac{\varpi^{1/\beta-2}}{2}\left[-\left(B - {}_{-\infty}^{RL}D_t^{2\beta-1} y_p(0)\right) - \varpi^{1/\beta}\left(A - {}_{-\infty}^{RL}D_t^{2\beta-2} y_p(0)\right)\right]. \tag{69} $$

Suppose that

$$ \rho = B - {}_{-\infty}^{RL}D_t^{2\beta-1} y_p(0), \quad \chi = A - {}_{-\infty}^{RL}D_t^{2\beta-2} y_p(0), \tag{70} $$

then

$$ c_1(\beta) = \frac{\varpi^{1/\beta-2}}{2}\left(-\rho + \varpi^{1/\beta}\chi\right), \tag{71} $$

$$ c_2(\beta) = \frac{\varpi^{1/\beta-2}}{2}\left(\rho + \varpi^{1/\beta}\chi\right). \tag{72} $$

Substituting (71) and (72) into (67), we obtain the solution of the system (64)–(65) in terms of the hyperbolic and trigonometric functions as

$$ y(t) = \varpi^{1/\beta-2}\left[\rho\sinh\left(\varpi^{1/\beta}t\right) + \chi\cosh\left(\varpi^{1/\beta}t\right)\right] + a\left[\frac{-\varpi^2\cos(\Omega t) + \Omega^{2\beta}\cos(\Omega t - \pi\beta)}{\varpi^4 + \Omega^{4\beta} - 2\varpi^2\Omega^{2\beta}\cos(\pi\beta)}\right], \tag{73} $$

where the coefficients ρ and χ are given explicitly in the forms:

$$ \rho = B - \Omega^{2\beta-1}[\lambda_1\sin(\pi\beta) - \lambda_2\cos(\pi\beta)], \tag{74} $$

$$ \chi = A + \Omega^{2\beta-2}[\lambda_1\cos(\pi\beta) + \lambda_2\sin(\pi\beta)], \tag{75} $$

and λ_1 and λ_2 are given by

$$ \lambda_1 = a\left(\frac{-\varpi^2 + \Omega^{2\beta}\cos(\pi\beta)}{\varpi^4 + \Omega^{4\beta} - 2\varpi^2\Omega^{2\beta}\cos(\pi\beta)}\right), \quad \lambda_2 = a\left(\frac{\Omega^{2\beta}\sin(\pi\beta)}{\varpi^4 + \Omega^{4\beta} - 2\varpi^2\Omega^{2\beta}\cos(\pi\beta)}\right). \tag{76} $$

It should be noted that the expression (76) also reduces to the solution of the ordinary version given in the previous section by Equation (63) as $\beta \to 1$.

5.3. Behavior of the Solution

It can be easily observed from Equation (73) that the solution is real at any given real values of the parameters ϖ and Ω provided that the denominator in Equation (73) does not vanish, i.e., $\varpi^4 + \Omega^{4\beta} - 2\varpi^2\Omega^{2\beta}\cos(\pi\beta) \neq 0, (1/2 < \beta < 1)$. The behavior of the solution (73) is examined at some selected values for the involved parameters. The influence of the fractional-order β on the solution is depicted in Figure 1 when $A = 1, B = 1, \varpi = \frac{1}{3}$, $\Omega = 3$, and $a = 2$. It is observed that the curves oscillate in the first part of the domain, however, such oscillations reduce as the value of β approaches one.

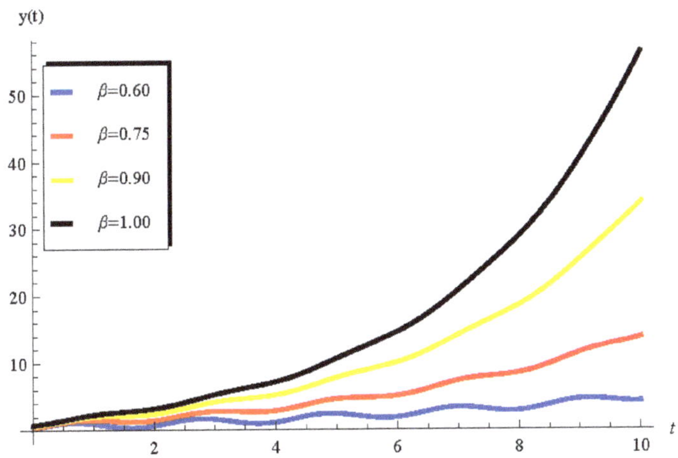

Figure 1. Plots of $y(t)$ in Equation (73) vs t when $A = 1, B = 1, \varpi = \frac{1}{3}, \Omega = 3$, and $a = 2$ at different values of β.

Figure 2 shows the variation of the solution (73) at different values of the coefficient $\varpi > 1$ when $A = 1$, $B = 1$, $\beta = \frac{3}{4}$, $\Omega = 3$, and $a = 2$. It is noticed in Figure 2 that the curves are smooth and have no oscillations. However, the oscillation of the solution $y(t)$ in Equation (73) returns to appear for another set of the ϖ values that are less than unity. This point is declared in Figure 3 which displays behavior for the solution when $A = 1, B = 1$, $\beta = \frac{3}{4}, \Omega = 3$, and $a = 2$ at different values of $\varpi < 1$.

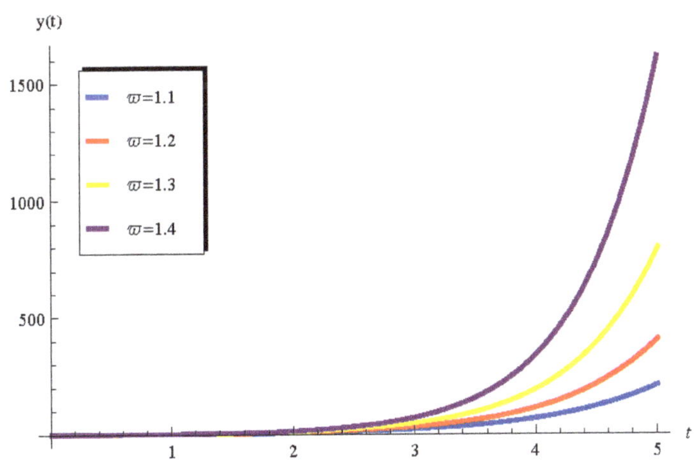

Figure 2. Plots of $y(t)$ in Equation (73) vs. t when $A = 1, B = 1, \beta = \frac{3}{4}, \Omega = 3$, and $a = 2$ at different values of $\varpi > 1$.

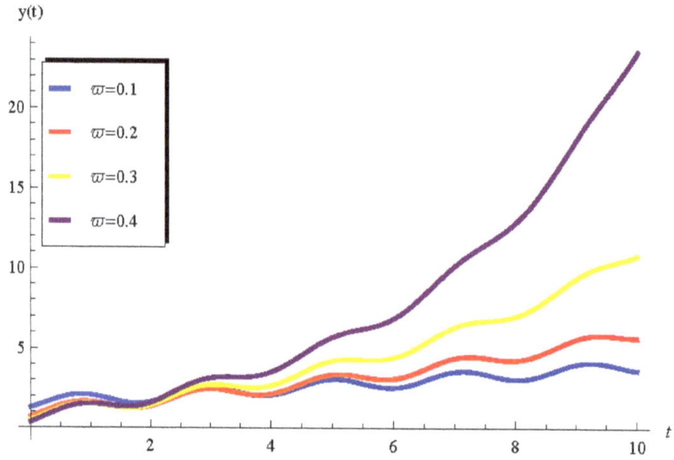

Figure 3. Plots of $y(t)$ in Equation (73) vs. t when $A = 1$, $B = 1$, $\beta = \frac{3}{4}$, $\Omega = 3$, and $a = 2$ at different values of $\varpi < 1$.

6. Conclusions

Two classes of fractional differential equations were solved in this paper by means of two different types of RLFD. The first type considered the lower bound of the integral involved in the RLFD as a zero. The second type treats the lower bound as negative infinity. It was also shown that the solution procedure depends mainly on the implemented type of the RLFD. For the first type of RLFD, the LT method was applied successfully to determine the solutions of the two classes in terms the Mittag–Leffler functions. In addition, a direct analysis was presented to obtain the solutions of the two classes governed by the second type of RLFD, where the solutions were obtained in explicit forms and expressed in terms of trigonometric and hyperbolic functions. Features of the obtained solutions are theoretically discussed and explained. The current analysis may deserve further extension to include other classes of fractional differential equations which describe applications in engineering and physical sciences. In future investigations, other kinds of the fractional derivatives such as Caputo [12,15,16], modified Riemann–Liouville derivative [25], and Atangana–Baleanu derivative [26] will be addressed to solve more complex models such as the nonlinear duffing-oscillator and the nonlinear relativistic oscillator.

Funding: The author would like to thank Deanship of Scientific Research at Majmaah University for supporting this work under Project Number No. R-2023-846.

Data Availability Statement: Data is contained within the article.

Conflicts of Interest: The author declares no conflict of interest.

References

1. Miller, K.S.; Ross, B. *An Introduction to the Fractional Calculus and Fractional Differential Equations*; John Wiley & Sons: New York, NY, USA, 1993.
2. Podlubny, I. *Fractional Differential Equations*; Academic Press: San Diego, CA, USA, 1999.
3. Hilfer, R. *Applications of Fractional Calculus in Physics*; World Scientific Publishing Company: Singapore, 2000.
4. Narahari Achar, B.N.; Hanneken, J.W.; Enck, T.; Clarke, T. Dynamics of the fractional oscillator. *Phys. A* **2001**, *297*, 361–367. [CrossRef]
5. Sebaa, N.; Fellah, Z.E.A.; Lauriks, W.; Depollier, C. Application of fractional calculus to ultrasonic wave propagation in human cancellous bone. *Signal Process.* **2006**, *86*, 2668–2677. [CrossRef]
6. Tarasov, V.E. Fractional Heisenberg equation. *Phys. Lett. A* **2008**, *372*, 2984–2988. [CrossRef]
7. Ding, Y.; Yea, H. A fractional-order differential equation model of HIV infection of CD4+T-cells. *Math. Comput. Model.* **2009**, *50*, 386–392. [CrossRef]

8. Wang, S.; Xu, M.; Li, X. Green's function of time fractional diffusion equation and its applications in fractional quantum mechanics. *Nonlinear Anal. Real World Appl.* **2009**, *10*, 1081–1086. [CrossRef]
9. Song, L.; Xu, S.; Yang, J. Dynamical models of happiness with fractional order. *Commun. Nonlinear Sci. Numer. Simul.* **2010**, *15*, 616–628. [CrossRef]
10. Gómez-Aguilara, J.F.; Rosales-García, J.J.; Bernal-Alvarado, J.J. Fractional mechanical oscillators. *Rev. Mex. Física* **2012**, *58*, 348–352.
11. Machado, J.T.; Kiryakova, V.; Mainardi, F. Recent history of fractional calculus. *Commun. Nonlinear Sci. Numer. Simul.* **2011**, *16*, 1140–1153. [CrossRef]
12. Garcia, J.J.R.; Calderon, M.G.; Ortiz, J.M.; Baleanu, D. Motion of a particle in a resisting medium using fractional calculus approach. *Proc. Rom. Acad. Ser. A* **2013**, *14*, 42–47.
13. Machado, J.T. A fractional approach to the Fermi-Pasta-Ulam problem. *Eur. Phys. J. Spec. Top.* **2013**, *222*, 1795–1803. [CrossRef]
14. Liaqat, M.I.; Akgül, A.; De la Sen, M.; Bayram, M. Approximate and Exact Solutions in the Sense of Conformable Derivatives of Quantum Mechanics Models Using a Novel Algorithm. *Symmetry* **2023**, *15*, 744. [CrossRef]
15. Ebaid, A. Analysis of projectile motion in view of the fractional calculus. *Appl. Math. Model.* **2011**, *35*, 1231–1239. [CrossRef]
16. Ebaid, A.; El-Zahar, E.R.; Aljohani, A.F.; Salah, B.; Krid, M.; Machado, J.T. Analysis of the two-dimensional fractional projectile motion in view of the experimental data. *Nonlinear Dyn.* **2019**, *97*, 1711–1720. [CrossRef]
17. Ahmad, B.; Batarfi, H.; Nieto, J.J.; Oscar, O.-Z.; Shammakh, W. Projectile motion via Riemann-Liouville calculus. *Adv. Differ. Equ.* **2015**, 63. https://doi.org/10.1186/s13662-015-0400-3. [CrossRef]
18. Kumar, D.; Singh, J.; Baleanu, D.; Rathore, S. Analysis of a fractional model of the Ambartsumian equation. *Eur. Phys. J. Plus* **2018**, *133*, 133–259. [CrossRef]
19. Ebaid, A.; Cattani, C.; Al Juhani, A.S.; El-Zahar, E.R. A novel exact solution for the fractional Ambartsumian equation. *Adv. Differ. Equ.* **2021**, *2021*, 88. [CrossRef]
20. El-Zahar, E.R.; Alotaibi, A.M.; Ebaid, A.; Aljohani, A.F.; Gómez Aguilar, J.F. The Riemann-Liouville fractional derivative for Ambartsumian equation. *Results Phys.* **2020**, *19*, 103551. [CrossRef]
21. Aljohani, A.F.; Ebaid, A.; Algehyne, E.A.; Mahrous, Y.M.; Cattani, C.; Al-Jeaid, H.K. The Mittag-Leffler Function for Re-Evaluating the Chlorine Transport Model: Comparative Analysis. *Fractal Fract.* **2022**, *6*, 125. [CrossRef]
22. Ebaid, A.; Al-Jeaid, H.K. The Mittag–Leffler Functions for a Class of First-Order Fractional Initial Value Problems: Dual Solution via Riemann–Liouville Fractional Derivative. *Fractal Fract.* **2022**, *6*, 85. [CrossRef]
23. Seddek, L.F.; Ebaid, A.; El-Zahar, E.R.; Aljoufi, M.D. Exact Solution of Non-Homogeneous Fractional Differential System Containing 2n Periodic Terms under Physical Conditions. *Mathematics* **2023**, *11*, 3308. [CrossRef]
24. Algehyne, E.A.; Aldhabani, M.S.; Areshi, M.; El-Zahar, E.R.; Ebaid, A.; Al-Jeaid, H.K. A Proposed Application of Fractional Calculus on Time Dilation in Special Theory of Relativity. *Mathematics* **2023**, *11*, 3343. [CrossRef]
25. Jumarie, G. Fractional partial differential equations and modified Riemann-Liouville derivative new methods for solution. *J. Appl. Math. Comput.* **2007**, *24*, 31–48. [CrossRef]
26. Atangana, A.; Gómez-Aguilar, J.F. Numerical approximation of Riemann-Liouville definition of fractional derivative: From Riemann-Liouville to Atangana-Baleanu. *Numer. Methods Partial. Differ. Eq.* **2018**, *34*, 1502. [CrossRef]

fractal and fractional

MDPI

Article

Anomalous Diffusion Models Involving Regularized General Fractional Derivatives with Sonin Kernels

Maryam Alkandari [1,*], Dimitri Loutchko [2] and Yuri Luchko [3]

[1] Department of Mathematics, Kuwait University, Kuwait City 13060, Kuwait
[2] Institute of Industrial Science, The University of Tokyo, Tokyo 153-8505, Japan; d.loutchko@edu.k.u-tokyo.ac.jp
[3] Department of Mathematics, Physics, and Chemistry, Berlin University of Applied Sciences and Technology, 13353 Berlin, Germany; luchko@bht-berlin.de
* Correspondence: maryam.alkandari@ku.edu.kw

Abstract: In this paper, we introduce a general fractional master equation involving regularized general fractional derivatives with Sonin kernels, and we discuss its physical characteristics and mathematical properties. First, we show that this master equation can be embedded into the framework of continuous time random walks, and we derive an explicit formula for the waiting time probability density function of the continuous time random walk model in form of a convolution series generated by the Sonin kernel associated with the kernel of the regularized general fractional derivative. Next, we derive a fractional diffusion equation involving regularized general fractional derivatives with Sonin kernels from the continuous time random walk model in the asymptotical sense of long times and large distances. Another important result presented in this paper is a concise formula for the mean squared displacement of the particles governed by this fractional diffusion equation. Finally, we discuss several mathematical aspects of the fractional diffusion equation involving regularized general fractional derivatives with Sonin kernels, including the non-negativity of its fundamental solution and the validity of an appropriately formulated maximum principle for its solutions on the bounded domains.

Keywords: anomalous diffusion; continuous time random walks; fractional master equation; regularized general fractional derivative; Sonin kernels; fractional diffusion equation; mean squared displacement; maximum principle

MSC: 26A33 (primary); 33E12; 35A22; 35B50; 45K05; 60E99; 60J60; 60J65

1. Introduction

Today, mathematical models involving fractional integrals, derivatives, and fractional differential equations are actively employed in various fields such as physics [1–3], financial economics [4,5], engineering [6–8], linear viscoelasticity [9,10], and bioengineering and medicine [11], to mention only a few of many relevant research areas. One of the most discussed and well investigated case studies of Fractional Calculus (FC) applications is the modeling of anomalous diffusion or anomalous transport processes that can be roughly characterized as those that do not follow the Gaussian statistics on long times, see, e.g., [12–14] and the references therein. In particular, the mean squared displacement (MSD) of diffusing particles is not a linear function of time, unlike in the case of conventional diffusion. For anomalous diffusion, this linear dependence is replaced by other relationships, such as power law functions of time, or the MSD is not finite.

The most popular mathematical descriptions of anomalous diffusion processes are the Continuous Time Random Walk (CTRW) models at the micro-level and fractional differential equations involving different types of fractional derivatives at the macro-level. The CTRW models were first introduced in [15] for the description of some transport processes which could be intepreted as a result of multiparticle motion. Assuming the particles are independent, their behavior can be described by the waiting time and jump length probability density functions (PDFs) of individual particles. A strong connection between the CTRW model and fractional differential equations was first established in [16], where a fractional master equation involving the Caputo fractional derivative was embedded into the framework of the general CTRW model. This equation was derived for a special waiting time PDF given in terms of the Mittag-Leffler function depending on a parameter (order of the fractional derivative in the fractional diffusion equation). It is worth mentioning that for this waiting time PDF, the fractional master equation was shown to be rigorously equivalent to the corresponding CTRW model and not just asymptotically as in the subsequent publications, see, e.g., [13,14]. In [17], a closed-form formula for solutions to the fractional master equation involving the Caputo fractional derivative was derived in terms of a special case of the Fox H-function, and its properties were investigated. In particular, the MSD of the diffusing particles governed by this fractional master equation was shown to be proportional to a power law function of time with the exponent being equal to the order of the fractional derivative.

Another significant result on the fractional diffusion equation with the Caputo fractional derivative with order between zero and one and the spatial Laplace operator was presented in [18], independently of the CTRW models and prior to publications [16,17]. In [18], the fundamental solution to this equation was derived in terms of the Fox H-function, and its properties were analyzed. In particular, it was shown that the fundamental solution to the fractional diffusion equation is non-negative and normalized and thus that it can be interpreted as a probability density function evolving in time.

The results presented in [16–18] demonstrated that the fractional diffusion equation involving the Caputo fractional derivative can serve as a model for a class of anomalous diffusion processes where the MSD of the diffusing particles is proportional to a power law. However, in many applications, deviations of the MSD from the power law with a fixed exponent are observed [19–21]. Thus, one needs other, more general fractional master equations that would lead to an extension of the class of functions that describe the MSD of the diffusing particles governed by these equations. Two important classes of such models suggested so far are the fractional differential equations with distributed order derivatives [22,23] and the fractional differential equations with variable order fractional derivatives [24,25]. However, in both cases, no direct connection to the CTRW model has been established until now.

For fractional differential equations with distributed order derivatives, the fundamental solution can be interpreted in some important cases as a PDF [26]. Moreover, the asymptotics of the MSD of diffusing particles governed by this equation has been derived in terms of power-logarithmic functions [22,23]. These properties of solutions to the fractional differential equations with distributed order derivatives suggested their usage as models of the so-called ultra-slow diffusion. Regarding fractional differential equations with variable order fractional derivatives, their mathematical properties and potential physical interpretation as models for anomalous diffusion are still under investigation.

Thus, fractional differential equations with distributed order derivatives and fractional differential equations with variable order derivatives do not provide a satisfactory solution to the problem mentioned above, i.e., a construction of a framework for anomalous diffusion models that would directly follow from the CTRW model, and would lead to some general classes of expressions for the MSD of the diffusing particles governed by these equations.

In this paper, we introduce and investigate a fractional master equation involving regularized general fractional derivatives (GFDs) with Sonin kernels. GFDs with various classes of Sonin kernels have been discussed in several publications, including [27–29]. These derivatives encompass most time-fractional derivatives as special cases. Due to the diversity of Sonin kernels [30,31], fractional differential equations with GFDs have became an important tool in applied mathematics. In many recent publications (PDFs, [32–34]), the GFDs with Sonin kernels and fractional differential equations with these derivatives were employed for modeling various physical processes and systems.

A key result presented in this paper is derivation of the fractional master equation involving the regularized GFDs with Sonin kernels from the general CTRW model. We show that the waiting time PDF of the CTRW model can be expressed in terms of a convolution series generated by the Sonin kernel associated with the kernel of the regularized GFD. Therefore, this master equation can be explicitly embedded within the CTRW model framework. Moreover, we show that the CTRW model is connected to the fractional diffusion equation involving regularized GFDs with Sonin kernels in the asymptotical sense of long times and large distances.

Another significant finding is a compact formula for the MSD of diffusing particles governed by the fractional diffusion equation involving regularized GFDs, expressed in terms of the Sonin kernels associated with the kernels of the regularized GFDs. Considering various specific cases of Sonin kernels and general formulas for constructing Sonin kernels [30,31], this equation can be adapted to available measurement data describing the MSD of diffusing particles within a certain diffusion process framework. Thus, our approach provides substantially more flexibility needed for the modeling of different kinds of anomalous diffusion processes compared to the fractional diffusion equations introduced so far.

In the last part of the paper, we present some relevant mathematical properties of solutions to the fractional diffusion equation involving regularized GFDs with Sonin kernels. Specifically, we discuss conditions on Sonin kernels that ensure normalization and non-negativity of its fundamental solution, as well as the validity of the maximum principle for solutions on bounded domains.

The rest of the paper is organized as follows. In Section 2, we discuss definitions and basic properties of the GFDs and the corresponding general fractional integrals (GFIs) with Sonin kernels. Section 3 is devoted to the derivation of the general fractional master equation involving regularized GFDs with Sonin kernels from the CTRW model. In doing so, the waiting time PDF of the CTRW model is expressed in terms of a convolution series generated by the Sonin kernel associated with the kernel of the GFD from the fractional master equation. Section 4 focuses on the fractional diffusion equation involving regularized GFDs with Sonin kernels, derived from the CTRW model in the asymptotical sense of long times and large distances. The main result of this section is an explicit formula for the MSD of the diffusing particles governed by this equation, expressed in terms of the Sonin kernel associated with the kernel of the regularized GFD. Finally, we discuss relevant mathematical properties of solutions to the Cauchy problem and to the initial-boundary-value problem formulated for the fractional diffusion equation with regularized GFDs with Sonin kernels.

2. Definitions and Basic Properties of the GFDs and GFIs

The general fractional master equation we are dealing with in this paper involves the GFDs with Sonin kernels. This derivative in different forms and with Sonin kernels from different classes was treated in a series of recent publications, including [27–29]. In this paper, we employ the general fractional integral (GFI), the GFD, and the regularized GFD that are defined as follows, respectively:

$$(\mathbb{I}_{(\kappa)}\, f)(t) := (\kappa * f)(t) = \int_0^t \kappa(t-\tau) f(\tau)\, d\tau,\ t>0, \tag{1}$$

$$(\mathbb{D}_{(k)}\, f)(t) := \frac{d}{dt}(k * f)(t) = \frac{d}{dt}(\mathbb{I}_{(k)}\, f)(t),\ t>0, \tag{2}$$

$$({}_*\mathbb{D}_{(k)}\, f)(t) := (\mathbb{D}_{(k)}\, f)(t) - f(0)k(t),\ t>0, \tag{3}$$

where the operation $*$ stands for the Laplace convolution and the kernels κ and k satisfy the condition

$$(\kappa * k)(t) \equiv 1,\ t>0. \tag{4}$$

Condition (4) was first introduced by Sonin in [35] and is referred to as the Sonin condition. The functions that satisfy the Sonin condition are called Sonin kernels. For a given Sonin kernel κ, the kernel k is referred to as its associated Sonin kernel.

The power law functions

$$\kappa(t) = h_\alpha(t),\ k(t) = h_{1-\alpha}(t),\ 0<\alpha<1 \ \text{ with } \ h_\alpha(t) := \frac{t^{\alpha-1}}{\Gamma(\alpha)},\ \alpha>0 \tag{5}$$

constitute the most known and probably most important pair of Sonin kernels. Originally, these kernels were introduced by Abel in [36,37] for the analytical treatment of the tautochrone problem.

The GFI (1), the GFD (2), and the regularized GFD (3) with the power law Sonin kernels (5) are reduced to the Riemann-Liouville fractional integral (6) and to the Riemann-Liouville and Caputo fractional derivatives (7) and (8) of the order α ($0<\alpha<1$), respectively:

$$(I^\alpha_{0+}\, f)(t) := (h_\alpha * f)(t) = \frac{1}{\Gamma(\alpha)}\int_0^t (t-\tau)^{\alpha-1} f(\tau)\, d\tau,\ t>0, \tag{6}$$

$$(D^\alpha_{RL}\, f)(t) := \frac{d}{dt}(I^{1-\alpha}_{0+}\, f)(t) = \frac{d}{dt}(h_{1-\alpha} * f)(t),\ t>0, \tag{7}$$

$$(D^\alpha_{C}\, f)(t) := (D^\alpha_{RL}\, f)(t) - f(0)h_{1-\alpha}(t). \tag{8}$$

The Formula (6) defines the Riemann-Liouville fractional integral for any $\alpha>0$ or more generally for any $\alpha\in\mathbb{C}$ with $\Re(\alpha)>0$ and the operator I^0_{0+} is interpreted as the identity. As to the Caputo fractional derivative, in most FC publications it is defined by the expression

$$(D^\alpha_{C}\, f)(t) := (h_{1-\alpha} * f')(t) = (I^{1-\alpha}_{0+}\, f')(t), \tag{9}$$

that follows from (8) for any absolutely continuous function f.

Another important pair of Sonin kernels that will be used in this paper is given by the formula [38–40]

$$\kappa(t) = h_{1-\alpha+\beta}(t) + h_{1-\alpha}(t),\ 0<\beta<\alpha<1, \tag{10}$$

$$k(t) = t^{\alpha-1}\, E_{\beta,\alpha}(-t^\beta), \tag{11}$$

where $E_{\beta,\alpha}$ stands for the two-parameters Mittag-Leffler function that is defined by the following convergent series:

$$E_{\beta,\alpha}(z) = \sum_{k=0}^{+\infty} \frac{z^k}{\Gamma(\beta k+\alpha)},\ \beta>0,\ \alpha,\ z\in\mathbb{C}. \tag{12}$$

More examples of Sonin kernels can be found in [30,31,38].

It is worth mentioning that the properties of the GFIs and the regularized GFDs essentially depend on the classes of functions that their kernels belong to. In the rest of this section, we focus on the GFIs and the regularized GFDs with Sonin kernels κ, k that belong to the space $C_{-1}(0,+\infty)$ defined as follows:

$$C_{-1}(0,+\infty) := \{f : f(t) = t^p f_1(t),\ t > 0,\ p > -1,\ f_1 \in C[0,+\infty)\}. \tag{13}$$

In [38,39] and subsequent publications, the class of Sonin kernels from the space $C_{-1}(0,+\infty)$ was referred to as $\mathcal{L}_1$. It is a very broad class that includes most of the known Sonin kernels. Still, it is worth mentioning that there exist some Sonin kernels with power-logarithmic asymptotics at the origin that do not belong to this class; see [41] for examples of such kernels.

In further discussions, we need some properties of the GFIs, the GFDs, and the regularized GFDs. As shown in [38,39], the GFIs and the GFDs with Sonin kernels that belong to the class $\mathcal{L}_1$ build a kind of calculus. In particular, the following analogies of the first and second fundamental theorems of calculus hold valid for the GFI, the GFD, and the regularized GFD:

(1) The GFD (2) is a left inverse operator to the GFI (1) on the space $C_{-1}(0,+\infty)$ defined as in (13):

$$(\mathbb{D}_{(k)}\, \mathbb{I}_{(\kappa)}\, f)(t) = f(t),\ f \in C_{-1}(0,+\infty),\ t > 0, \tag{14}$$

and the regularized GFD (3) is a left inverse operator to the GFI (1) on the space $\mathbb{I}_{(k)}(C_{-1}(0,+\infty))$:

$$({}_*\mathbb{D}_{(k)}\, \mathbb{I}_{(\kappa)}\, f)(t) = f(t),\ f \in \mathbb{I}_{(k)}(C_{-1}(0,+\infty)),\ t > 0, \tag{15}$$

where $\mathbb{I}_{(k)}(C_{-1}(0,+\infty)) := \{f : f(t) = (\mathbb{I}_{(k)}\, \phi)(t),\ \phi \in C_{-1}(0,+\infty)\}$.

(2) The relations

$$(\mathbb{I}_{(\kappa)}\, \mathbb{D}_{(k)}\, f)(t) = f(t) - (\mathbb{I}_{(k)}\, f)(0)\, \kappa(t),\ t > 0,\ f \in C^1_{-1,(k)}(0,+\infty), \tag{16}$$

and

$$(\mathbb{I}_{(\kappa)}\, {}_*\mathbb{D}_{(k)}\, f)(t) = f(t) - f(0),\ t > 0,\ f \in C^1_{-1}(0,+\infty), \tag{17}$$

hold valid, where

$$C^1_{-1,(k)}(0,+\infty) = \{f \in C_{-1}(0,+\infty) : (\mathbb{D}_{(k)}\, f) \in C_{-1}(0,+\infty)\}, \tag{18}$$

and

$$C^1_{-1}(0,+\infty) := \{f \in C_{-1}(0,+\infty) : f' \in C_{-1}(0,+\infty)\}. \tag{19}$$

For the Riemann-Liouville fractional integral with the kernel $\kappa(t) = h_\alpha(t)$ and the Riemann-Liouville and Caputo fractional derivatives with the kernel $k(t) = h_{1-\alpha}(t)$, $0 < \alpha < 1$, the relations (16) and (17) take the following well-known form:

$$(I^\alpha_{0+}\, D^\alpha_{0+}\, f)(t) = f(t) - (I^{1-\alpha}_{0+}\, f)(0)\, h_\alpha(t),\ t > 0, \tag{20}$$

and

$$(I^\alpha_{0+}\, {}_*D^\alpha_{0+}\, f)(t) = f(t) - f(0),\ t > 0. \tag{21}$$

3. The General Fractional Master Equation Involving Regularized GFDs

In this section, we apply the method suggested in [16] to demonstrate that the general fractional master equation involving regularized GFDs with Sonin kernels can be embedded into the framework of the CTRW model. More precisely, we show that this general fractional master equation is equivalent to the CTRW model with a certain waiting time PDF that can be expressed in terms of a convolution series generated by the Sonin kernel associated with the kernel of the regularized GFD.

3.1. The CTRW Model

In this subsection, we briefly present the main equations of the CTRW model. This model is based on the idea that the displacement $\mathbf{x} \in \mathbb{R}^n$ of a random walker by each single jump and the waiting times between two successive jumps are governed by certain PDFs that we denote by $\lambda(\mathbf{x})$ and $\psi(t)$, respectively. In what follows, we assume that there is no correlation between displacements and waiting times, that at time $t = 0$ the random walker is located at position $\mathbf{x} = \mathbf{0}$, and that the locations $\mathbf{x}$ of the random walker are either some discrete points from $\mathbb{R}^n$ or the whole $\mathbb{R}^n$. In the last case, the sums in the Formulas (22) and (26) have to be interpreted as the integrals over $\mathbb{R}^n$.

Denoting by $u(\mathbf{x},t)$ the unknown probability to find the random walker at the location $\mathbf{x}$ at time t, the law of total probability leads to the following integral equation [42]:

$$u(\mathbf{x},t) = \int_0^t \psi(t-t') \sum_{\mathbf{x}'} \lambda(\mathbf{x}-\mathbf{x}')\, u(\mathbf{x}',t')\, dt' \; + \; \delta(\mathbf{x})\Psi(t), \tag{22}$$

where $\Psi = \Psi(t)$ stands for the survival probability at the initial position that is defined by the formula

$$\Psi(t) = 1 - \int_0^t \psi(t')\, dt'. \tag{23}$$

Applying the Fourier and the Laplace transforms to the relation (22), we obtain the equation

$$\widehat{\widetilde{u}}(\zeta,s) = \widetilde{\psi}(s)\widehat{\lambda}(\zeta)\widehat{\widetilde{u}}(\zeta,s) + \widetilde{\Psi}(s), \tag{24}$$

that can be solved for the Fourier-Laplace transform $\widehat{\widetilde{u}}(\zeta,s)$ of solution $u(\mathbf{x},t)$ to the integral Equation (22), and we arrive at the formula

$$\widehat{\widetilde{u}}(\zeta,s) = \frac{\widetilde{\Psi}(s)}{1-\widetilde{\psi}(s)\widehat{\lambda}(\zeta)}. \tag{25}$$

We remind the readers that the Fourier and Laplace transforms are defined by the following formulas, respectively:

$$\widehat{f}(\zeta) = \mathcal{F}\{f(\mathbf{x});\zeta\} = \sum_{\mathbf{x}} e^{i\zeta\mathbf{x}} f(\mathbf{x})\,,\; \zeta \in \mathbb{R}^n\,, \tag{26}$$

$$\widetilde{f}(s) = \mathcal{L}\{f(t);s\} = \int_0^\infty e^{-st} f(t)\, dt,\; \Re(s) > C_f. \tag{27}$$

The Formula (23) in the Laplace domain takes the form

$$\widetilde{\Psi}(s) = \frac{1}{s} - \frac{1}{s}\widetilde{\psi}(s). \tag{28}$$

Substituting this relation into the right-hand side of the expression (25), we obtain the following solution formula to the integral Equation (22) in the Fourier-Laplace domain:

$$\widehat{\widetilde{u}}(\zeta,s) = \frac{1-\widetilde{\psi}(s)}{s}\frac{1}{1-\widetilde{\psi}(s)\widehat{\lambda}(\zeta)}. \tag{29}$$

3.2. The General Fractional Master Equation

In this subsection, we introduce a general fractional master equation involving the regularized fractional GFD with the Sonin kernel k in the form

$$({}_*\mathbb{D}_{(k)}\, u(\mathbf{x},\cdot))(t) = \sum_{\mathbf{x}'} \omega(\mathbf{x}-\mathbf{x}')u(\mathbf{x}',t), \tag{30}$$

equipped with the initial condition

$$u(\mathbf{x},0) = \delta(\mathbf{x}), \tag{31}$$

where the fractional transition rates $\omega(\mathbf{x})$ satisfy the relation $\sum_{\mathbf{x}'} \omega(\mathbf{x}') = 0$ and the domain of the variable $\mathbf{x}'$ is either a discrete subset of $\mathbb{R}^n$ or the whole $\mathbb{R}^n$. In the last case, the sums in the Equations (30) and (32) have to be interpreted as integrals over $\mathbb{R}^n$.

Due to the Formula (17), Equations (30) and (31) can be transformed to the integral equation

$$u(\mathbf{x},t) = (\mathbb{I}_{(\kappa)} \sum_{\mathbf{x}'} \omega(\mathbf{x}-\mathbf{x}')u(\mathbf{x}',\cdot))(t) + \delta(\mathbf{x}), \tag{32}$$

where $\mathbb{I}_{(\kappa)}$ is the GFI with the Sonin kernel κ associated with the Sonin kernel k of the regularized GFD in Equation (30).

Applying the Fourier and the Laplace transforms to the Formula (32) leads to the equation

$$\widehat{\widetilde{u}}(\zeta,s) = \widetilde{\kappa}(s)\widehat{\omega}(\zeta)\widehat{\widetilde{u}}(\zeta,s) + \frac{1}{s}, \tag{33}$$

that can be solved for the Fourier-Laplace transform $\widehat{\widetilde{u}}(\zeta,s)$ of the unknown function $u(\mathbf{x},t)$ as follows:

$$\widehat{\widetilde{u}}(\zeta,s) = \frac{1}{s}\frac{1}{1-\widetilde{\kappa}(s)\widehat{\omega}(\zeta)}. \tag{34}$$

3.3. The General Fractional Master Equation as a CTRW Model

For embedding of the general fractional master Equation (30) along with the initial condition (31) into the framework of the CTRW model provided by the Equations (22) and (23), we suppose that their solutions and thus their Fourier-Laplace transforms given by the Formulas (29) and (34), respectively, are identically equal, i.e., the following relation holds valid:

$$\frac{1-\widetilde{\psi}(s)}{s}\frac{1}{1-\widetilde{\psi}(s)\widehat{\lambda}(\zeta)} = \frac{1}{s}\frac{1}{1-\widetilde{\kappa}(s)\widehat{\omega}(\zeta)}. \tag{35}$$

By elementary transformations, the variables ζ and s in the relation (35) can be separated and we arrive at the formula

$$\frac{\widehat{\lambda}(\zeta)-1}{\widehat{\omega}(\zeta)} = \frac{\widetilde{\kappa}(s)(1-\widetilde{\psi}(s))}{\widetilde{\psi}(s)}. \tag{36}$$

Because the variables ζ and s are independent from each other, the functions on the left- and the right-hand sides of the Equation (36) have to be equal to the same constant and thus we get two important relations:

$$\frac{\widehat{\lambda}(\zeta)-1}{\widehat{\omega}(\zeta)} = C,\ C \in \mathbb{R},\ C \neq 0, \tag{37}$$

$$\frac{\widetilde{\kappa}(s)(1-\widetilde{\psi}(s))}{\widetilde{\psi}(s)} = C,\ C \in \mathbb{R},\ C \neq 0. \tag{38}$$

In what follows, without loss of generality, we set $C = 1$ in the Formulas (37) and (38).

Solving the Equation (38) with $C = 1$ for $\widetilde{\psi}$, we arrive at the following relation between the Laplace transforms of the waiting time PDF ψ from the CTRW model and the Sonin kernel κ associated with the kernel k of the regularized GFD from the general fractional master Equation (30):

$$\widetilde{\psi}(s) = \frac{\widetilde{\kappa}(s)}{1+\widetilde{\kappa}(s)}. \tag{39}$$

Now we assume that $\widetilde{\kappa}(s) \to 0$ as $s \to +\infty$ (see the condition K3 for Sonin kernels from the class $\mathcal{K}$ presented in Section 4.3) and obtain the series representation of the Laplace transform of the waiting time PDF ψ in the form

$$\widetilde{\psi}(s) = \widetilde{\kappa}(s) \sum_{n=0}^{\infty} (-\widetilde{\kappa}(s))^n = \sum_{n=0}^{\infty} (-1)^n \, (\widetilde{\kappa}(s))^{n+1}, \tag{40}$$

that holds valid for $\Re(s) > C(\kappa)$, where $C(\kappa)$ is a constant which depends on the kernel κ.

Applying the inverse Laplace transform to the Equation (40), we arrive at the formula

$$\psi(t) = \sum_{n=0}^{\infty} (-1)^n \, \kappa^{<n+1>}(t), \tag{41}$$

where the notation $f^{<n>}$ stands for the convolution power defined as follows:

$$f^{<n>}(t) := \begin{cases} f(t), & n = 1, \\ (\underbrace{f * \ldots * f}_{n \text{ times}})(t), & n = 2, 3, \ldots. \end{cases} \tag{42}$$

The series as on the right-hand side of the Formula (41) was introduced for the first time in [39] (see also [43] for more details) and was there called the convolution series. As has been shown in [39,43], for any kernel $\kappa \in C_{-1}(0, +\infty)$, this convolution series is convergent for all $t > 0$ and defines a function that belongs to the space $C_{-1}(0, +\infty)$.

In the FC literature, the convolution series of the type as in the right-hand side of the Formula (41) is denoted by $l_{\kappa,\mu}$ and defined as follows:

$$l_{\kappa,\mu}(t) := \sum_{n=0}^{+\infty} \mu^n \kappa^{<n+1>}(t). \tag{43}$$

Using this notation, we can represent the Formula (41) in the form

$$\psi(t) = l_{\kappa,-1}(t), \tag{44}$$

where the convolution series $l_{\kappa,-1}(t)$ is defined as in (43).

In the case of the kernel $\kappa(t) = h_\alpha(t),\ 0 < \alpha < 1$ of the Riemann-Liouville fractional integral, the formula $\kappa^{<n+1>}(t) = h_\alpha^{<n+1>}(t) = h_{(n+1)\alpha}(t)$ is valid (see, e.g., [39,43]) and the convolution series (43) takes the form

$$l_{\kappa,\mu}(t) = \sum_{j=0}^{+\infty} \mu^j h_{(j+1)\alpha}(t) = t^{\alpha-1} \sum_{j=0}^{+\infty} \frac{\mu^j \, t^{j\alpha}}{\Gamma(j\alpha + \alpha)} = t^{\alpha-1} E_{\alpha,\alpha}(\mu \, t^\alpha), \tag{45}$$

where the two-parameters Mittag-Leffler function $E_{\alpha,\alpha}$ is defined as in the Equation (12).

For the Sonin kernel $\kappa(t) = h_{1-\alpha+\beta}(t) + h_{1-\alpha}(t)$, $0 < \beta < \alpha < 1$ (see Formula (10)), the convolution series (43) takes the following form [39]:

$$l_{\kappa,\mu}(t) = \frac{1}{\mu t}\sum_{j=0}^{+\infty}\sum_{l_1+l_2=j}\frac{j!}{l_1!l_2!}\frac{(\mu t^{1-\alpha+\beta})^{l_1}(\mu t^{1-\alpha})^{l_2}}{\Gamma(l_1(1-\alpha+\beta)+l_2(1-\alpha))} =$$

$$\frac{1}{\mu t}E_{(1-\alpha,1-\alpha+\beta),0}(\mu t^{1-\alpha}, \mu t^{1-\alpha+\beta}),$$

where $E_{(1-\alpha,1-\alpha+\beta),0}$ is a particular case of the multinomial Mittag-Leffler function defined by the expression [44]:

$$E_{(\alpha_1,\ldots,\alpha_m),\gamma}(z_1,\ldots,z_m) := \sum_{j=0}^{+\infty}\sum_{l_1+\cdots+l_m=j}\frac{j!}{l_1!\times\cdot\times l_m!}\frac{\prod_{i=1}^{m} z_i^{l_i}}{\Gamma(\gamma+\sum_{i=1}^{m}\alpha_i l_i)}. \tag{46}$$

It is also worth mentioning that the Sonin condition (4) in the Laplace domain takes the form

$$\tilde{\kappa}(s)\cdot\tilde{k}(s) = \frac{1}{s},\ \Re(s) > 0, \tag{47}$$

that leads to another representation of the relation (39):

$$\tilde{\psi}(s) = \frac{1}{1+s\tilde{k}(s)}, \tag{48}$$

where k is the Sonin kernel of the GFD from the fractional master Equation (30).

Another important feature of the convolution series $l_{\kappa,\mu}(t)$ defined by (43) is that this function is the main component of the solution formulas for linear fractional differential equations with GFDs and constant coefficients [39,45]. In particular, it is the unique solution to the following initial-value problem for the fractional differential equation involving the GFD with the kernel k [45]:

$$\begin{cases} (\mathbb{D}_{(k)}\, y)(t) = \mu\, y(t),\ t > 0, \\ (\mathbb{I}_{(k)}\, y)(0) = 1. \end{cases} \tag{49}$$

Taking into account the representation (44) of the waiting time PDF ψ in terms of the convolution series $l_{\kappa,-1}(x)$, the function ψ can be also interpreted as the eigenfunction of the GFD $\mathbb{D}_{(k)}$ to the eigenvalue $\mu = -1$ that satisfies the non-local initial condition in terms of the GFI with the Sonin kernel k:

$$\begin{cases} (\mathbb{D}_{(k)}\, \psi)(t) = -\psi(t),\ t > 0, \\ (\mathbb{I}_{(k)}\, \psi)(0) = 1. \end{cases} \tag{50}$$

As an example, let us discuss the case of the power law Sonin kernels $\kappa(t) = h_\alpha(t)$ and $k(t) = h_{1-\alpha}(t), 0 < \alpha < 1$ that was analyzed for the first time in [16]. As mentioned in Section 2, the GFI with the kernel $\kappa(t) = h_\alpha(t)$ is the Riemann-Liouville fractional integral and the regularized GFD with the kernel $k(t) = h_{1-\alpha}(t)$ is the Caputo fractional derivative. Thus, the fractional master Equation (30) takes the form

$$(\,_*D_{0+}^{\alpha}\, u(\mathbf{x},\cdot))(t) = \sum_{\mathbf{x}'}\omega(\mathbf{x}-\mathbf{x}')u(\mathbf{x}',t),\ 0 < \alpha < 1. \tag{51}$$

Equipped with the initial condition

$$u(\mathbf{x},0) = \delta(\mathbf{x}), \tag{52}$$

this equation is equivalent to the integral equation with the Riemann-Liouville fractional integral in the form

$$u(\mathbf{x},t) = (\mathbb{I}^{\alpha}_{0+} \sum_{\mathbf{x}'} \omega(\mathbf{x}-\mathbf{x}')u(\mathbf{x}',\cdot))(t) + \delta(\mathbf{x}),\ 0 < \alpha < 1. \tag{53}$$

Due to the well-known formula

$$\mathcal{L}\{h_{\alpha}(\cdot);s\} = \widetilde{h}_{\alpha}(s) = s^{-\alpha},\ \alpha > 0,\ \Re(s) > 0, \tag{54}$$

our derivations demonstrate that the fractional master equation in its integral form (53) is a particular case of the CTRW model with the Laplace transform of the waiting time PDF given by the formula (see the Equation (48))

$$\widetilde{\psi}(s) = \frac{1}{1+s\widetilde{h}_{1-\alpha}(s)} = \frac{1}{1+s^{\alpha}},\ 0 < \alpha < 1,\ \Re(s) > 0. \tag{55}$$

The inverse Laplace transform of the right-hand side of the Formula (55) is well-known (see, e.g., [16]) and we arrive at the following representation of the waiting time PDF ψ of the CTRW model in terms of the two-parameters Mittag-Leffler function defined as in (12):

$$\psi(t) = t^{\alpha-1}E_{\alpha,\alpha}(-t^{\alpha}),\ 0 < \alpha < 1. \tag{56}$$

Of course, the relation (56) immediately follows also from the general Formula (44) and the Formula (45) for the convolution series $l_{\kappa,\mu}(t)$ generated by the Sonin kernel $\kappa(t) = h_{\alpha}(t),\ 0 < \alpha < 1$.

It is also worth mentioning that the function on the right-hand side of Formula (56) can be interpreted as a PDF for all values of $\alpha \in (0, 1]$ (see, e.g., [46]) and that this function is the eigenfunction of the Riemann-Liouville fractional derivative to the eigenvalue $\mu = -1$ that satisfies the non-local initial condition $(I^{\alpha}_{0+}\,\psi)(0) = 1$ (see the Formula (50)).

Finally, we remark that the Formulas (37) and (38) provide a two-sided relation between the displacement PDF λ and waiting time PDF ψ of the CTRW model (22) and the fractional transition rates ω and the Sonin kernel k of the regularized GFD from the general fractional master Equation (30). Using this connection, the general fractional master equation can be interpreted as a CTRW model and vice versa, the CTRW model can be represented in the form of a general fractional master equation.

4. The Fractional Diffusion Equation with Regularized GFDs

In this section, we derive the fractional diffusion equation involving regularized GFDs with Sonin kernels from the CTRW model in the asymptotical sense of long times and large distances. Then we establish a formula for the MSD of a random walker (diffusing particle) governed by this equation in terms of the Sonin kernel associated with the kernel of the regularized GFD and demonstrate this formula on several known and new examples. We also discuss some relevant mathematical properties of solutions to the Cauchy and initial-boundary value problems for the fractional diffusion equation involving regularized GFDs with Sonin kernels.

4.1. Derivation of the Fractional Diffusion Equation Involving Regularized GFDs

The Formula (37) with $C = 1$ provides a relation between the Fourier transforms of the displacement PDF λ of the CTRW model and the fractional transition rates ω of the general fractional master Equation (30) in the form

$$\widehat{\lambda}(\zeta) = 1 + \widehat{\omega}(\zeta). \tag{57}$$

Let us suppose that the displacement PDF λ possesses finite variance σ^2. Without loss of generality, we set $\sigma^2 = 2$ and obtain the asymptotical relation [17]

$$\widehat{\lambda}(\zeta) \sim 1 - \zeta^2,\ \zeta \to 0. \tag{58}$$

The last formula combined with (57) yields the representation

$$\widehat{\omega}(\zeta) = \widehat{\lambda}(\zeta) - 1 \sim -\zeta^2,\ \zeta \to 0. \tag{59}$$

On the other hand, the Formula (48) leads to the asymptotical relation

$$\widetilde{\psi}(s) \sim 1 - s\widetilde{k}(s),\ s \to 0, \tag{60}$$

where k is the Sonin kernel of the regularized GFD from the fractional master Equation (30) that satisfies $s\widetilde{k}(s) \to 0$ as $s \to 0$ (see the condition K3 for the Sonin kernels from the class $\mathcal{K}$ presented in Section 4.3).

Substituting the asymptotical relations (58) and (60) into the right-hand side of the Formula (29) for solution of the CTRW integral Equation (22) in the Fourier-Laplace domain, we obtain the equation

$$\widehat{\widetilde{u}}(\zeta, s) \sim \frac{s\,\widetilde{k}(s)}{s}\,\frac{1}{1-(1-\zeta^2)(1-s\,\widetilde{k}(s))} \sim \frac{\widetilde{k}(s)}{s\,\widetilde{k}(s)\,+\,\zeta^2},\ \zeta \to 0,\ s \to 0. \tag{61}$$

The Laplace transform formula [27]

$$\mathcal{L}\{(\,_*\mathbb{D}_{(k)}\,f)(t);s\} = s\,\widetilde{k}(s)\widetilde{f}(s) - \widetilde{k}(s)f(0) \tag{62}$$

for the regularized GFD (3) implicates the representation

$$\widehat{\widetilde{u}}(\zeta, s) = \frac{\widetilde{k}(s)}{s\,\widetilde{k}(s)\,+\,\zeta^2} \tag{63}$$

for the Fourier-Laplace transform of solution to the Cauchy problem for the fractional diffusion equation with the regularized GFD with the Sonin kernel k in the form

$$(\,_*\mathbb{D}_{(k)}\,u(\mathbf{x},\cdot))(t) = \Delta\,u(\mathbf{x},t),\ t > 0,\ \mathbf{x} \in \mathbb{R}^n, \tag{64}$$

equipped with the initial condition

$$u(\mathbf{x},0) = \delta(\mathbf{x}). \tag{65}$$

Thus, the asymptotical relation (61) means that the Cauchy problem for the fractional diffusion Equation (64) involving regularized GFD can be obtained from the CTRW model (22) with the waiting time PDF in the form (48) and with displacement PDFs with finite variances in the asymptotical sense of long times and large distances.

On the other hand, in the case of displacement PDFs with finite variances, one can derive the fractional diffusion Equation (64) directly from the general fractional master Equation (30) in the asymptotical sense of large distances. Indeed, substituting the asymptotic relation (59) into the Formula (34) for the solution of the general fractional master Equation (30) in the Fourier-Laplace domain and using the Sonin condition in the Laplace domain in the form (47), we obtain the formula

$$\widehat{\widetilde{u}}(\zeta, s) \sim \frac{1}{s}\,\frac{1}{1+\widetilde{\kappa}(s)\zeta^2} = \frac{\widetilde{k}(s)}{s\,\widetilde{k}(s)+\zeta^2},\ \zeta \to 0, \tag{66}$$

and the result follows from comparison of the Formulas (63) and (66).

It is also worth mentioning that the asymptotical relation (66) is valid for any s and not just for $s \to 0$ as the relation (61).

Summarizing the findings of this subsection, the fractional diffusion Equation (64) is closely related to both the CTRW model (22) and to the general fractional master Equation (30), and thus it can serve as a new and very general framework for modeling anomalous diffusion processes. In the rest of this section, we present some additional arguments that confirm this thesis.

4.2. MSD of a Random Walker Governed by the Fractional Diffusion Equation with Regularized GFDs

For a general Sonin kernel κ, a closed form formula for the inverse Laplace and inverse Fourier transforms of the right-hand side of Formula (63) is not known and probably does not exist at all. However, this formula can be used to calculate the MSD of a random walker governed by the fractional diffusion Equation (64) subject to the initial condition (65).

Indeed, the Laplace transform $\widetilde{\langle \mathbf{x}^2\rangle}(s)$ of the MSD $\langle \mathbf{x}^2\rangle(t)$ satisfies the relation (see, e.g., [17])

$$\widetilde{\langle \mathbf{x}^2\rangle}(s) = \int_{\mathbb{R}^n} \mathbf{x}^2\, \tilde{u}(\mathbf{x},s)\, d\mathbf{x} = -\left(\nabla_\zeta^2\, \widehat{\tilde{u}}(\zeta,s)\right)\Big|_{\zeta=\mathbf{0}}. \tag{67}$$

For the function $\widehat{\tilde{u}}(\zeta,s)$ given by the right-hand side of the Equation (63), routine calculations lead to the formula

$$\nabla_\zeta^2\, \widehat{\tilde{u}}(\zeta,s) = -\frac{2}{s}\tilde{\kappa}(s)\left(-4\tilde{\kappa}(s)(1+\zeta^2\tilde{\kappa}(s))^{-3}\zeta^2 + (1+\zeta^2\tilde{\kappa}(s))^{-2}\right). \tag{68}$$

Combining the Formulas (67) and (68), we get the representation

$$\widetilde{\langle \mathbf{x}^2\rangle}(s) = \frac{2}{s}\,\tilde{\kappa}(s), \tag{69}$$

where κ is the Sonin kernel associated with the kernel k of the regularized GFD from the fractional diffusion Equation (64).

The inverse Laplace transform of the right-hand side of the Formula (69) leads to a simple and elegant formula for the MSD of the random walker governed by the fractional diffusion Equation (64) in the form

$$\left\langle \mathbf{x}^2\right\rangle(t) = 2\int_0^t \kappa(\tau)\, d\tau = 2(1\, *\, \kappa)(t) = 2(h_1\, *\, \kappa)(t). \tag{70}$$

Now let us consider some known and new examples of the fractional diffusion Equation (64) with different Sonin kernels and calculate the corresponding MSDs of the random walkers governed by this equation.

We start with the case of the power law Sonin kernels $k(t) = h_{1-\alpha}(t)$, $\kappa(t) = h_\alpha(t)$ $(0 < \alpha < 1)$ that has been considered in [16,17]. As already mentioned, the fractional diffusion Equation (64) involving the regularized GFD with the Sonin kernel k takes the form of the fractional diffusion Equation (51) with the Caputo fractional derivative of order α, $0 < \alpha < 1$. Applying the relation (70), we obtain the known formula (see, e.g., [17]) for the MSD of the random walker governed by the fractional diffusion Equation (51):

$$\left\langle \mathbf{x}^2\right\rangle(t) = 2(h_1\, *\, h_\alpha)(t) = 2h_{1+\alpha}(t) = \frac{2\, t^\alpha}{\Gamma(1+\alpha)}. \tag{71}$$

The next example is the pair of Sonin kernels $k(t) = h_{1-\alpha+\beta}(t) + h_{1-\alpha}(t)$, $\kappa(t) = t^{\alpha-1}\, E_{\beta,\alpha}(-t^\beta)$ $(0 < \beta < \alpha < 1)$ (see the Formulas (10) and (11)). In this case, the fractional diffusion Equation (64) with the regularized GFD with the Sonin kernel k contains two Caputo fractional derivatives:

$$({}_*D^{\alpha}_{0+}\, u(\mathbf{x},\cdot))(t) + ({}_*D^{\alpha-\beta}_{0+}\, u(\mathbf{x},\cdot))(t) = \Delta u(\mathbf{x},t),\ t>0,\ \mathbf{x}\in\mathbb{R}^n,\ 0<\beta<\alpha<1. \quad (72)$$

According to the Formula (70), the MSD of the random walker governed by the Equation (72) takes the form

$$\left\langle \mathbf{x}^2 \right\rangle(t) = 2(h_1(\tau) * \tau^{\alpha-1}\, E_{\beta,\alpha}(-\tau^{\beta}))(t) = 2\, t^{\alpha} E_{\beta,\alpha+1}(-t^{\beta}). \quad (73)$$

The known asymptotic behavior of the two-parameters Mittag-Leffler function (see, e.g., [46]) leads to the formula

$$\left\langle \mathbf{x}^2 \right\rangle(t) \sim \begin{cases} \frac{2\,t^{\alpha}}{\Gamma(1+\alpha)}, & t\to 0+, \\ \frac{2\,t^{\alpha-\beta}}{\Gamma(1+\alpha-\beta)}, & t\to +\infty. \end{cases} \quad (74)$$

According to the Formula (74), the behavior of the MSD changes in the course of time between power laws with two different exponents that allows its tuning to anomalous diffusion processes with characteristics that vary in time.

Finally, we discuss the case of Sonin kernels $k(t) = t^{-\alpha}\, E_{\beta,1-\alpha}(-t^{\beta}), \kappa(t) = h_{\alpha}(t) + h_{\alpha+\beta}(t)$, $(\alpha,\beta > 0,\ \alpha+\beta < 1)$ that are kernels given by the Formulas (10) and (11) in reverse sequence.

For the kernel k, the fractional diffusion Equation (64) takes the form

$$({}_*D^{\alpha,\beta}_{ML}\, u(\mathbf{x},\cdot))(t) = \Delta u(\mathbf{x},t),\ t>0,\ \mathbf{x}\in\mathbb{R}^n,\ \alpha,\beta>0,\ \alpha+\beta<1, \quad (75)$$

where ${}_*D^{\alpha,\beta}_{ML}$ stands for the regularized GFD with the Sonin kernel in terms of the two-parameters Mittag-Leffler function defined as follows:

$$({}_*D^{\alpha,\beta}_{ML}\, f)(t) := (\tau^{-\alpha}\, E_{\beta,1-\alpha}(-\tau^{\beta}) * f'(\tau))(t),\ \alpha,\beta>0,\ \alpha+\beta<1. \quad (76)$$

The MSD of the random walker governed by Equation (75) is given by the formula

$$\left\langle \mathbf{x}^2 \right\rangle(t) = 2(h_1 * \kappa)(t) = 2(h_1 * (h_{\alpha} + h_{\alpha+\beta}))(t) =$$

$$2(h_{1+\alpha}(t) + h_{1+\alpha+\beta}(t)) = \frac{2\,t^{\alpha}}{\Gamma(1+\alpha)} + \frac{2\,t^{\alpha+\beta}}{\Gamma(1+\alpha+\beta)}. \quad (77)$$

The asymptotic behavior of the right-hand side of the Formula (77) is similar to one presented in the Formula (74):

$$\left\langle \mathbf{x}^2 \right\rangle(t) \sim \begin{cases} \frac{2\,t^{\alpha}}{\Gamma(1+\alpha)}, & t\to 0+, \\ \frac{2\,t^{\alpha+\beta}}{\Gamma(1+\alpha+\beta)}, & t\to +\infty. \end{cases} \quad (78)$$

However, the essential difference between the Formulas (74) and (78) is the sign of the parameter β. As a result, the fractional diffusion Equations (72) and (75) can be employed for modelling of the anomalous diffusion processes with the time-dependent MSD growth rate (the exponent in its power law asymptotics) that becomes both smaller (Equation (72)) and bigger (Equation (75)) in the course of time.

It is also worth mentioning that in the framework of our model, the behavior of the MSD depends on the Sonin kernel κ associated with the kernel k of the GFD from the fractional diffusion Equation (64), see the Formula (70). In its turn, the kernel κ determines the behavior of the waiting time PDF ψ from the corresponding CTRW model (see the Formula (39)). Thus, the crossover behavior of MSD from short to long times is provoked by variation in the waiting time PDF ψ in the course of time that can be induced by different physical reasons depending on the kind of the anomalous diffusion processes.

4.3. Mathematical Properties of Solutions to the Fractional Diffusion Equation with Regularized GFDs

In this subsection, we discuss some mathematical properties of solutions to the fractional diffusion equation involving regularized GFDs with Sonin kernels that are relevant to its interpretation as a model of the anomalous diffusion processes.

First, following [27], we present an important result regarding the fundamental solution to the fractional diffusion equation involving the regularized GFD with the Sonin kernel k that satisfies the following conditions:

(K1) The Laplace transform $\tilde{k}(s)$ of k exists for all real $s > 0$.
(K2) The Laplace transform $\tilde{k}(s)$ is a Stieltjes function (see [47] for definition and properties of the Stieltjes functions).
(K3) The Laplace transform $\tilde{k}(s)$ meets the asymptotical relations $\tilde{k}(s) \to 0$ and $s\tilde{k}(s) \to +\infty$ as $s \to +\infty$ and $\tilde{k}(s) \to +\infty$ and $s\tilde{k}(s) \to 0$ as $s \to 0$.

The class of Sonin kernels that satisfy the conditions (K1)–(K3) was introduced by Kochubei in [27], see also [48]. We denote this class by $\mathcal{K}$ and refer to it as to the Kochubei class of Sonin kernels.

In [27], Kochubei studied the Cauchy problems for ordinary and partial fractional differential equations involving the regularized GFD (3). In particular, he proved that the fundamental solution to the fractional diffusion equation involving the regularized GFD with the Sonin kernel k from the class $\mathcal{K}$ in the form

$$({}_*\mathbb{D}_{(k)}\, u(\mathbf{x},\cdot))(t) = \Delta u(\mathbf{x},t),\ t > 0,\ x \in \mathbb{R}^n, \tag{79}$$

equipped with the initial condition

$$u(\mathbf{x},0) = u_0(\mathbf{x}),\ \mathbf{x} \in \mathbb{R}^n, \tag{80}$$

is locally integrable in t, infinitely differentiable for $\mathbf{x} \neq 0$, and can be interpreted as a spatial PDF evolving in time.

We note that the fundamental solution to the Cauchy problem (79) and (80) is exactly the solution to the fractional diffusion Equation (64) subject to the initial condition (65). Thus, the solution $u(\mathbf{x},t)$ to the fractional diffusion Equation (64) involving the regularized GFD with the Sonin kernel $k \in \mathcal{K}$ is a spatial PDF evolving in time. In its turn, this means that this equation can be interpreted as a model for anomalous diffusion processes. In the framework of this model, Formula (48) provides an explicit relation between the waiting time PDF ψ of the general CTRW model and the Sonin kernel k of the regularized GFD. The MSD of the diffusing particles governed by this equation is given by Formula (70).

Another important aspect of the fractional diffusion equation involving regularized GFDs with Sonin kernels related to its interpretation as a mathematical model for anomalous diffusion processes is the maximum principle for its solutions on the bounded spatial domains. For the first time, this maximum principle was proved in [49].

The results presented in [49] were formulated for the initial-boundary value problems for the fractional diffusion equation involving regularized GFDs with Sonin kernels and a general second-order spatial differential operator. In what follows, we restate the relevant results for the case of the fractional diffusion equation in the form

$$({}_*\mathbb{D}_{(k)}\, u(\mathbf{x},\cdot))(t) = \Delta u(\mathbf{x},t), \;\; (x,t) \in \Omega \times (0,T], \tag{81}$$

subject to the initial condition

$$u(x,t)\big|_{t=0} = u_0(x), \; x \in \bar{\Omega}, \tag{82}$$

and the boundary condition

$$u(x,t)\big|_{(x,t)\in\partial\Omega\times(0,T]} = v(x,t), \; (x,t) \in \partial\Omega \times (0,T]. \tag{83}$$

In Equations (81)–(83), Ω is an open and bounded domain in $\mathbb{R}^n$ with a smooth boundary $\partial\Omega$, $T > 0$, and the Sonin kernel k of the regularized GFD from the left-hand side of Equation (81) satisfies the following conditions:

(L1) $k \in C^1(\mathbb{R}_+) \cap L_1^{loc}(\mathbb{R}_+)$,
(L2) $k(\tau) > 0$ and $k'(\tau) < 0$ for $\tau > 0$,
(L3) $k(\tau) = o(\tau^{-1}), \; \tau \to 0$.

Now we apply Theorem 3.2 from [49] and arrive at the following result:

Let a function $u(x,t)$, $(x,t) \in \bar{\Omega} \times [0,T]$ satisfy the inclusions $u \in C(\bar{\Omega} \times [0,T])$, $u(\cdot,t) \in C^2(\Omega)$ for any $t > 0$, and $\partial_t u(x,\cdot) \in C(0,T] \cap L_1(0,T)$ for any $x \in \Omega$, and the inequality

$$({}_*\mathbb{D}_{(k)}\, u(\mathbf{x},\cdot))(t) - \Delta u(\mathbf{x},t) \le 0, \; (x,t) \in \Omega \times (0,T]. \tag{84}$$

Then the following maximum principle holds true:

$$\max_{(x,t)\in\, \bar{\Omega}\times[0,T]} u(x,t) \le \max\{\max_{x\in\bar{\Omega}} u(x,0), \max_{(x,t)\in\, \partial\Omega\times[0,T]} u(x,t), \; 0\}. \tag{85}$$

For further results regarding the Cauchy and initial-boundary value problems for the fractional diffusion Equation (64) we refer to [27] and to [49], respectively.

5. Discussion and Conclusions

In this paper, for the first time in the FC literature, we introduced a general fractional master equation involving regularized GFDs with Sonin kernels and analyzed its mathematical properties and some of its physical characteristics.

GFDs with various Sonin kernels and more generally with different classes of Sonin kernels are nowadays a hot topic in the FC literature. These derivatives contain most of the time-fractional derivatives as particular cases. Due to diversity of Sonin kernels, the GFDs and the fractional differential equations with GFDs are actively employed for modeling of several physical processes and systems. In particular, such equations with the GFDs with the special Sonin kernels have been already suggested for modeling of anomalous diffusion processes. In this paper, we provided a background for employing the fractional differential equations with the GFDs involving arbitrary Sonin kernels for modeling of anomalous diffusion processes by establishing their connection to the CTRW model.

One of the main results derived in the paper is a close relation between the conventional CTRW model and the general fractional master equation involving regularized GFDs with Sonin kernels. It turns out that this equation can be embedded into the framework of the CTRW model with the waiting time PDFs expressed in terms of the convolution series generated by the Sonin kernels associated with the kernels of the regularized GFDs. In the case of the fractional master equation with the Caputo fractional derivative involving a power law Sonin kernel, this convolution series is reduced to the known waiting time PDF in terms of the two-parameters Mittag-Leffler function.

Another component of the theory presented in the paper is derivation of the fractional diffusion equation involving regularized GFDs with Sonin kernels from the CTRW model in the asymptotical sense of long times and large distances. This connection suggests employing the fractional diffusion equation with regularized GFDs for modeling of the anomalous diffusion processes. In the framework of this model, the MSD of the diffusing particles governed by the fractional diffusion equation involving regularized GFDs was derived in terms of the Sonin kernels associated with the kernels of the regularized GFDs.

Until now, only some particular cases of this anomalous diffusion model with the power law Sonin kernels were discussed in the literature. The power law Sonin kernels in the fractional diffusion equation induce the MSD of the diffusing particles in form of the power law functions with fixed exponents. In the framework of our model, one can employ any Sonin kernels that lead to a variety of possible expressions for the MSD of the diffusing particles governed by the fractional diffusion equation involving regularized GFDs with Sonin kernels. For a given anomalous diffusion process, the MSD of diffusing particles can be measured in the course of time and in some cases its behavior cannot be imitated by a power law with a fixed exponent. In the framework of our model in form of the fractional diffusion equation involving regularized GFDs with Sonin kernels, this behavior can be fitted and simulated more precisely by selecting an appropriate Sonin kernel. As an example, we presented two particular cases of our model with the crossover behavior of MSD from short to long times. Thus, our approach provides substantially more flexibility, which is needed for modeling of different kinds of anomalous diffusion processes, as compared to the fractional diffusion equations introduced so far.

As to the mathematical properties of solutions to the fractional diffusion equation involving regularized GFDs with Sonin kernels, we discussed conditions on Sonin kernels that ensure some important characteristics of any diffusion-type process. These are non-negativity of the fundamental solution to this fractional diffusion equation and validity of the maximum principle for its solutions on the bounded domains.

Author Contributions: Conceptualization, M.A., D.L. and Y.L.; methodology, M.A., D.L. and Y.L.; validation, M.A. and D.L.; formal analysis, M.A., D.L. and Y.L.; investigation, D.L. and Y.L.; writing—original draft preparation, Y.L.; writing—review and editing, M.A., D.L. and Y.L.; supervision, Y.L.; project administration, M.A.; funding acquisition, M.A. All authors have read and agreed to the published version of the manuscript.

Funding: This research was funded by the Kuwait Foundation for the Advancement of Sciences (KFAS) grant number PN23-16SM-1809.

Data Availability Statement: The original contributions presented in this study are included in the article. Further inquiries can be directed to the corresponding author.

Conflicts of Interest: The authors declare no conflicts of interest.

References

1. Atanacković, T.M.; Pilipović, S.; Stanković, B.; Zorica, D. *Fractional Calculus with Applications in Mechanics: Vibrations and Diffusion Processes, Mechanical Engineering and Solid Mechanics*, 1st ed.; Wiley-ISTE: London, UK, 2014.
2. Hilfer, R. *Applications of Fractional Calculus in Physics*, 1st ed.; World Scientific Publishing Company: Singapore, 2000.
3. Tarasov, V.E. *Fractional Dynamics: Applications of Fractional Calculus to Dynamics of Particles, Fields and Media, Nonlinear Physical Science*, 1st ed.; Springer: Heidelberg, Germany, 2011.
4. Tarasov, V.E. Mathematical Economics: Application of Fractional Calculus. *Mathematics* **2020**, *8*, 660. [CrossRef]
5. Fallahgoul, H.; Focardi, S.M.; Fabozzi, F. *Fractional Calculus and Fractional Processes with Applications to Financial Economics*, 1st ed.; Academic Press: London, UK, 2016.

6. Atanacković, T.M.; Pilipović, S. Zener Model with General Fractional Calculus: Thermodynamical Restrictions. *Fractal Fract.* **2022**, *6*, 617. [CrossRef]
7. Obembe, A.D.; Al-Yousef, H.Y.; Hossain, M.E.; Abu-Khamsin, S.A. Fractional derivatives and their applications in reservoir engineering problems: A review. *J. Pet. Sci. Eng.* **2017**, *157*, 312–327. [CrossRef]
8. Povstenko, Y. *Fractional Thermoelasticity*, 1st ed.; Birkhäuser: Basel, Switzerland, 2015.
9. Freed, A.; Diethelm, K.; Luchko, Y. *Fractional-Order Viscoelasticity (FOV): Constitutive Development Using the Fractional Calculus*, 1st ed.; NASA's Glenn Research Center: Brook Rark, OH, USA, 2002.
10. Mainardi, F. *Fractional Calculus and Waves in Linear Viscoelasticity: An Introduction to Mathematical Models*, 2nd ed.; World Scientific Publishing Company: Singapore, 2022.
11. Magin, R.L. *Fractional Calculus in Bioengineering*, 1st ed.; Begell House Inc.: Redding, CT, USA, 2006.
12. Klages, R.; Radons, G.; Sokolov, I.M. *Anomalous Transport: Foundations and Applications*, 1st ed.; Wiley-VCH: Weinheim, Germany, 2008.
13. Metzler, R.; Klafter, J. The random walk's guide to anomalous diffusion: A fractional dynamics approach. *Phys. Rep.* **2000**, *339*, 1–77. [CrossRef]
14. Metzler, R.; Klafter, J. The restaurant at the end of the random walk: Recent developments in the description of anomalous transport by fractional dynamics. *J. Phys. A* **2004**, *37*, 161–208. [CrossRef]
15. Montroll, E.; Weiss, G. Random walks on lattices II. *J. Math. Phys.* **1965**, *6*, 167–181. [CrossRef]
16. Hilfer, R.; Anton, L. Fractional Master Equations and Fractal Time Random Walk. *Phys. Rev. E* **1995**, *51*, R848. [CrossRef]
17. Hilfer, R. Exact Solutions for a Class of Fractal Time Random Walks. *Fractals* **1995**, *3*, 211–216. [CrossRef]
18. Schneider, W.R.; Wyss, W. Fractional Diffusion and Wave Equations. *J. Math. Phys.* **1989**, *30*, 134–144. [CrossRef]
19. Schiessel, H.; Sokolov, I.M.; Blumen, A. Dynamics of a polyampholyte hooked around an obstacle. *Phys. Rev. E* **1997**, *56*, R2390. [CrossRef]
20. Igloi, F.; Turban, L.; Rieger, H. Anomalous diffusion in aperiodic environments. *Phys. Rev. E* **1999**, *59*, 1465. [CrossRef]
21. Prosen, T.; Znidaric, M. Anomalous diffusion and dynamical localization in polygonal billiards. *Phys. Rev. Lett.* **2001**, *87*, 114101. [CrossRef]
22. Chechkin, A.V.; Gorenflo, R.; Sokolov, I.M. Retarding subdiffusion and accelerating superdiffusion governed by distributed-order fractional diffusion equations. *Phys. Rev. E* **2002**, *66*, 046129. [CrossRef] [PubMed]
23. Chechkin, A.V.; Gorenflo, R.; Sokolov, I.M.; Gonchar, V.Y. Distributed order time fractional diffusion equation. *Fract. Calc. Appl. Anal.* **2003**, *6*, 259–280.
24. Garrappa, R.; Giusti, A.; Mainardi, F. Variable-order fractional calculus: A change of perspective. *Commun. Nonlinear Sci. Numer. Simul.* **2021**, *102*, 105904. [CrossRef]
25. Beghin, L.; Cristofaro, L.; Garrappa, R. Renewal processes linked to fractional relaxation equations with variable order. *J. Math. Anal. Appl.* **2024**, *531*, 127795. [CrossRef]
26. Gorenflo, R.; Luchko, Y.; Stojanovic, M. Fundamental solution of a distributed order time-fractional diffusion-wave equation as probability density. *Fract. Calc. Appl. Anal.* **2013**, *16*, 297–316. [CrossRef]
27. Kochubei, A.N. General fractional calculus, evolution equations, and renewal processes. *Integral Equ. Oper. Theory* **2011**, *71*, 583–600. [CrossRef]
28. Luchko, Y. General fractional integrals and derivatives and their applications. *Phys. D Nonlinear Phenom.* **2023**, *455*, 133906. [CrossRef]
29. Tarasov, V.E. General fractional calculus: Multi-kernel approach. *Mathematics* **2021**, *9*, 1501. [CrossRef]
30. Luchko, Y. On Symmetrical Sonin Kernels in Terms of Hypergeometric-Type Functions. *Mathematics* **2024**, *12*, 3943. [CrossRef]
31. Samko, S.G.; Cardoso, R.P. Integral equations of the first kind of Sonine type. *Int. J. Math. Math. Sci.* **2003**, *57*, 3609–3632. [CrossRef]
32. Mišković-Stanković, V., Atanacković, T.M. On a System of Equations with General Fractional Derivatives Arising in Diffusion Theory. *Fractal Fract.* **2023**, *7*, 518. [CrossRef]
33. Tarasov, V.E. Nonlocal statistical mechanics: General fractional Liouville equations and their solutions. *Phys. A Stat. Mech. Its Appl.* **2023**, *609*, 128366. [CrossRef]
34. Tarasov, V.E. Nonlocal classical theory of gravity: Massiveness of nonlocality and mass shielding by nonlocality. *Eur. Phys. J. Plus.* **2022**, *137*, 1336. [CrossRef]
35. Sonine, N. Sur la généralisation d'une formule d'Abel. *Acta Math.* **1884**, *4*, 171–176. [CrossRef]
36. Abel, N.H. Oplösning af et Par Opgaver ved Hjelp af bestemte Integraler. *Mag. Naturvidenskaberne* **1823**, *2*, 55–68.
37. Abel, N.H. Auflösung einer mechanischen Aufgabe. *J. Reine Angew. Math.* **1826**, *1*, 153–157.
38. Luchko, Y. General fractional integrals and derivatives with the Sonine kernels. *Mathematics* **2021**, *9*, 594. [CrossRef]
39. Luchko, Y. Operational calculus for the general fractional derivatives with the Sonine kernels. *Fract. Calc. Appl. Anal.* **2021**, *24*, 338–375. [CrossRef]

40. Hanyga, A. A comment on a controversial issue: A Generalized Fractional Derivative cannot have a regular kernel. *Fract. Calc. Anal. Appl.* **2020**, *23*, 211–223. [CrossRef]
41. Rubin, B.S.; Volodarskaja, G.F. An embedding theorem for convolutions on a finite interval and its application to integral equations of the first kind. *Sov. Math. Dokl.* **1979**, *20*, 234–239.
42. Klafter, J.; Blumen, A.; Shlesinger, M. Stochastic pathway to anomalous diffusion. *Phys. Rev. A* **1987**, *35*, 3081. [CrossRef] [PubMed]
43. Luchko, Y. Convolution series and the generalized convolution Taylor formula. *Fract. Calc. Appl. Anal.* **2022**, *25*, 207–228. [CrossRef]
44. Hadid, S.B.; Luchko, Y. An operational method for solving fractional differential equations of an arbitrary real order. *Panam. Math. J.* **1996**, *6*, 57–73.
45. Luchko, Y. Fractional Differential Equations with the General Fractional Derivatives of Arbitrary Order in the Riemann–Liouville Sense. *Mathematics* **2022**, *10*, 849. [CrossRef]
46. Haubold, H.J.; Mathai, A.M.; Saxena, R.K. Mittag–Leffler Functions and Their Applications. *J. Appl. Math.* **2011**, *2011*, 298628. [CrossRef]
47. Schilling, R.L.; Song, R.; Vondracek, Z. *Bernstein Functions. Theory and Application*, 1st. ed.; De Gruyter: Berlin, Germany, 2010.
48. Kochubei, A.N. General fractional calculus. In *Handbook of Fractional Calculus with Applications, Volume 1: Basic Theory*; Kochubei, A., Luchko, Y., Eds.; De Gruyter: Berlin, Germany, 2019; pp. 111–126.
49. Luchko, Y.; Yamamoto, M. General time-fractional diffusion equation: Some uniqueness and existence results for the initial-boundary-value problems. *Fract. Calc. Appl. Anal.* **2016**, *19*, 675–695. [CrossRef]

fractal and fractional

MDPI

Article

Approximate Solutions of Fractional Differential Equations Using Optimal q-Homotopy Analysis Method: A Case Study of Abel Differential Equations

Süleyman Şengül [1], Zafer Bekiryazici [1] and Mehmet Merdan [2,*]

[1] Department of Mathematics, Recep Tayyip Erdogan University, Rize 53100, Turkey; suleyman.sengul@erdogan.edu.tr (S.Ş.); zafer.bekiryazici@erdogan.edu.tr (Z.B.)

[2] Department of Mathematical Engineering, Gümüşhane University, Gümüşhane 29100, Turkey

* Correspondence: mmerdan@gumushane.edu.tr

Abstract: In this study, the optimal q-Homotopy Analysis Method (optimal q-HAM) has been used to investigate fractional Abel differential equations. This article is designed as a case study, where several forms of Abel equations, containing Bernoulli and Riccati equations, are given with ordinary derivatives and fractional derivatives in the Caputo sense to present the application of the method. The optimal q-HAM is an improved version of the Homotopy Analysis Method (HAM) and its modification q-HAM and focuses on finding the optimal value of the convergence parameters for a better approximation. Numerical applications are given where optimal values of the convergence control parameters are found. Additionally, the correspondence of the approximate solutions obtained for these optimal values and the exact or numerical solutions are shown with figures and tables. The results show that the optimal q-HAM improves the convergence of the approximate solutions obtained with the q-HAM. Approximate solutions obtained with the fractional Differential Transform Method, q-HAM and predictor–corrector method are also used to highlight the superiority of the optimal q-HAM. Analysis of the results from various methods points out that optimal q-HAM is a strong tool for the analysis of the approximate analytical solution in Abel-type differential equations. This approach can be used to analyze other fractional differential equations arising in mathematical investigations.

Keywords: Abel differential equation; optimal q-homotopy analysis method; Caputo fractional derivative; fractional differential transform method

1. Introduction

Mathematical modeling has been instrumental for people in a variety of ways for centuries. The roots of today's modeling studies in economy, medicine and engineering can be traced back to the first applications of algebraic equations for analyzing inheritance and trade problems. Recent studies in modeling focus on the use of differential equations using the tools of calculus to analyze changes in certain components of various systems. In most of these studies, fractional calculus has become the center of attention.

Certain events or systems in nature can be modeled more efficiently using non-integer order derivation. Dating back to the letter of Leibniz in the late 17th century, studies on fractional calculus improved constantly with a certain increase in the numbers in the last few decades. Riemann–Liouville, Grünwald–Letnikov and Caputo fractional derivative definitions have been extensively studied in the literature. More recent definitions, such as the Atangana–Baleanu fractional derivative and Caputo–Fabrizio fractional derivative, are also popular tools in modeling studies. Katugampola, Hilfer and many other derivatives have been given in the literature (see reference [1]) along with conformable fractional derivative which has become the basis of conformable calculus [2,3].

A certain number of studies on fractional calculus focus on numerical or approximate analytical approaches rather than analytical techniques. Some of the well-known methods such as the Differential Transformation Method (DTM) and the Variational Iteration Method (VIM) have fractional counterparts that are frequently used in applications [4,5]. He's Homotopy Perturbation Method [6] and the Homotopy Analysis Method proposed by Liao [7] share a common relation with the homotopy concept in topology [8] and are both among the most studied methods in the literature. Liao [8] showed that the Homotopy Perturbation Method (HPM) is a special case of the Homotopy Analysis Method (HAM), and the former has many applications in fractional calculus. HAM and its modifications such as the optimal q-HAM [9], which is based on the improvement of the convergence by using auxiliary convergence parameters, have been used in the literature for several applications. Some of these applications include the investigation of heat transfer [10], option pricing [11], the convection–diffusion equation [12], the fractional order logistic equation [13] and non-Newtonian fluid flow [14] in their ordinary and fractional forms. A more general form of HAM, the q-Homotopy Analysis Method (q-HAM), has been proposed by El-Tawil and Huseen and the method uses two parameters to achieve faster convergence in comparison to HAM [15,16]. The q-HAM and the q-HATM, which is a combination of q-HAM and the Laplace transform method, have also been applied to many modeling problems such as Burger's equation [17], non-Darcy Flow problem [18], the fractional vibration equation [19] and the fractional heat equation [20]. Recent studies on HAM, q-HAM and their modifications focus mostly on fractional applications such as the fractional KdV equation [21], the fractional Sawada-Kotera equation [22] and the fractional Fisher's equation [23]. Some other examples of the most recent studies for the method can be exemplified as follows. Biswas and Ghosh have used the q-HAM to analyze the time-fractional Harry Dym equation [24]. Hussein et al. have analyzed the Cahn-Hilliard equation using the q-HAM [25]. Cheng et al. have used the q-HAM to solve the time-fractional Keller–Segel-type equations. In the mentioned study, the authors have also performed a symmetry analysis alongside the implementation of the q-HAM [26]. Sunita et al. have used the q-HAM with Elzaki transform to investigate the two-dimensional solute transform problem [27]. One modification of the q-HAM, called the optimal q-HAM (or Oq-HAM), focuses on finding the optimal values for the auxiliary parameter. This method uses the optimal value for the parameter, controlling the rate and region of convergence, and hence offers a better approximation to the solution. This method has been recently used to investigate the Kaup–Kupershmidt equation [28] and various fractional partial differential equations [29]. Another problem that can be investigated using the fractional optimal q-HAM is the Abel differential equation.

The Abel equation is named after the Norwegian mathematician Niels Henrik Abel who lived in the 19th century. The Abel differential equation of the first kind is a generalization of the Riccati equation, and the Abel differential equation of the second kind is a further generalization [30]. Abel equations have been used to describe the relativistic evolution of a causal dissipative cosmological fluid in conformally flat space–time [31], magnetostatic problems [32] or inflationary dynamics [33]. Abel equations are ordinary differential equations and several studies on their general or periodic solutions have been given in the literature (see references [34,35]). These equations have also been studied recently in the fractional sense using various fractional derivatives. The use of the short memory principle for the solution of the fractional equation [36], a numerical analysis of the equation with a Caputo–Fabrizio derivative [37], a numerical approach using Genocchi polynomials for the fractional model with a Caputo derivative [38] and a numerical investigation of the fractional Abel equation using generalized Bessel functions [39] are some of the recent fractional studies.

In this study, optimal q-HAM will be used to investigate the fractional Abel equation in the Caputo sense. The motivation of this study is the existing literature on the HAM method and the improvements in the convergence achieved by the Oq-HAM modification of the scheme. In accordance with the focus of the recent literature on mathematical modeling using tools of fractional calculus, it is aimed at achieving such improvement for Abel differential equations within the fractional framework. Although the Caputo fractional derivative has been used for this study, other definitions of fractional derivation could also be employed, whenever it is checked that they satisfy the necessary conditions to apply these methods. This approach enables an investigation taking advantage of non-integer order derivation, such as a more generalized investigation and the ability to provide a more accurate modeling of real phenomena. This article adds to the current literature on fractional Abel equations, such as the study by Jafari et al. which uses HAM to demonstrate numerical results [40]. Several numerical examples are given with a variety of coefficients for Abel equations of the first type or equations that are reduced to Bernoulli or Riccati equations in the ordinary and fractional forms. Exact solutions of the equations are, whenever available, compared with the results from optimal q-HAM to demonstrate that the method is a valuable tool to analyze the fractional Abel differential equation. It should be noted that, as mentioned above, optimal q-HAM is a well-established method, and this manuscript is structured as a case study for the analysis of fractional Abel equations using the method. This case study concentrates on the improvement of the approximation obtained with q-HAM through determining the optimal values of the auxiliary parameter. A comprehensive comparison of the improved approximation is presented using results from various methods to verify the benefits of the application of optimal q-HAM in the case of fractional Abel equations. Key contributions of this study can be given as the following bullet points for a clearer presentation:

- A fractional optimal q-HAM has been presented and the approximate solutions for several ordinary and fractional Abel differential equations have been given.
- The approximate solutions have been graphically presented for examples and comparisons of the approximations have been made with exact or numerical solutions.
- The optimal values of h and the convergence regions have been given for various selections of the auxiliary parameters.
- Relative errors, h-curves and numerical comparisons of solutions have been given to underline the suitability of the method and the improvements achieved by using Oq-HAM.
- Approximate analytical solutions from fractional DTM and q-HAM have been compared with solutions obtained with Oq-HAM to underline the superiority of the method.
- Results from q-HAM have been used to point out that a better approximation is achieved as the value of the auxiliary parameter h approaches its optimal value, verifying the improvement through Oq-HAM.

2. Abel Differential Equation of the First Kind and Its Analysis with Optimal q-HAM

The Abel differential equation of the first kind is given by the following:

$$y'(x) = f_3(x)y^3(x) + f_2(x)y^2(x) + f_1(x)y(x) + f_0(x) \tag{1}$$

where $f_3(x) \neq 0$, $f_2(x)$, $f_1(x)$ and $f_0(x)$ are meromorphic functions. A Riccati equation will be obtained in the case where $f_3(x) = 0$, and a Bernoulli equation can also be obtained in the case where $f_0(x) = 0$ and $f_2(x) = 0$ or $f_3(x) = 0$. An Abel equation of the second kind can be given by the following:

$$[g_0(x) + g_1(x)y(x)]y'(x) = f_3(x)y^3(x) + f_2(x)y^2(x) + f_1(x)y(x) + f_0(x)$$

which is a generalization of the equation of the first kind. The equation of the second kind reduces to the equation of the first kind for $g_0(x) = 1$ and $g_1(x) = 0$ [30].

In order to apply q-HAM to analyze the Abel equation of the first kind, Equation (1) is rewritten as follows:

$$y'(x) - f_3(x)y^3(x) - f_2(x)y^2(x) - f_1(x)y(x) - f_0(x) = 0 \tag{2}$$

or

$$N[y(x)] = 0 \tag{3}$$

where $N[y(x)] = \frac{d}{dx}y(x) - f_3(x)y^3(x) - f_2(x)y^2(x) - f_1(x)y(x) - f_0(x)$ is the nonlinear operator. The zero-order deformation of q-HAM is given as follows:

$$(1 - nq)L[\phi(x;q) - y(0)] = qhH(x)N[\phi(x;q)] \tag{4}$$

where $0 \leq q \leq \frac{1}{n}, n \geq 1$ is the embedded parameter, $L[\phi(x;q)] = \frac{d}{dx}\phi(x)$ is the linear operator, $h \neq 0$ is an auxiliary parameter and $H(x) \neq 0$ is an auxiliary function [15]. Equation (4) becomes the following:

$$\phi(x;0) = y(0)$$

for $q = 0$ and similarly the following:

$$\phi\left(x;\frac{1}{n}\right) = y(x)$$

for $q = \frac{1}{n}$. Hence, the solution $\phi(x;q)$ approaches the solution $y(x)$ from the initial condition $y(0)$ as q changes from 0 to $\frac{1}{n}$ [12].

Using the Taylor series expansion for $\phi(x;q)$, we obtain the following:

$$\phi(x;q) = y(0) + \sum_{m=1}^{\infty} u_m(x)q^m \tag{5}$$

where

$$u_m(x) = \frac{1}{m!}\frac{\partial^m \phi(x;q)}{\partial q^m}\bigg|_{q=0}. \tag{6}$$

Assuming the auxiliary linear parameter h, the auxiliary function $H(x)$ and the initial condition $y(0)$ are properly selected such that the series (5) converges as $q \to \frac{1}{n}$, the approximate solution is given as follows:

$$y(x) = \phi\left(x;\frac{1}{n}\right) = y(0) + \sum_{m=1}^{\infty} u_m(x)\left(\frac{1}{n}\right)^m. \tag{7}$$

Define the vector as follows:

$$\vec{u}_r(x) = \{u_0(x), u_1(x), \ldots, u_r(x)\}. \tag{8}$$

If Equation (4) is differentiated m times with respect to q and divided by $m!$ and q is set to zero, the m -th order deformation equation is obtained as follows:

$$L[u_m(x) - \chi_m u_{m-1}(x)] = hH(x)R_m\left(\vec{u}_{m-1}(x)\right) \tag{9}$$

with the initial condition as follows:

$$u_m^{(k)}(x) = 0, k = 0,1,2,\ldots,m-1 \tag{10}$$

where

$$R_m\left(\vec{u}_{m-1}(x)\right) = \frac{1}{(m-1)!}\frac{\partial^{m-1}N[\phi(x;q)]}{\partial q^{m-1}}\bigg|_{q=0} \tag{11}$$

and

$$\chi_m = \begin{cases} 0, & if\ m \leq 1 \\ n, & if\ m > 1 \end{cases}. \tag{12}$$

Note that, for $n = 1$ in Equation (7), the method reduces to the standard HAM. However, if $n \neq 1$, the existence of the factor $\left(\frac{1}{n}\right)^m$ in Equation (7) enables a much faster convergence for q-HAM compared to the standard HAM.

Considering the Abel equation of the first kind (1), differentiation of Equation (4) with respect to $q = 0$ gives the following first order deformation equation:

$$\frac{du_1}{dx}(x) = hH(x)\left[\frac{du_0}{dx}(x) - f_3(x)u_0^3(x) - f_2(x)u_0^2(x) - f_1(x)u_0(x) - f_0(x)\right]. \tag{13}$$

The general form of the m -th order deformation equation can be given as follows:

$$\frac{du_m}{dx}(x) = n\frac{d}{dx}[u_{m-1}(x)] + hH(x)\left[\frac{du_{m-1}}{dx}(x) - f_3(x)\sum_{i=0}^{m-1} u_{m-1-i}\sum_{j=0}^{i} u_j u_{i-j} - f_2(x)\sum_{k=0}^{m-1} u_k u_{m-1-k} - f_1(x)u_{m-1}(x)\right]. \quad (14)$$

The solution of Equation (14) considering the initial condition (10) gives $u_m(x)$ and the numerical solution is obtained through Equation (7).

Improving the Convergence through Minimizing the Residual Error

Several studies by Liao and others [9,41] have presented a methodology for obtaining the optimal convergence control parameters by minimizing the square residual errors over the whole region [42]. The method, up to the stage where the solution $u_m(x)$ is obtained, is called q-HAM. The naming "optimal q-HAM" is based on the idea of selecting the optimal h value for better convergence. A limited number of studies, such as [40], focus on the use of the analysis of Abel equations with HAM or other methods. The main goal of this study is to improve the convergence of solutions obtained by HAM and q-HAM through optimizing the auxiliary parameter. The methodology used to obtain this improvement works in a similar manner to the least-squares approach. If the square residual error is denoted as follows:

$$\Delta_m(h) = \int_{\Omega} (N(u_m(x)))^2 d\Omega, \quad (15)$$

then the optimal value of the auxiliary parameter h will be the value minimizing the square residual error, which can be obtained by solving the equation below:

$$\frac{d}{dh}\Delta_m(h) = 0. \quad (16)$$

This study presents results for a case study of the application of optimal q-HAM for the analysis of Abel equations and focuses on the determination of the optimal values of the auxiliary parameter for analyzing fractional Abel differential equations defined in the Caputo sense. Hence, the definitions of Riemann–Liouville and Caputo fractional derivative [43] operators needed for the fractional analysis are given in this section.

Definition 1. [44] *Let $n \in \mathbb{R}_+$. The operator J_a^n, defined on $L_1[a,b]$ by*

$$J_a^n f(x) = \frac{1}{\Gamma(n)}\int_a^x (x-t)^{n-1} f(t)dt$$

for $a \leq x \leq b$, is called the Riemann–Liouville fractional integral operator of the order n. It is also known that when $n = 0$, $J_a^0 = I$ is obtained (where I is the identity operator).

Definition 2. [44] *Let $n \in \mathbb{R}_+$ and $m = \lceil n \rceil$. The operator D_a^n, defined by following:*

$$D_a^n f(x) = D^m J_a^{m-n} f(x)$$

is called the Riemann–Liouville fractional derivative operator of the order n (where $\lceil n \rceil$ is the ceiling function and denotes the smallest integer that is larger than n). Once again, for $n = 0$, $D_a^0 = I$ is obtained.

Definition 3. [44] *Let $n = \lceil \alpha \rceil$. Then, the Caputo fractional derivative operator ${}^C D_t^\alpha$ is given as follows:*

$${}^C D_t^\alpha f(t) = \frac{1}{\Gamma(n-\alpha)}\int_0^t \frac{f^{(n)}(\tau)}{(t-\tau)^{\alpha+1-n}} d\tau.$$

Properties of the Riemann–Liouville fractional integral and derivative operators and the Caputo fractional derivative operator can be found in the literature. We will be denoting the Caputo fractional derivative as D_x^α, where α is the order or derivation, in correspondence with the general notation in the literature.

3. Numerical Examples

In this section, various forms of the (ordinary) Abel differential equation of the first kind, including Bernoulli and Riccati equations with varying coefficients, are given as numerical examples in addition to fractional Abel differential equations with a fractional Caputo derivative.

Example 1 (Riccati Differential Equation). *In Equation (1), if we take* $f_3(x) = 0$, $f_2(x) = 1 - x$, $f_1(x) = 2x - 1$ *and* $f_0(x) = -x$, *the following Riccati differential equation is obtained, where* $0 \le x \le 1$.

$$y'(x) = (1-x)y^2(x) + (2x-1)y(x) - x$$

Putting the initial condition $y(0) = 2$, the analytical solution can be formulated as follows:

$$y(x) = \frac{3 - e^x + xe^x}{3 - 2e^x + xe^x}.$$

Using $H(x) = 1$ in q-HAM, the first three terms are obtained as follows:

$$\begin{aligned}
u_1(x) &= h\left(-2x + \tfrac{x^2}{2}\right),\\
u_2(x) &= hn\left(-2x + \tfrac{x^2}{2}\right) + h\left(-2hx + \tfrac{7hx^2}{2} - \tfrac{11hx^3}{6} + \tfrac{hx^4}{4}\right),\\
u_3(x) &= h\left(-2h^2x - 2hnx + \tfrac{13h^2x^2}{2} + \tfrac{7}{2}hnx^2 - 8h^2x^3 - \tfrac{11}{6}hnx^3 + \tfrac{39h^2x^4}{8} + \tfrac{1}{4}hnx^4 - \tfrac{4h^2x^5}{3} + \tfrac{h^2x^6}{8}\right)\\
&\quad + n\left(hn\left(-2x + \tfrac{x^2}{2}\right) + h\left(-2hx + \tfrac{7hx^2}{2} - \tfrac{11hx^3}{6} + \tfrac{hx^4}{4}\right)\right).
\end{aligned}$$

Solution (7) from the q-HAM can be given as a finite series as follows:

$$y_k(x) = \sum_{m=1}^{\infty} u_m(x)\left(\frac{1}{n}\right)^m \cong \sum_{m=1}^{k} u_m(x)\left(\frac{1}{n}\right)^m. \tag{17}$$

This solution depends on the value of the auxiliary parameter h. Some of the relative errors have been given below in Table 1 with the corresponding n and h values used for obtaining the approximate solutions (Table 1).

Table 1. Relative errors obtained for the Riccati differential equation with q-HAM.

x	$n = 1, h = -0.5$	$n = 1, h = -1$	$n = 1, h = -1.25$	$n = 20, h = -1$
0.1	0.00037533	$2.74631072 \times 10^{-10}$	$2.54314884 \times 10^{-9}$	0.06599027
0.2	0.00220035	$3.68633053 \times 10^{-7}$	$1.16212931 \times 10^{-9}$	0.14343628
0.3	0.00791511	0.00002018	$1.08409111 \times 10^{-7}$	0.23032080
0.4	0.02150092	0.00029051	0.00001266	0.32344195
0.5	0.04762474	0.00196197	0.00024490	0.41849102
0.6	0.08942998	0.00800457	0.00184491	0.51032883
0.7	0.14554139	0.02243673	0.00758219	0.59345618
0.8	0.20780964	0.04627964	0.01987730	0.66261677
0.9	0.26161939	0.07256799	0.03572155	0.71341999
1.0	0.28971143	0.08673558	0.04471525	0.74285215

The values in Table 1 represent approximate solutions with growing relative errors. It is also seen that the amount of error in these solutions, obtained with q-HAM, change with respect to the changes in the value of the auxiliary parameter h. The use of optimal q-HAM offers a methodology for determining the approximate solution from q-HAM that has the least error, through the analysis of the optimal h.

The square residual error for the Riccati differential equation is written below to obtain the optimum value of the auxiliary parameter h.

$$\Delta_m = \int_{\Omega} \left[y_k'(x) - (1-x)y_k^2(x) - (2x-1)y(x) + x \right]^2 dx. \tag{18}$$

The optimal value of h is obtained by minimizing the square residual error given in Equation (18). The h-curves for various values of the parameter n at $x = 1$ for $k = 10$ have been shown in Figure 1. The convergence regions have been determined from these graphs using the intervals where the lines are parallel to the x-axis. The optimal values of h are selected in these regions through the roots of the nonlinear equation as follows:

$$\frac{d\Delta_m}{dh} = 0. \tag{19}$$

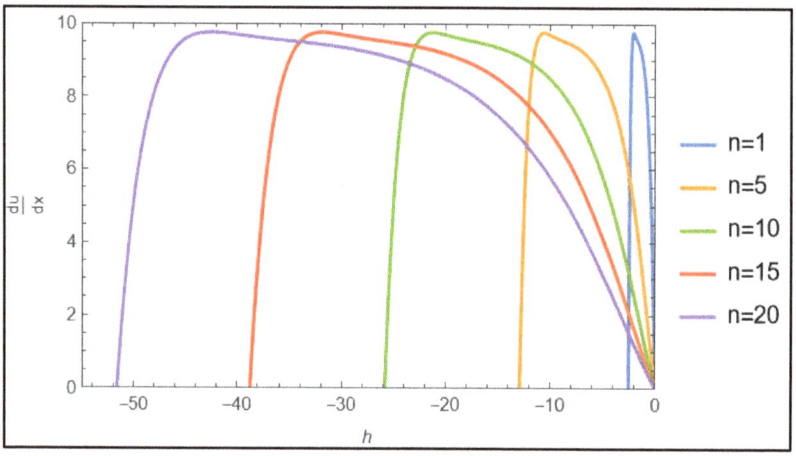

Figure 1. The h-curve of $u\prime(x)$ at $x = 1$ for $k = 10$.

The convergence regions, the optimal h values and the minimum values of Equation (18) for $k = 10$ are given in Table 2 for the Riccati differential equation.

Table 2. Optimal h and the convergence region of h for the Riccati differential equation.

n	Convergence Region	Optimal h	Δ_m
1	$-2.1793 \leq h \leq -1.4460$	-1.87312216	0.00946045
5	$-11.0632 \leq h \leq -5.8422$	-9.36561082	0.01025391
10	$-21.7929 \leq h \leq -14.4595$	-18.73122164	0.01025391
15	$-32.6281 \leq h \leq -22.3157$	-28.09683247	0.00982666
20	$-43.2345 \leq h \leq -34.4072$	-37.46244329	0.01025391

The approximation solution and the analytical solution with the optimal h values are shown in Figure 2. The figure contains the exact solution, the solution obtained with q-HAM and the solution obtained by using Optimal q-HAM with $n = 1$. Note that the solution curve for $n = 20$ is inseparable from the curve for $n = 1$ in this example and hence, not plotted additionally.

Figure 2 shows that the analytical solution and the approximate solution (17) are similar for optimal h values. The figure also contains the solution curve obtained with q-HAM for $h = -1$. Note that all of the solution curves obtained with optimal q-HAM are plotted similarly in all figures for a consistent presentation. In addition, these two solutions have been numerically compared in the following table for the various values of the independent variable (Table 3).

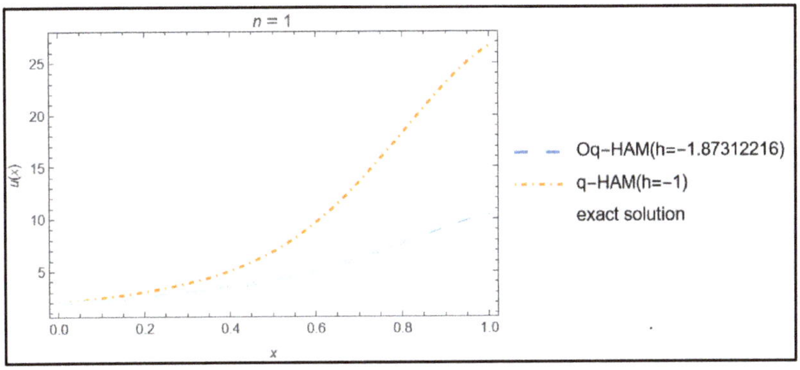

Figure 2. The analytical and approximate solutions for optimal h values for the Riccati equation.

Table 3. The exact and optimal q-HAM approximate solutions compared for $k = 10$.

x	Relative Error (n = 1)	Relative Error (n = 20)
0.1	0.00011073	0.00011073
0.2	0.00142025	0.00142025
0.3	0.00143402	0.00143402
0.4	0.00096602	0.00096602
0.5	0.00021452	0.00021452
0.6	0.00057228	0.00057228
0.7	0.00138279	0.00138279
0.8	0.00299686	0.00299686
0.9	0.00593229	0.00593229
1.0	0.00767123	0.00767123

Table 3 shows that, considering the relative errors shown in the last column, which all satisfy $\varepsilon_{Relative} < 0.8\%$ in the analyzed interval, it can be concluded that the approximate solution is a suitable approximation of the analytical solution. It can also be seen that, for $n = 1$ and $n = 20$, the relative errors in the solutions obtained with q-HAM decrease as the value of the auxiliary parameter h approaches the optimal value used for Oq-HAM.

Example 2 (Abel Differential Equation). *In Equation (1), if we take* $f_3(x) = -x^2$, $f_2(x) = 5x$, $f_1(x) = -2x$ *and* $f_0(x) = x^3$, *the following Abel differential equation of the first kind is obtained, where* $0 \leq x \leq 0.7$.

$$y'(x) = -x^2y^3(x) + 5xy^2(x) - 2xy(x) + x^3.$$

The initial condition will be used as $\mathrm{y}(0) = 1$. The approximate solution from q-HAM will be compared to the numerical solution obtained with Mathematica using NDSolve.

Using $\mathrm{H}(\mathrm{x}) = 1$ in the q-HAM, the first three terms are obtained as follows:

$$u_1(x) = h\left(-\frac{3x^2}{2} + \frac{x^3}{3} - \frac{x^4}{4}\right),$$
$$u_2(x) = hn\left(-\frac{3x^2}{2} + \frac{x^3}{3} - \frac{x^4}{4}\right) + h\left(-\frac{3hx^2}{2} + \frac{hx^3}{3} + \frac{11hx^4}{4} - \frac{43hx^5}{30} + \frac{hx^6}{2} - \frac{3hx^7}{28}\right),$$
$$u_3(x) = h\left(-\frac{3}{2}h^2x^2 - \frac{3}{2}hnx^2 + \frac{h^2x^3}{3} + \frac{1}{3}hnx^3 + \frac{23h^2x^4}{4} + \frac{11}{4}hnx^4 - \frac{43h^2x^5}{15} - \frac{43}{30}hnx^5 - \frac{39h^2x^6}{8} + \frac{1}{2}hnx^6\right.$$
$$\left.+ \frac{1843h^2x^7}{420} - \frac{3}{28}hnx^7 - \frac{2809h^2x^8}{1440} + \frac{485h^2x^9}{756} - \frac{127h^2x^{10}}{1120} + \frac{3h^2x^{11}}{176}\right)$$
$$+n\left(hn\left(-\frac{3x^2}{2} + \frac{x^3}{3} - \frac{x^4}{4}\right) + h\left(-\frac{3hx^2}{2} + \frac{hx^3}{3} + \frac{11hx^4}{4} - \frac{43hx^5}{30} + \frac{hx^6}{2} - \frac{3hx^7}{28}\right)\right).$$

Similarly, the q-HAM solution for this problem is given in the form of Equation (17). To calculate the optimal h values, the derivative of Δ_m in the equation is calculated with respect to h and set to zero. The h-curves for different n values and $k = 6$ are obtained at $x = 0.6$ as shown in Figure 3.

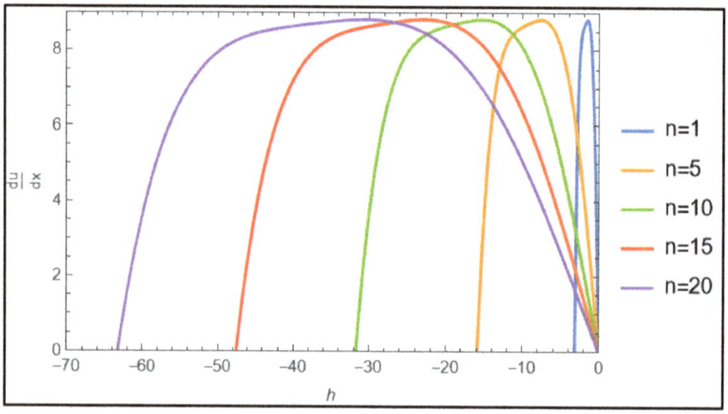

Figure 3. The h-curve of $u'(x)$ with $x = 0.6$, $k = 6$.

The convergence regions, the optimal h values and the minimum values of Equation (1) for $k = 6$ for the Abel differential equation are given in Table 4. Also, the optimal q-HAM solution and the NDSolve solution with the optimal h values are shown in Figure 4 for $n = 20$. Once again, the solution curve for $n = 1$ has been omitted to prevent repeated use of an inseparable plot. Figure 4 shows that the approximate solution is in accordance with the solution obtained with NDSolve for $k = 6$.

Table 4. Optimal h and the convergence region of h for the Abel differential equation.

n	Convergence Region	Optimal h	Δ_m
1	$-2.4872 \leq h \leq -1.0394$	-1.17183989	0.00427890
5	$-12.4361 \leq h \leq -5.1972$	-5.83815009	0.00468601
10	$-22.1298 \leq h \leq -10.9513$	-11.68006881	0.00465427
15	$-24.8946 \leq h \leq -15.5917$	-17.60030257	0.00399791
20	$-30.9369 \leq h \leq -22.6137$	-23.36013762	0.00465427

Example 3 (Fractional Bernoulli Differential Equation). *A fractional Bernoulli differential equation can be obtained from the ordinary Abel differential equation using fractional derivatives and suitable coefficient functions. The following fractional Bernoulli initial value problem will be considered for* $x \in (0, 1)$.

$$D_x^{\alpha} y = x^4 y - x^2 y^2, \; y(0) = 1 \tag{20}$$

The m-th order deformation can be obtained for fractional differential equations in similarity to the q-HAM approximation approach for ordinary differential equations. In this case, the ordinary derivation in Equation (14) needs to be replaced with fractional derivatives. The Caputo derivative (Definition 3) is used in this regard to obtain a fractional differential equation.

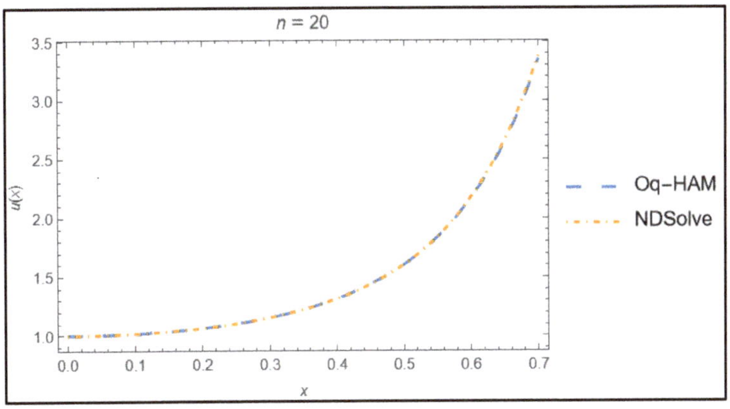

Figure 4. The Oq-HAM and NDSolve solutions for $n = 20$.

Using $\mathrm{H(x)} = 1, \alpha = 0.5$ in the q-HAM, the first three terms are obtained as

$$
\begin{aligned}
&u_1(x) = 0.5641895835477563h(1.0666666666666667x^{2.5} - 0.8126984126984127x^{4.5}),\\
&u_2(x) = 0.5641895835477563h^2(0.9305382717253959x^5 - 0.9995109922628649x^7\\
&+0.2671648878690047x^9)\\
&+(h+n)(0.5641895835477563h(1.0666666666666667x^{2.5} - 0.8126984126984127x^{4.5})),\\
&u_3(x) = 0.5641895835477563h^2(n(0.930538271725396x^5 - 0.9995109922628648x^7\\
&+0.2671648878690047x^9) + h(0.930538271725396x^5 - 0.9995109922628648x^7\\
&+0.8988704875870189x^{7.5} + 0.2671648878690047x^9 - 1.2512690912236168x^{9.5}\\
&+0.5561133343471595x^{11.5} - 0.07204306295221984x^{13.5})) + (h+n)\\
&(0.5641895835477563h^2(0.9305382717253959x^5 - 0.9995109922628649x^7\\
&+0.2671648878690047x^9) + (h+n)(0.5641895835477563h(1.0666666666666667x^{2.5}\\
&-0.8126984126984127x^{4.5}))).
\end{aligned}
$$

The approximate results from the q-HAM will be compared to the numerical results obtained with the Predictor–Corrector method for fractional differential equations given in [45]. The numerical method is an improved version of the Adams–Bashforth–Moulton algorithm and will be referred to as the Predictor–Corrector (PC) method throughout the study.

To calculate the optimal value of the auxiliary parameter h, the h-curve graphs are drawn for $\alpha = 0.5$ and $\alpha = 1$ with $k = 4$, which is the number of terms taken in the q-HAM solution at $x = 1$ in Figure 5a,b.

For the fractional Bernoulli differential equation, the exact square residual error is obtained as follows:

$$
\Delta_m = \int_\Omega \left[D_x^\alpha y_k(x) - x^4 y_k(x) + x^2 y_k^2(x) \right]^2 dx.
$$

If the derivative of Δ_m with respect to h is calculated and solved for zero, the tables of optimal h values obtained for $\alpha = 0.5$ and $\alpha = 1$ are given in Tables 5 and 6, respectively.

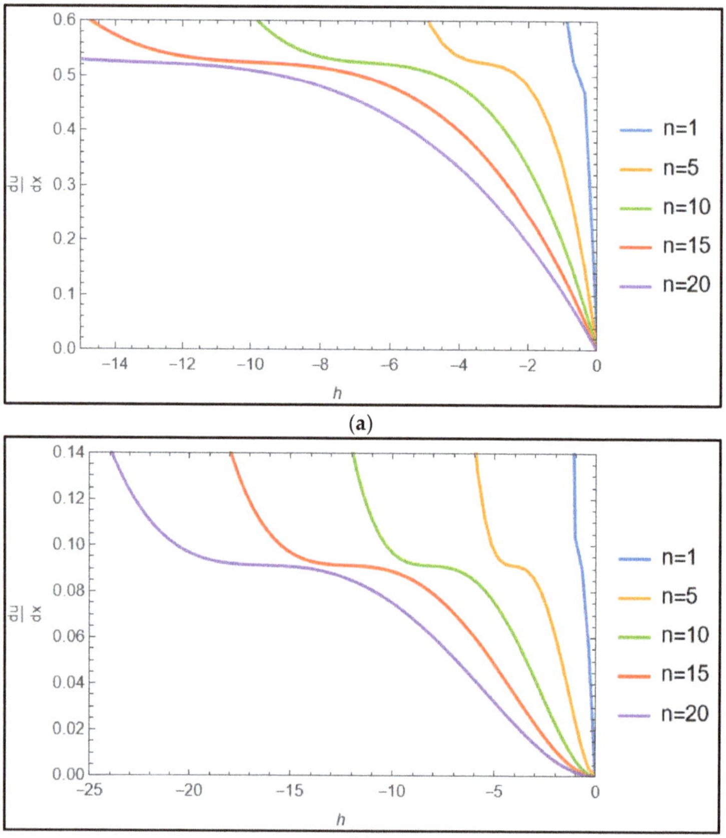

Figure 5. (**a**) h-curve graphs for $\alpha = 0.5$ at $x = 1$. (**b**) h-curve graphs for $\alpha = 1$ at $x = 1$.

Table 5. The optimal h and the convergence region of h for $\alpha = 0.5$.

n	Convergence Region	Optimal h	Δ_m
1	$-0.7635 \leq h \leq -0.5590$	−0.71310376	$3.37203607 \times 10^{-8}$
5	$-3.8175 \leq h \leq -2.7950$	−3.56551974	$3.37178963 \times 10^{-8}$
10	$-8.0043 \leq h \leq -5.2082$	−7.13103948	$3.37178963 \times 10^{-8}$
15	$-12.0063 \leq h \leq -7.8123$	−10.69655936	$3.37170178 \times 10^{-8}$
20	$-16.5847 \leq h \leq -9.8154$	−14.26207897	$3.37178963 \times 10^{-8}$

From Tables 5 and 6, it is seen that, for the optimal values of h, the square residual errors are minimal. In addition, the solutions for the optimal h values obtained with optimal q-HAM have been found to be similar to the solutions from the PC method (for $\alpha = 0.5$), as shown in Figure 6, and the exact solutions (for $\alpha = 1$), as shown in Figure 7. Hence, it can be concluded that the optimal h-values given in Tables 5 and 6 are suitable for the fractional Bernoulli differential equation. Note that $n = 1$ and $n = 20$ produce inseparable curves for Figures 6 and 7, hence, only the figures for $n = 1$ have been given.

Table 6. The optimal h and the convergence region of h for $\alpha = 1$.

n	Convergence Region	Optimal h	Δ_m
1	$-0.9087 \leq h \leq -0.7178$	-0.86488950	$3.40577788 \times 10^{-10}$
5	$-4.5790 \leq h \leq -3.5435$	-4.30383827	$3.40577233 \times 10^{-10}$
10	$-8.6973 \leq h \leq -7.6468$	-8.60767655	$3.40577233 \times 10^{-10}$
15	$-12.9723 \leq h \leq -11.5535$	-12.91151482	$3.40577955 \times 10^{-10}$
20	$-18.0723 \leq h \leq -15.8497$	-17.21535309	$3.40577233 \times 10^{-10}$

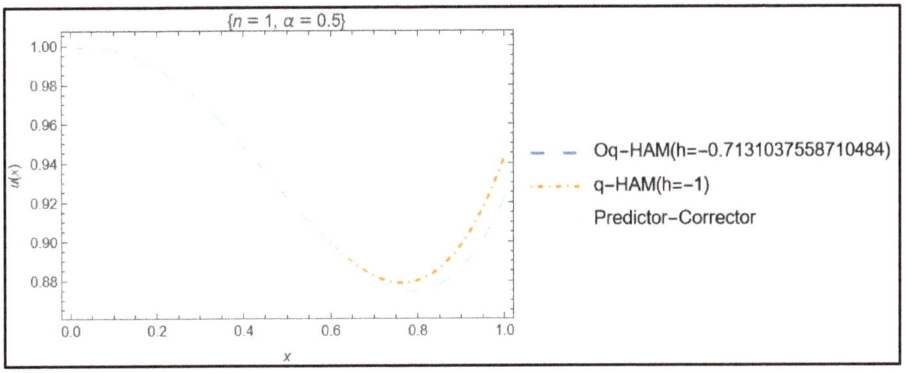

Figure 6. The approximate solutions from fractional Oq-HAM and q-HAM compared for $\alpha = 0.5$, $n = 1$.

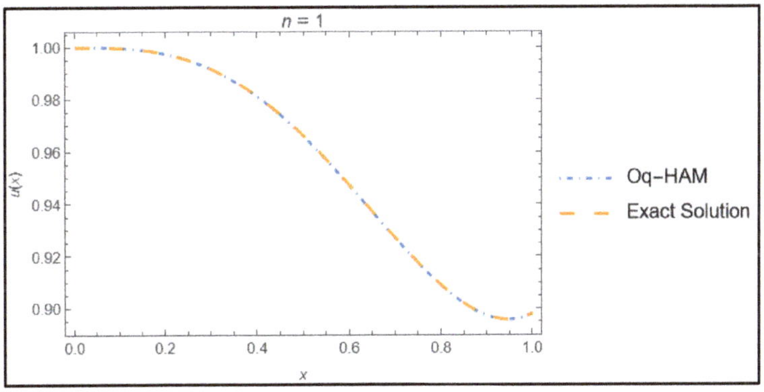

Figure 7. The approximate solutions for optimal h values for $\alpha = 1$, $n = 1$.

In order to give a comparison of the solutions obtained with the optimal q-HAM and the solutions from another approximation method for fractional differential equations, we use the fractional Differential Transform Method [46]. The fractional counterpart of the Differential Transform Method (DTM) has been another widely used tool for analyzing equations with fractional order derivatives and has been applied to study projectile motion [47] and COVID-19 transmission [48]. The reader is advised to refer to the study of Arikoglu and Ozkol for the theorems and properties of fractional DTM [46]. The solution of the fractional Bernoulli differential Equation (20) using fractional DTM has been shown below (Figure 8).

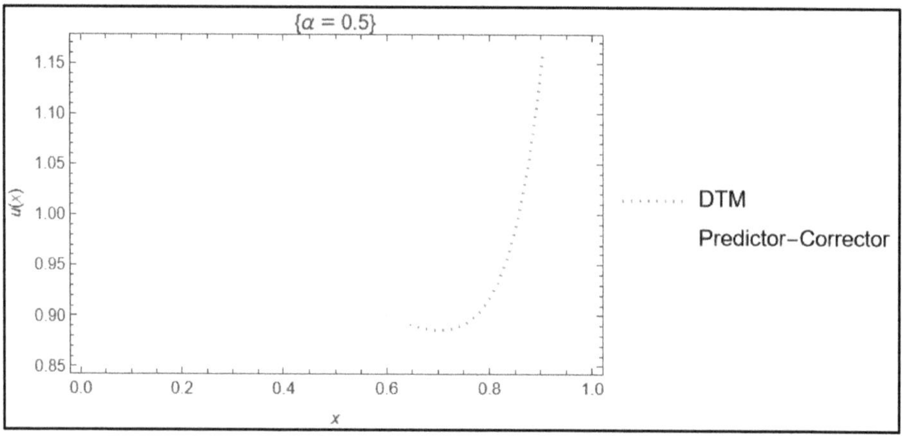

Figure 8. The fractional DTM solution for (20) compared to the numerical solution.

The values for the numerical solution (PC method) and the approximate solutions have been compared for $x \in [0,1]$ in the table below (Table 7).

Table 7. Numerical and approximate solutions of (20) compared for $x \in [0,1]$ and $n = 1$.

x	PC Method	DTM	Oq-HAM	q-HAM ($h = -0.5$)	q-HAM ($h = -1$)	q-HAM ($h = -1.25$)
0.1	0.99809477	0.99811661	0.99812903	0.99823303	0.99811661	0.99812438
0.2	0.98968409	0.98972089	0.98978053	0.99032479	0.98972089	0.98977507
0.3	0.97341252	0.97347280	0.97358992	0.97487314	0.97347292	0.97369769
0.4	0.95054829	0.95063802	0.95077595	0.95282813	0.95064119	0.95145505
0.5	0.92440765	0.92453475	0.92462529	0.92713087	0.92456096	0.92725681
0.6	0.89960938	0.90008460	0.89976706	0.90220525	0.90002374	0.90798397
0.7	0.88137849	0.88596782	0.88143340	0.88332823	0.88287250	0.90323390
0.8	0.87523525	0.91332540	0.87512733	0.87617499	0.87987603	0.92411447
0.9	0.88720130	1.13112410	0.88689226	0.88683630	0.89823968	0.97849497
1.0	0.92444239	2.18855686	0.92399200	0.92244773	0.94414273	1.06294033

Note that the approximate solutions for fractional DTM have been obtained with 30 terms in the approximation. Although a detailed approximation has been obtained for (20) with fractional DTM, the results show that the optimal q-HAM provides a better approximation with optimal h values. Hence, it can be concluded that the convergence is improved in comparison to the classical q-HAM and the DTM method as well by optimizing the value of the auxiliary parameter. The relative errors in Table 8 show how the approximation obtained with optimal q-HAM has incomparably smaller relative errors. For instance, at $x = 0.9$, the relative error for DTM (0.274935128211391) is more than 700 times larger than the relative error for optimal q-HAM ($0.348329311959152 \times 10^{-3}$).

The solutions obtained with q-HAM have varying relative errors, depending on the choice of the value of the auxiliary parameter h. Figure 6 presents the solution curve obtained by using the optimal h value in comparison to the solution curve obtained with q-HAM using $h = -1$. As the value of the parameter h approaches its optimal value, the relative errors are expected to decrease, which also means the curves from Oq-HAM and q-HAM become closer. The results in Tables 7 and 8 and the curves in Figure 6 are a clear indicator of the importance of using the optimal h value. This value, obtained by analyzing the square errors to obtain the minimal error, clearly results in a better approximation to the exact solution.

Table 8. Relative errors in approximate solutions of (20) compared.

x	DTM	q-HAM ($h=-0.5$)	q-HAM ($h=-1$)	q-HAM ($h=-1.25$)	Oq-HAM
0.1	0.00002188	0.00013853	0.00002188	0.00002967	$0.03431887 \times 10^{-3}$
0.2	0.00003718	0.00064738	0.00003718	0.00009193	$0.09744808 \times 10^{-3}$
0.3	0.00006192	0.00150051	0.00006204	0.00029295	$0.18224420 \times 10^{-3}$
0.4	0.00009440	0.00239845	0.00009774	0.00095394	$0.23951227 \times 10^{-3}$
0.5	0.00013749	0.00294591	0.00016584	0.00308215	$0.23543438 \times 10^{-3}$
0.6	0.00052825	0.00288554	0.00046059	0.00930913	$0.17527668 \times 10^{-3}$
0.7	0.00520699	0.00221215	0.00169508	0.02479686	$0.06229900 \times 10^{-3}$
0.8	0.04351990	0.00107370	0.00530232	0.05584695	$0.12330404 \times 10^{-3}$
0.9	0.27493513	0.00041140	0.01244180	0.10290074	$0.34832931 \times 10^{-3}$
1.0	1.36743456	0.00215768	0.02131052	0.14981782	$0.48719902 \times 10^{-3}$

Example 4 (Fractional Abel Differential Equation). *Consider the following fractional Abel differential equation of the first kind.*

$$D_x^{\alpha} y = x^4 y - x^2 y^2 - x y^3 + x, \; y(0) = 1.$$

Using $\mathrm{H(x)} = 1$ and $\alpha = 0.5$ in the q-HAM, the first three terms are obtained as

$$\begin{aligned}
&u_1(x) = 0.5641895835477563h(1.0666666666666667x^{2.5} - 0.8126984126984127x^{4.5}),\\
&u_2(x) = 0.5641895835477563h^2(1.550897119542327x^4 + 0.930538271725396x^5\\
&-0.974849617998034x^6 - 0.999510992262865x^7 + 0.2671648878690047x^9)\\
&+(h+n)(0.5641895835477563h(1.0666666666666667x^{2.5} - 0.8126984126984127x^{4.5})),\\
&u_3(x) = \tfrac{1}{x^{0.5}}0.5641895835477563h^2(n(1.550897119542327x^{4.5} + 0.930538271725396x^{5.5}\\
&-0.974849617998034x^{6.5} - 0.999510992262865x^{7.5} + 0.2671648878690048x^{9.5})\\
&+h(1.550897119542327x^{4.5} + 0.930538271725396x^{5.5} + 1.9393939393939406x^6\\
&-0.974849617998034x^{6.5} + 3.0085738865913085x^7 - 0.999510992262865x^{7.5}\\
&-0.1513859226693921 3x^8 - 3.1885000918855044x^9 + 0.2671648878690048x^{9.5}\\
&-1.2512690912236175x^{10} + 0.882618761181763x^{11} + 0.5561133343471595x^{12}\\
&-0.07204306295221984x^{14})) + (h+n)(0.5641895835477563h^2(1.550897119542327x^4\\
&+0.930538271725396x^5 - 0.974849617998034x^6 - 0.999510992262865x^7\\
&+0.2671648878690047x^9) + (h+n)(0.5641895835477563h(1.0666666666666667x^{2.5}\\
&-0.8126984126984127x^{4.5}))).
\end{aligned}$$

The h-curve graphs for $\alpha = 0.5$ and $\alpha = 1$ at $x = 1$ are given in Figure 9a,b. Here, four terms ($k = 4$) are used for the q-HAM solution. The optimal h values can be determined in the convergence region where $u''_m(x) = 0$.

The convergence regions, the optimal h-values and square residual errors for $\alpha = 0.5$ and $\alpha = 1$ are given, in Tables 9 and 10, respectively.

The numerical solution graphs of the optimal q-HAM and the PC method for the h values obtained are shown in Figures 10 and 11. Only one plot has been given for $n = 1$ and $n = 20$ in both figures, since these values of the parameter produce inseparable solution curves.

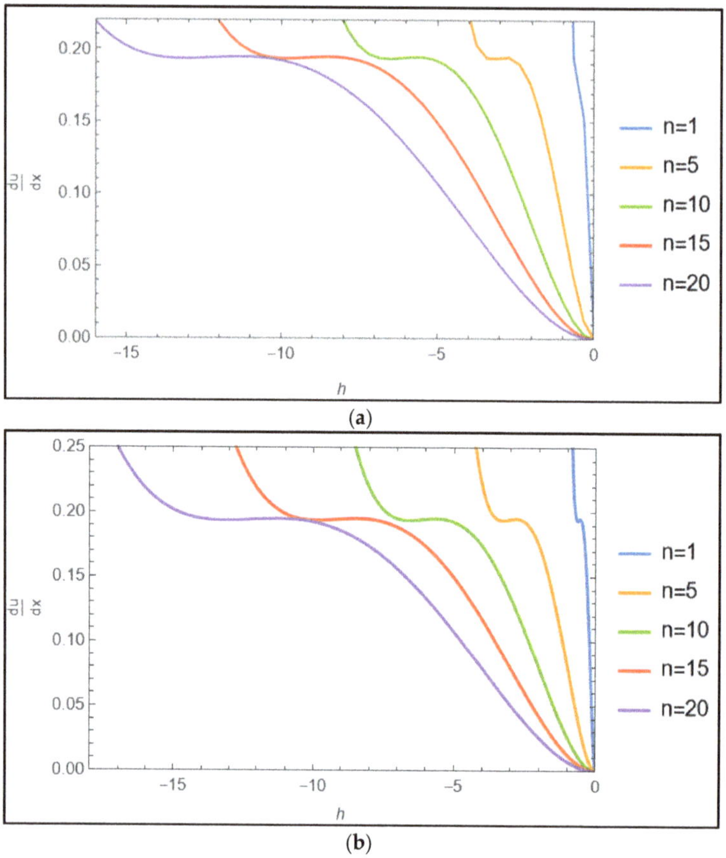

Figure 9. (**a**) h-curve graphs for $\alpha = 0.5$ at $x = 1$. (**b**) h-curve graphs for $\alpha = 1$ at $x = 1$.

Table 9. The optimal h and the convergence region of h for $\alpha = 0.5$.

n	Convergence Region	Optimal h	Δ_m
1	$-0.4733 < h < -0.3412$	−0.44457431	0.00001744
5	$-1.7703 < h < -3.0819$	−2.22287156	0.00001744
10	$-4.7330 < h < -3.5605$	−4.44574312	0.00001744
15	$-7.8677 < h < -5.2408$	−6.66861468	0.00001744
20	$-7.0409 < h < -11.4363$	−8.89148624	0.00001744

It is seen from Figure 10 that the Oq-HAM solution and the PC method exhibit similar behaviors. To analyze the graphs numerically, the relative errors at several points can be analyzed. The relative errors are given in the following table for $\alpha = 0.5$ and $\alpha = 1$ (Table 11).

Once again, the tables and figures show that for the optimal h values, minimal square residual errors are obtained and the solutions from the PC and Oq-HAM methods are almost identical within the interval of interest.

Table 10. The optimal h and the convergence region of h for $\alpha = 1$.

n	Convergence Region	Optimal h	Δ_m
1	$-0.8361 < h < -0.5755$	-0.66406054	0.00000287
5	$-3.9465 < h < -2.9461$	-3.32030272	0.00000287
10	$-8.3606 < h < -6.0067$	-6.64060545	0.00000287
15	$-11.8395 < h < -9.0364$	-9.96090817	0.00000287
20	$-14.7504 < h < -12.0772$	-13.28121090	0.00000287

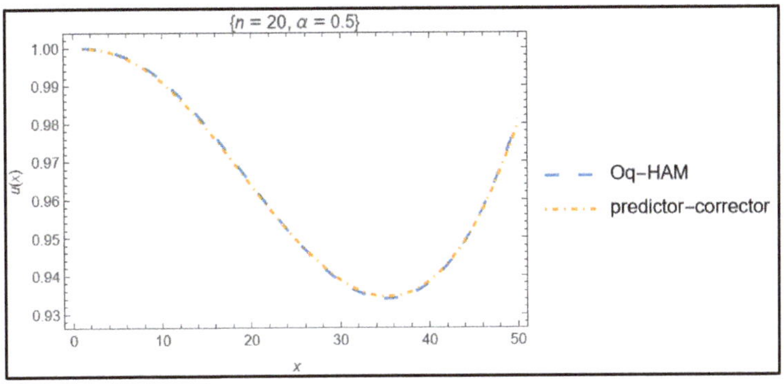

Figure 10. The approximate solutions for optimal h values for $\alpha = 0.5$, $n = 20$.

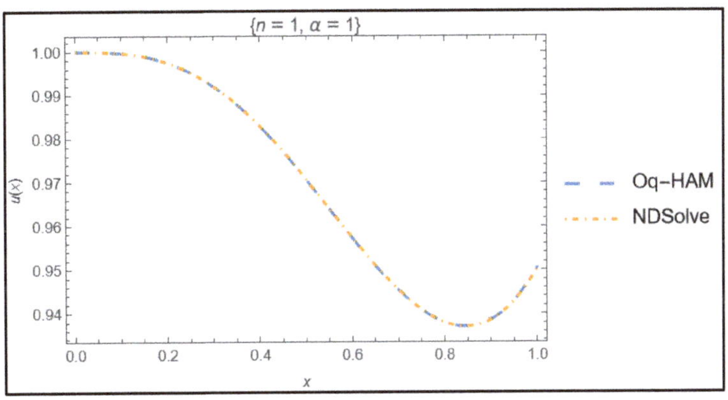

Figure 11. The approximate solutions for optimal h values for $\alpha = 1$ and $n = 1$.

The approximate solution of the fractional Abel differential equation obtained with fractional DTM using 30 terms in the approximation is shown below (Figure 12).

Several values of $x \in [0, 1]$ have been compared below for the numerical solutions and the approximate solutions of the fractional Abel differential equation (Table 12).

The relative errors (relative to the numerical solution) for the approximate solutions obtained with the fractional DTM and optimal q-HAM methods have been compared below (Table 13).

Table 11. Relative errors from Oq-HAM compared for various values of α and n.

x	$n = 1, \alpha = 0.5$	$n = 20, \alpha = 0.5$	$n = 1, \alpha = 1$
0.1	0.00018036	0.00018036	0.00000398
0.2	0.00061307	0.00061307	0.00002582
0.3	0.00084274	0.00084274	0.00005754
0.4	0.00058553	0.00058553	0.00006133
0.5	0.00003805	0.00003805	0.00000251
0.6	0.00040642	0.00040642	0.00010365
0.7	0.00055971	0.00055971	0.00018170
0.8	0.00046573	0.00046573	0.00014956
0.9	0.00008034	0.00008034	0.00003481
1.0	0.00077584	0.00077584	0.00044462

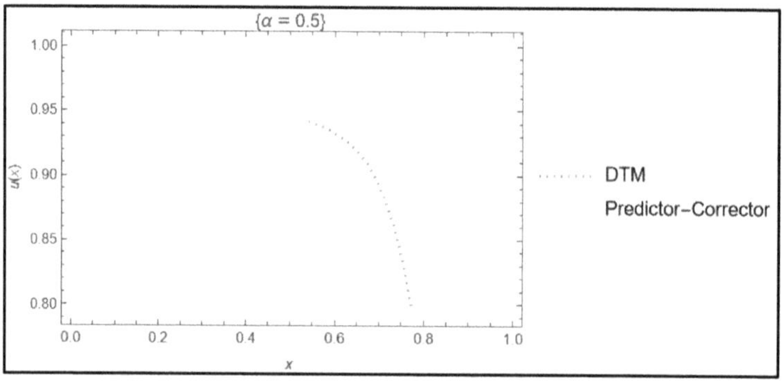

Figure 12. The approximate solutions from fractional DTM compared to the numerical solutions.

Table 12. Solutions of the fractional Abel equation compared.

x	PC Method	DTM	Optimal q-HAM (n = 1)
0.1	0.99816551	0.99819974	0.99834554
0.2	0.99081774	0.99090882	0.99142519
0.3	0.97841889	0.97858007	0.97924344
0.4	0.96353307	0.96378185	0.96409724
0.5	0.94931777	0.94939298	0.94935389
0.6	0.93876790	0.93435200	0.93838637
0.7	0.93448129	0.89709713	0.93395826
0.8	0.93869199	0.74365559	0.93825481
0.9	0.95338380	0.17671416	0.95330720
1.0	0.98037835	−1.58723431	0.98113897

Note that the improved convergence obtained through the use of the optimal value for the auxiliary parameter in the optimal q-HAM can be observed in the figures. The relative error for the optimal q-HAM is more than 1000 times smaller compared to the relative error for the fractional DTM method at $x = 0.9$. The results in Tables 12 and 13 and Figures 10–12 also underline that optimal q-HAM provides a better approximation for this equation.

Table 13. Relative errors for the fractional Abel equation compared.

x	DTM	Oq-HAM
0.1	0.00003430	0.00018036
0.2	0.00009192	0.00061307
0.3	0.00016474	0.00084274
0.4	0.00025820	0.00058553
0.5	0.00007923	0.00003805
0.6	0.00470394	0.00040642
0.7	0.04000525	0.00055971
0.8	0.20777465	0.00046573
0.9	0.81464531	0.00008034
1.0	2.61900180	0.00077584

4. Discussion

There are only a limited number of studies on the approximate solutions of fractional Abel differential equations in the literature. One study that might be considered related, by Jafari et al. [40], presents the application of HAM for the analysis of Abel equations of fractional order. This study improves the mentioned study and the following related studies in a way that adds to the current literature with a detailed presentation of Oq-HAM for Abel-type differential equations. The convergence analysis and the resulting optimality investigation for the auxiliary parameter h, comparison of the results with q-HAM, DTM, PC methods and exact solutions, etc. provide an in-depth analysis that extends the existing methodology. Some of the numerical results found in the literature are given below to compare the findings of this article with the existing literature numerically as well. The study by Al-Smadi et al. presents numerical values for the residual errors in the numerical solution of Abel differential equations analyzed fractionally with a Caputo–Fabrizio derivative using the reproducing kernel method [37]. The results of this study show that, for $t \in [0,1]$, the residual errors have a minimal value of 2.675×10^{-3} for $\alpha = 0.9$ and 2.679×10^{-3} for $\alpha = 0.85$. Although the error decreases for non-integer orders of derivation that are closer to 1, considering that the relative errors in Table 8 are given for $\alpha = 0.5$, it can be said that the results in our study are better in some regions. For instance, the Oq-HAM relative error at $x = 1.0$ (the highest amount in the inspected interval) is 0.487×10^{-3}. This relative error is also better than the error obtained with fractional DTM as well. The similarity between the approximate solutions of the optimal q-HAM and the exact/numerical solutions for the examples is also in accordance with the similarity of the results from the reproducing kernel method and the exact solutions given in Al-Smadi et al. [37]. Another study by Rigi and Tajadodi presents numerical results obtained for fractional Abel differential equations in the Caputo sense using Genocchi polynomials [38]. Results are given for $x \in [0,1]$ for two examples, and it can be said that the similarity of the approximate solutions to the exact/numerical solutions in this study matches the similarity between the approximate and exact solutions presented in the study by Rigi and Tajadodi [38]. For instance, the relative error in Example 4, for $n = 1, \alpha = 0.5$ is around 0.776×10^{-3} at $x = 1$ in our study, whereas the absolute error for $\alpha = 1$ with $N = 4$ in the Genocchi polynomials method is obtained as 8.56552×10^{-3} at $x = 1$ for the first example in the referred study. Results from existing numerical approximation methods are also found to be similar to the findings presented in our study. However, considering that Oq-HAM is an approximate analytical method, it can be said that the method provides better results in comparison to the other approximate analytical solution methods available for fractional Abel equations in the literature.

5. Conclusions

In this study, the optimal q-Homotopy Analysis Method (Oq-HAM) has been used to analyze Abel differential equations with various coefficient functions. Bernoulli and Riccati equations, which are special forms of Abel differential equations, are used, along with the general case in ordinary and fractional frameworks, to demonstrate the application of q-HAM. The Caputo fractional derivative is used to obtain fractional Abel differential equations from ordinary equations, and applications of optimal q-HAM are given for ordinary Abel equations and fractional Abel equations. This flow has been specifically designed to start from the application of q-HAM for ordinary Abel equations and finally reach the application of the optimal method for fractional equations. Four numerical examples have been given to present the method for obtaining the approximate solutions of the equations using q-HAM. The solutions are then analyzed to determine the optimal value of the convergence control parameter by minimizing the square residual errors. A theoretical analysis of the improvement in the convergence obtained using the auxiliary parameter in optimal q-HAM has been given by Liao [9] for the case with ordinary derivatives. Hence, this study is structured to present the improvement gained for the analysis of fractional Abel equations by focusing on comparisons of the application of optimal q-HAM with various other schemes. The optimal values of the auxiliary parameter h have been given to show the convergence regions, and the approximate solutions corresponding to these optimal values have been compared with the exact or numerical solutions of the problems. The results show that the use of Oq-HAM enables finding the optimal values of h and, thus, finding better approximations than those obtained by using q-HAM. The exact solutions or numerical solutions obtained with the NDSolve function are shown to be almost identical to the approximate solutions from Oq-HAM when the optimal values of the auxiliary parameter are used. The specific aim of this study is to analyze the approximations with q-HAM for Abel equations and to improve the convergence through optimizing auxiliary parameters. This is verified through the presentation of the results showing that Oq-HAM enhances the convergence of the solutions that would be obtained by using HAM, q-HAM or similar other methods.

The first example, the ordinary Riccati equation, has been analyzed with q-HAM and Oq-HAM and the solutions have been compared with the exact solution. Relative error analysis shows that, for $n = 1$, the optimal value of the auxiliary parameter h is obtained as $h = -1.87312216$. This is verified by the analysis of approximate solutions obtained with q-HAM, where the solutions were analyzed for $h = -0.5, -1$ and -1.25 when $n = 1$. Results show that the relative errors (relative to the exact solution) are growing along with the increase in x and for $x = 1$, the relative errors are obtained as 0.28971143 $(h = -0.5)$, 0.08673558 $(h = -1)$, 0.04471525 $(h = -1.25)$ and 0.00767123 (optimal h). This shows that the relative error for optimal h is at least 170 times smaller for Oq-HAM. The improvement in the approximation using the optimal h value can also be seen for the case where $n = 20$. Figure 2 shows the similarity of the solution curves for the exact solution and the Oq-HAM solution. The improvement from q-HAM to Oq-HAM is further analyzed for the fractional Bernoulli equation in the third example. The relative errors in Table 8, shown for various selections of the parameters, are better than the relative errors given for the solutions from q-HAM in all cases analyzed for this example.

Approximate solutions of fractional Abel equations have also been obtained with fractional DTM to highlight the improved convergence obtained with optimal q-HAM. A similar growth in relative errors, along with the increase in x, is seen for both methods. However, as Figure 12 suggests, the relative error of DTM at $x = 1$ (2.61900180) is almost 3375 times more than the relative error obtained with Oq-HAM (0.00077584). Further discussion of Oq-HAM is given in comparison to the exact solutions and numerical solutions obtained with the predictor–corrector method. Figures and tables provide results that verify that optimal q-HAM is a reliable tool for the investigation of fractional Abel differential equations.

This manuscript presents a case study for the application of the well-established optimal q-HAM to achieve improved approximations for fractional Abel differential equations. A detailed comparison of the approximate results obtained by using the optimal values of the auxiliary parameter determined with Oq-HAM justifies the advantages of the method. This methodology can be generalized to other fractional equations containing different fractional derivatives for a wider range of applications. Many differential equations and mathematical models can be evaluated through the use of optimal q-HAM to obtain better approximations of the solutions. Possible future studies can be made for the comparison of the solutions obtained with the q-HAM and optimal q-HAM methods with other approximation methods such as the VIM method for fractional Abel differential equations. Comparison of the approximate solutions with numerical schemes, such as the fractional Euler method, to investigate the convergence of solutions could also form the basis for new studies. The use of random components and other definitions of fractional derivation are among the possible ideas for future investigations.

Author Contributions: Conceptualization, S.Ş., Z.B. and M.M.; methodology, M.M.; software, S.Ş.; validation, S.Ş., Z.B. and M.M.; formal analysis, S.Ş., Z.B. and M.M.; investigation, S.Ş. and Z.B.; resources, S.Ş. and Z.B.; data curation, S.Ş. and Z.B.; writing—original draft preparation, S.Ş. and Z.B.; writing—review and editing, Z.B.; visualization, S.Ş. and Z.B.; supervision, M.M.; project administration, M.M.; funding acquisition, S.Ş. All authors have read and agreed to the published version of the manuscript.

Funding: This study has been supported by the Recep Tayyip Erdoğan University Development Foundation. Grant Number: 02024007019018.

Data Availability Statement: Data are contained within the article.

Conflicts of Interest: The authors declare no conflicts of interest.

References

1. Teodoro, G.S.; Machado, J.T.; De Oliveira, E.C. A review of definitions of fractional derivatives and other operators. *J. Comput. Phys.* **2019**, *388*, 195–208. [CrossRef]
2. Khalil, R.; Al Horani, M.; Yousef, A.; Sababheh, M. A new definition of fractional derivative. *J. Comput. Appl. Math.* **2014**, *264*, 65–70. [CrossRef]
3. Abdeljawad, T. On conformable fractional calculus. *J. Comput. Appl. Math.* **2015**, *279*, 57–66. [CrossRef]
4. Molliq, Y.; Noorani, M.S.M.; Hashim, I. Variational iteration method for fractional heat-and wave-like equations. *Nonlinear Anal. Real World Appl.* **2009**, *10*, 1854–1869. [CrossRef]
5. Srivastava, H.M.; Günerhan, H. Analytical and approximate solutions of fractional-order susceptible-infected-recovered epidemic model of childhood disease. *Math. Methods Appl. Sci.* **2019**, *42*, 935–941. [CrossRef]
6. He, J.H. Homotopy perturbation technique. *Comput. Methods Appl. Mech. Eng.* **1999**, *178*, 257–262. [CrossRef]
7. Liao, S.J. The Proposed Homotopy Analysis Technique for the Solution of Nonlinear Problems. Ph.D. Thesis, Shanghai Jiao Tong University, Shanghai, China, 1992.
8. Liao, S. Comparison between the homotopy analysis method and homotopy perturbation method. *Appl. Math. Comput.* **2005**, *169*, 1186–1194. [CrossRef]
9. Liao, S. An optimal homotopy-analysis approach for strongly nonlinear differential equations. *Commun. Nonlinear Sci. Numer. Simul.* **2010**, *15*, 2003–2016. [CrossRef]
10. Abbasbandy, S. The application of homotopy analysis method to nonlinear equations arising in heat transfer. *Phys. Lett. A* **2006**, *360*, 109–113. [CrossRef]
11. Park, S.H.; Kim, J.H. Homotopy analysis method for option pricing under stochastic volatility. *Appl. Math. Lett.* **2011**, *24*, 1740–1744. [CrossRef]
12. Mohamed, M.S.; Hamed, Y.S. Solving the convection-diffusion equation by means of the optimal q-homotopy analysis method (Oq-HAM). *Results Phys.* **2016**, *6*, 20–25. [CrossRef]
13. Mohamed, M.S. Application of optimal HAM for solving the fractional order logistic equation. *Appl. Comput. Math.* **2014**, *3*, 27–31. [CrossRef]
14. Lee, C.; Nadeem, S. Numerical study of non-Newtonian fluid flow over an exponentially stretching surface: An optimal HAM validation. *J. Braz. Soc. Mech. Sci. Eng.* **2017**, *39*, 1589–1596.
15. El-Tawil, M.A.; Huseen, S.N. The q-Homotopy Analysis Method (qHAM). *Int. J. Appl. Math. Mech.* **2012**, *8*, 51–75.
16. El-Tawil, M.A.; Huseen, S.N. On convergence of the q-homotopy analysis method. *Int. J. Contemp. Math. Sci.* **2013**, *8*, 481–497. [CrossRef]

17. Shah, K. Solution of Burger's Equation in a One-Dimensional Groundwater Recharge by Spreading Using q-Homotopy Analysis Method. *Eur. J. Pure Appl. Math.* **2016**, *9*, 114–124.
18. Adebanjo, F.O.; Samueal, O. Application of Homotopy Analysis Method for Solving Non-Darcy Flow Problem in Porous Media. *Int. J. Res. Rev. Appl. Sci.* **2016**, *28*, 26–43.
19. Srivastava, H.M.; Kumar, D.; Singh, J. An efficient analytical technique for fractional model of vibration equation. *Appl. Math. Model.* **2017**, *45*, 192–204. [CrossRef]
20. Iyiola, O.S.; Zaman, F.D. A note on analytical solutions of nonlinear fractional 2D heat equation with non-local integral terms. *Pramana* **2016**, *87*, 51. [CrossRef]
21. Akinyemi, L.; Iyiola, O.S. A reliable technique to study nonlinear time-fractional coupled Korteweg-de Vries equations. *Adv. Differ. Equ.* **2020**, *2020*, 169. [CrossRef]
22. Akinyemi, L. q-Homotopy analysis method for solving the seventh-order time-fractional Lax's Korteweg-de Vries and Sawada-Kotera equations. *Comput. Appl. Math.* **2019**, *38*, 191. [CrossRef]
23. Veeresha, P.; Prakasha, D.G.; Baskonus, H.M. Novel simulations to the time-fractional Fisher's equation. *Math. Sci.* **2019**, *13*, 33–42. [CrossRef]
24. Biswas, S.; Ghosh, U. Formulation of Conformable Time Fractional Differential Equation and q-HAM Solution Comparison with ADM. *J. Phys. Soc. Jpn.* **2022**, *91*, 044007. [CrossRef]
25. Hussain, S.; Shah, A.; Ullah, A.; Haq, F. The q-homotopy analysis method for a solution of the Cahn-Hilliard equation in the presence of advection and reaction terms. *J. Taibah Univ. Sci.* **2022**, *16*, 813–819. [CrossRef]
26. Cheng, X.; Wang, L.; Hou, J. Solving time fractional Keller-Segel type diffusion equations with symmetry analysis, power series method, invariant subspace method and q-homotopy analysis method. *Chin. J. Phys.* **2022**, *77*, 1639–1653. [CrossRef]
27. Sunitha, M.; Gamaoun, F.; Abdulrahman, A.; Malagi, N.S.; Singh, S.; Gowda, R.J.; Gowda, R.P. An efficient analytical approach with novel integral transform to study the two-dimensional solute transport problem. *Ain Shams Eng. J.* **2023**, *14*, 101878. [CrossRef]
28. Kadir, S.M.E.A.; Taha, W.M.; Hameed, R.A.; Jameel, A. Efficient approximate analytical methods to solve Kaup-Kupershmidt (KK) equation. In Proceedings of the 2022 International Symposium on Multidisciplinary Studies and Innovative Technologies (ISMSIT), Ankara, Turkey, 20–22 October 2022; pp. 206–211.
29. Darzi, R.; Agheli, B. Analytical approach to solving fractional partial differential equation by optimal q-homotopy analysis method. *Numer. Anal. Appl.* **2018**, *11*, 134–145. [CrossRef]
30. Murphy, G.M. *Ordinary Differential Equations and Their Solutions*; Dover Publications: Mineola, NY, USA, 2011.
31. Harko, T.; Mak, M.K. Relativistic dissipative cosmological models and Abel differential equation. *Comput. Math. Appl.* **2003**, *46*, 849–853. [CrossRef]
32. Lebrun, J.P.M. On two coupled Abel-type differential equations arising in a magnetostatic problem. *Il Nuovo C. A (1965–1970)* **1990**, *103*, 1369–1379. [CrossRef]
33. García, A.; Macías, A.; Mielke, E.W. Stewart-Lyth second-order approach as an Abel equation for reconstructing inflationary dynamics. *Phys. Lett. A* **1997**, *229*, 32–36. [CrossRef]
34. Alwash, M.A.M. Periodic solutions of Abel differential equations. *J. Math. Anal. Appl.* **2007**, *329*, 1161–1169. [CrossRef]
35. Mak, M.K.; Harko, T. New method for generating general solution of Abel differential equation. *Comput. Math. Appl.* **2002**, *43*, 91–94. [CrossRef]
36. Xu, Y.; He, Z. The short memory principle for solving Abel differential equation of fractional order. *Comput. Math. Appl.* **2011**, *62*, 4796–4805. [CrossRef]
37. Al-Smadi, M.; Djeddi, N.; Momani, S.; Al-Omari, S.; Araci, S. An attractive numerical algorithm for solving nonlinear Caputo-Fabrizio fractional Abel differential equation in a Hilbert space. *Adv. Differ. Equ.* **2021**, *2021*, 271. [CrossRef]
38. Rigi, F.; Tajadodi, H. Numerical approach of fractional Abel differential equation by Genocchi polynomials. *Int. J. Appl. Comput. Math.* **2019**, *5*, 134. [CrossRef]
39. Parand, K.; Nikarya, M. New numerical method based on generalized Bessel function to solve nonlinear Abel fractional differential equation of the first kind. *Nonlinear Eng.* **2019**, *8*, 438–448. [CrossRef]
40. Jafari, H.; Sayevand, K.; Tajadodi, H.; Baleanu, D. Homotopy analysis method for solving Abel differential equation of fractional order. *Open Phys.* **2013**, *11*, 1523–1527. [CrossRef]
41. Abbasbandy, S.; Jalili, M. Determination of optimal convergence-control parameter value in homotopy analysis method. *Numer. Algorithms* **2013**, *64*, 593–605. [CrossRef]
42. Saad, K.M.; Al-Shareef, E.H.; Mohamed, M.S.; Yang, X.J. Optimal q-homotopy analysis method for time-space fractional gas dynamics equation. *Eur. Phys. J. Plus* **2017**, *132*, 23. [CrossRef]
43. Caputo, M. Linear models of dissipation whose Q is almost frequency independent-II. *Geophys. J. Int.* **1967**, *13*, 529–539. [CrossRef]
44. Diethelm, K. *The Analysis of Fractional Differential Equations: An Application-Oriented Exposition Using Differential Operators of Caputo Type*; Springer Science & Business Media: Berlin/Heidelberg, Germany, 2010.
45. Faieghi, M.R.; Delavari, H. Chaos in fractional-order Genesio-Tesi system and its synchronization. *Commun. Nonlinear Sci. Numer. Simul.* **2012**, *17*, 731–741. [CrossRef]
46. Arikoglu, A.; Ozkol, I. Solution of fractional differential equations by using differential transform method. *Chaos Solitons Fractals* **2007**, *34*, 1473–1481. [CrossRef]

47. El-Sayed, A.M.A.; Nour, H.M.; Raslan, W.E.; El-Shazly, E.S. A study of projectile motion in a quadratic resistant medium via fractional differential transform method. *Appl. Math. Model.* **2015**, *39*, 2829–2835. [CrossRef]
48. Baleanu, D.; Mohammadi, H.; Rezapour, S. A fractional differential equation model for the COVID-19 transmission by using the Caputo-Fabrizio derivative. *Adv. Differ. Equ.* **2020**, *2020*, 299. [CrossRef]

fractal and fractional

MDPI

Article

Comparative Study of the Nonlinear Fractional Generalized Burger-Fisher Equations Using the Homotopy Perturbation Transform Method and New Iterative Transform Method

Mashael M. AlBaidani

Department of Mathematics, College of Science and Humanities, Prince Sattam bin Abdulaziz University, Al Kharj 11942, Saudi Arabia; m.albaidani@psau.edu.sa

Abstract: The time-fractional generalized Burger–Fisher equation (TF-GBFE) is utilized in many physical applications and applied sciences, including nonlinear phenomena in plasma physics, gas dynamics, ocean engineering, fluid mechanics, and the simulation of financial mathematics. This mathematical expression explains the idea of dissipation and shows how advection and reaction systems can work together. We compare the homotopy perturbation transform method and the new iterative method in the current study. The suggested approaches are evaluated on nonlinear TF-GBFE. Two-dimensional (2D) and three-dimensional (3D) figures are displayed to show the dynamics and physical properties of some of the derived solutions. A comparison was made between the approximate and accurate solutions of the TF-GBFE. Simple tables are also given to compare the integer-order and fractional-order findings. It has been verified that the solution generated by the techniques given converges to the precise solution at an appropriate rate. In terms of absolute errors, the results obtained have been compared with those of alternative methods, including the Haar wavelet, OHAM, and q-HATM. The fundamental benefit of the offered approaches is the minimal amount of calculations required. In this research, we focus on managing the recurrence relation that yields the series solutions after a limited number of repetitions. The comparison table shows how well the methods work for different fractional orders, with results getting closer to precision as the fractional-order numbers get closer to integer values. The accuracy of the suggested techniques is greatly increased by obtaining numerical results in the form of a fast-convergent series. Maple is used to derive the approximate series solution's behavior, which is graphically displayed for a number of fractional orders. The computational stability and versatility of the suggested approaches for examining a variety of phenomena in a broad range of physical science and engineering fields are highlighted in this work.

Keywords: elzaki transform; caputo derivative; time fractional generalized Burger–Fisher equation (TF-GBFE); new iterative method; homotopy perturbation method

1. Introduction

A unique area of applied analysis, fractional calculus, deals with real or complex derivatives of any order. Therefore, we may generalise the formula from positive integer to any real-order differentiation because fractional-order calculus provides us with an understanding of differentiation and course integration. FC was founded by two mathematicians, Leibniz and L'Hospital, and its precise birthdate is thought to have been 30 September 1695. The extension of classical calculus known as fractional calculus is gaining popularity in various fields, including fluid mechanics, control theory, and signal processing. Although fractional calculus, particularly fractional differential equations, is a topic that is frequently addressed nowadays. In fact, the famous mathematician Abel first introduced the concept in 1823. Scientists from several fields have worked on fractional calculus for the past 200 years. Numerous definitions exist for fractional derivatives, but not all are frequently applied. The most commonly used operators are the Riemann-Liouville (R-L), Caputo-Fabrizio, Caputo, and conformable operators [1–5]. The R-L and Caputo fractional derivatives have singular kernels. The index law and other classical conditions were satisfied by this class of fractional differential operators. This singularity prevents the description of the entire physical structure of memory. The ability to simulate and analyse complex systems with intricate nonlinear processes and higher-order behaviours makes fractional derivatives better for modelling in some situations than integer-order derivatives. This has two primary reasons. First, the derivative operator does not have to be of an integer order; we can use any order. Second, non-integer-order derivatives are useful when the system has long-term memory, depending on the present and past situation. Non-classical differential equations are a generalisation of conventional differential equations with fractional derivatives. Fractional differential equations have been widely employed for their relaxation and oscillation models in physics, biology, engineering, chemistry, and other domains [6–10].

The study of fractional-order chaotic systems has gained popularity in recent years as chaotic theory research has advanced and gotten more refined. Specifically, the fractional-order chaotic systems' complexity is correlated with both the system's fractional order and parametric characteristics. The four-wing fractional chaotic system [11], fractional Lorenz hyperchaotic system [12], fractional Lorenz system [13], and other non-integer-order chaotic systems have been proposed by numerous scholars based on integer-order chaotic systems [14,15]. Many researchers have made some progress in the numerical finding of fractional chaotic systems, specifically in the discretisation of fractional chaotic systems, using the Adomian decomposition method (ADM) [11–13], the Adams-Bashforth-Moulton (ABM) algorithm [16,17], and the frequency-domain method (FDM) [18]. Using Laplace change, FDM employs a high-dimensional system that is nearly fractional-order, although the error is comparatively substantial [19]. Although ABM is the most widely employed technique, it operates slowly. In contrast, the ADM method is more accurate and uses less computing power than the ABM algorithm [11–13]. According to reference [20], complexity, the Lyapunov index, the bifurcation diagram, and other factors demonstrate that fractional-order chaotic systems exhibit more complicated chaotic behaviours than integer-order chaotic systems. The complexity of the system increases with decreasing system order [21].

The growing field of artificial intelligence provided new opportunities for estimating the parameters of dynamic systems. There have been attempts to include deep learning in dynamic system modelling, which uses neural networks to approximate unknown system dynamics, because of its powerful function approximation capabilities and end-to-end learning paradigm. ResNet is a highly important work that was proposed recently and has transformed deep learning with its deep residual learning, which allows networks to be trained deeper than previously utilised networks using shortcut connections [22–24]. Yan et al. [25] investigated how resilient neural ODEs were to input disturbances and offered strategies to improve their stability and dependability. Poli et al. [26] show how combining neural ODE with graph neural networks may efficiently simulate dynamic processes on networks, expanding the use of neural ODE to graph-structured data. Zhu et al. [27] worked on the neural ODE's numerical integration feature. Their study focused on a crucial element influencing the effectiveness and performance of neural ODEs in a range of applications. Recently, Yong Yang et al. [28] proposed a novel approach to parameter estimation that combines physical prior knowledge with neural ordinary differential equations (neural ODEs). This method can achieve robust and accurate parameter estimation under high noise and small sample conditions, particularly for complex nonlinear dynamic systems. These papers demonstrate the advancements made and the areas that require further research to reach the full potential of neural ODEs in dynamic system modelling.

Our everyday lives are filled with randomness and uncertainty [29], such as estimating the number of points before a dice roll, forecasting the weather, and projecting a company's stock price. These occurrences show how unpredictable and varied many facets of life are by nature. In recognition of this, scholars have long endeavoured to comprehend and measure uncertainty in a methodical manner. When only discrete observations are available, estimating unknown parameters is a critical problem in uncertain differential equations (UDE). Yao and Liu [30] first presented the method of moments, which was based on the Euler method. This approach was further expanded to parameter estimation for unknown delay differential equations by Liu and Jia [31]. A novel approach to estimating unknown parameters by creating a minimization optimization problem was presented by Wu [32]. In comparison to conventional UDE methods, this approach offers more parameter degrees of freedom, can better fit real data, and increases forecast accuracy. Jing Ning et al. [33] employ prediction-correction techniques to solve fractional UDEs and introduce rectangular and trapezoidal algorithms to numerically approximate the optimization problem in order to broaden its research on parameter estimation accuracy.

Fractional partial differential equations (FPDEs) have received a lot of attention in recent decades because of their rapidly expanding and wide-ranging applications in various scientific and technical fields, such as biology, chemistry, electrical engineering, medicine, and viscoelasticity. Further information on these and other uses can be found in earlier research [34–37]. In this perspective, including FPDE approximations and approximate solutions is crucial for perfectly describing the dynamics of basic physical processes. Given the previously discussed facts, mathematicians have created and applied a wide variety of approximate and analytical methods to solve several significant mathematical models related to real-world issues. Despite the difficulty of finding analytical or even close solutions to some nonlinear FPDEs and systems of FPDEs, mathematicians continue to work in this field [38–41]. Several approaches have been utilised for addressing FPDEs, including the optimal homotopy analysis method [42], the general residual power series method [43], the homotopy analysis method [44], the Galerkin finite element method [45], and the finite difference method [46].

Due to their ability to simulate tidal oscillations brought on by undersea landslides and tsunamis, nonlinear diffusion and convection equations are crucial to oceanography and fluid dynamics. Examples of nonlinear dispersive waves and travelling waves that frequently occur in oceanography, marine engineering, acoustics, and fluid dynamics include gravitational waves, surface water disturbances in shallow rivers and seas, ship bumps on water, and tsunami dispersion [47–49]. Burgers-type equations for various wave propagation processes have drawn a lot of interest in these fields. These models depict interface dynamics, non-equilibrium, and nonlinear turbulence in hydrodynamics and ocean sciences. This study aimed to better understand the mechanism dictated by nonlinear FPDEs by investigating TFGBFE. The response, dissipation mechanisms, and advection are combined in the nonlinear equation called the TF-GBFE. The Burgers and Fisher diffusion transfer qualities and reaction form properties are used in this nonlinear equation.

The TF-GBFE is an interesting fluid dynamic model that several researchers have studied to help examine various numerical techniques and the mathematical analysis of physical flows. Due to the inclusion of diffusion mechanisms, convection, and reaction, the TF-GBFE is highly nonlinear. It is called Burger–Fisher because it combines the diffusion and reaction qualities of Fisher's equation with the convective and diffusion properties of

Burger's equation. The TF-GBFE is an important nonlinear diffusion equation in ocean engineering since it depicts the distant field of wave propagation in the ocean. Strong turbulent diffusion leads to the travelling waves due to convection, turbulent diffusion, and nonlinear radiation's impact on the irregularity of sea surface temperature. The currents created by winds determine the travelling wavefronts' speed and direction of movement [50]. According to [51], the TF-GBFE is responsible for the convection-diffusion model that may replicate underwater landslides, which could lead to the most dangerous tsunamis in the coastal area.

The TF-GBFE can be expressed as follows using the fractional order η and any real constants a, b, and δ:

$$D_{\wp}^{\eta}\mathbb{P}(\delta,\wp) - \mathbb{P}_{\delta\delta}(\delta,\wp) + a\mathbb{P}^{\delta}(\delta,\wp)\mathbb{P}_{\delta}(\delta,\wp) + b\mathbb{P}(\delta,\wp)(\mathbb{P}^{\delta}(\delta,\wp) - 1) = 0, \ \ 0 < \eta \leq 1, \quad 0 \leq \delta \leq 1, \ \ \wp \geq 0 \tag{1}$$

here a, b, δ are positive parameters, having initial guess as:

$$\mathbb{P}(\delta,0) = \left[\frac{1}{2}\left(1 - \tanh\left(\frac{a\delta}{2(1+\delta)}\delta\right)\right)\right]^{\frac{1}{\delta}}. \tag{2}$$

having an exact solution:

$$\mathbb{P}(\delta,\wp) = \left[\frac{1}{2}\left(1 - \tanh\left(\frac{a\delta}{2(1+\delta)}\left(\delta - \left(\frac{a^2 + b(1+\delta)^2}{a(1+\delta)}\right)\wp\right)\right)\right)\right]^{\frac{1}{\delta}}. \tag{3}$$

Differential equations are usually solved with simple mathematical techniques such as the Fourier, Laplace, Sumudu, and Elzaki transforms. Khuri [52] uses the Laplace transform (LT) in combination with the Adomian decomposition approach to get the approximate solution of a class of ordinary differential equations that are nonlinear. Many scholars have used a variety of techniques in connection with the LT approach to solve partial differential equations in recent years. These include the homotopy perturbation transform method [53], laplace variational iteration strategy [54], the Laplace homotopy analysis method [55], and many more. The new iterative transform method (NITM) and the homotopy perturbation transform method (HPTM) are extended in this study to solve TF-GBFE. Guo created non-abelian extensions of Rota-Baxter algebras, which serve as the foundation for other decomposition techniques, such as the Adomian polynomials employed in NITM [56]. The Daftardar–Jafari and Adomian polynomials are combined in the NITM [57], which is a modified version of the Elzaki transform decomposition method. The offered method merges the New Iterative Method (NIM) and Elzaki transformation. Tarig ELzaki presented the Elzaki Transform (ET), a novel integral transform, in 2010. ET is a modified version of the Laplace and Sumudu transforms. It is important to note that some differential equations with variable coefficients may be difficult to solve using the Sumudu and Laplace transforms, but they can be quickly resolved with ET's help. He introduced HPM in 1998 [58,59]. His polynomials are used to decompose the nonlinear terms after the differential equations are transformed into algebraic equations with the aid of the ET. The result of this method is taken to be in series form, which quickly converges to the precise answer after a small number of terms. This method can be used to solve nonlinear PDEs effectively. A higher level of accuracy was verified when the HPTM results were compared with the real solution to the issues. The methods offered accurate solutions to challenging issues, resulting in remarkable outcomes. The fractional problem findings acquired by applying the given approaches are also utilised to assess the issues from a fractional perspective. In summary, the original FPDE is transformed into its corresponding

PDE by approximating the fractional Caputo derivative using the Elzaki transform method. The original FPDE may be solved quickly and easily by using the new iterative method and the homotopy perturbation method on the derived PDE. The current study is essential because it finds an approximate, fractional-order solution to the TF-GBFE equations by employing two relatively new and innovative methods. It also compares the accurate solution of the proposed models to fourth-order approximations for a range of values of the fractional derivative. The presentation of two novel strategies for TF-GBFE with minimal and progressive phases makes this work interesting. The outline of our work is given below: Important definitions of FC are given in Section 2. The main notion of NITM is presented in Section 3, and the basic concept of the HPTM approach is presented in Section 4. The convergence and uniqueness results were covered in Section 5. In Section 6, the suggested techniques with the validity of the error bound theorem are provided. Section 7 presents a numerical problem to demonstrate the significance of the approaches mentioned. A brief discussion of the core outcomes and conclusions is provided in Section 8.

2. Basic Definitions

Here, we give some important definitions related to the current study.

Definition 1. *The Abel–Riemann non-integer derivative is as [60]*

$$D^{\eta}\nu(\wp) = \begin{cases} \frac{d^{\varpi}}{d\wp^{\varpi}}\nu(\wp), \ \eta = \varpi, \\ \frac{1}{\Gamma(\varpi-\eta)}\frac{d}{d\wp^{\varpi}}\int_0^{\wp}\frac{\nu(\wp)}{(\wp-\delta)^{\eta-\varpi+1}}d\delta, \ \varpi - 1 < \eta < \varpi, \end{cases} \tag{4}$$

with $\varpi \in Z^{+}, \eta \in R^{+}$ *and*

$$D^{-\eta}\nu(\wp) = \frac{1}{\Gamma(\eta)}\int_0^{\wp}(\wp-\delta)^{\eta-1}\nu(\delta)d\delta, \ 0 < \eta \leq 1. \tag{5}$$

Definition 2. *The Abel-Riemann non-integer integration operator is as [60]*

$$J^{\eta}\nu(\wp) = \frac{1}{\Gamma(\eta)}\int_0^{\wp}(\wp-\delta)^{\eta-1}\nu(\wp)d\wp, \ \ \wp > 0, \ \eta > 0, \tag{6}$$

with given properties:

$$J^{\eta}\wp^{\varpi} = \frac{\Gamma(\varpi+1)}{\Gamma(\varpi+\eta+1)}\wp^{\varpi+\delta},$$
$$D^{\eta}\wp^{\varpi} = \frac{\Gamma(\varpi+1)}{\Gamma(\varpi-\eta+1)}\wp^{\varpi-\wp}.$$

Definition 3. *The Caputo non-integer derivative is as [61]*

$${}^{C}D^{\eta}\nu(\wp) = \begin{cases} \frac{1}{\Gamma(\varpi-\eta)}\int_0^{\wp}\frac{\nu^{\varpi}(\delta)}{(\wp-\delta)^{\eta-\varpi+1}}d\delta, \ \varpi - 1 < \eta < \varpi, \\ \frac{d^{\varpi}}{d\wp^{\varpi}}\nu(\wp), \ \varpi = \eta, \end{cases} \tag{7}$$

with given properties
$\varpi_{\wp}^{\eta}D_{\wp}^{\eta}g(\wp) = g(\wp) - \sum_{k=0}^{m} g^{k}(0^{+})\frac{\wp^{k}}{k!}, \ for \ \wp > 0, \ and \ \varpi - 1 < \eta \leq \varpi, \ \varpi \in N.$
$D_{\wp}^{\eta}\varpi_{\wp}^{\eta}g(\wp) = g(\wp).$

Lemma 1. *For* $n < \eta \leq 1$, $\wp \geq 0$ *and* $k \in R$, *we have*

$$(a)\quad D_{\wp}^{\eta}\wp^{k}=\frac{\Gamma(k+1)}{\Gamma(k+1-\eta)}\wp^{k-\eta}.$$
$$(b)\quad D_{\wp}^{\eta}I_{\wp}^{\eta}[\mathbb{P}(\delta,\wp)]=\mathbb{P}(\delta,\wp).$$
$$(c)\quad I_{\wp}^{\eta}\wp^{k}=\frac{\Gamma(k+1)}{\Gamma(k+1+\eta)}\wp^{k+\eta}.$$
$$(d)\quad I_{\wp}^{\eta}D_{\wp}^{\eta}[\mathbb{P}(\delta,\wp)]=\mathbb{P}(\delta,\wp)-\sum_{i=0}^{n-1}\partial^{i}\mathbb{P}(\delta,0)\frac{\wp^{i}}{i!}.$$

Definition 4. *The ET of a function is as [62]*

$$E[g(\wp)]=G(r)=r\int_{0}^{\infty}h(\wp)e^{\frac{-\wp}{r}}d\wp,\quad r>0. \tag{8}$$

Definition 5. *The ET of Caputo operator is stated as [62]*

$$E[D_{\wp}^{\eta}g(\wp)]=s^{-\eta}E[g(\wp)]-\sum_{k=0}^{\varpi-1}s^{2-\eta+k}g^{(k)}(0),\ \textit{where}\ \varpi-1<\eta<\varpi.$$

3. General Procedure of NITM

Here, we illustrated the general analysis of the offered approach as given.

$$D_{\wp}^{\eta}\mathbb{P}(\delta,\wp)+N\mathbb{P}(\delta,\wp)+M\mathbb{P}(\delta,\wp)=h(\delta,\wp),\quad \wp>0,\ 1<\eta\leq 0, \tag{9}$$

with

$$\mathbb{P}^{k}(\delta,0)=f(\delta), \tag{10}$$

with N, M indicates the linear and nonlinear terms.

By executing the ET to Equation (9), we may have

$$E[D_{\wp}^{\eta}\mathbb{P}(\delta,\wp)]+E[N\mathbb{P}(\delta,\wp)+M\mathbb{P}(\delta,\wp)]=E[h(\delta,\wp)]. \tag{11}$$

In terms of differentiation property

$$E[\mathbb{P}(\delta,\wp)]=\sum_{k=0}^{m}s^{2-\eta+k}\mathbb{P}^{(k)}(\delta,0)+s^{\eta}E[h(\delta,\wp)]-s^{\eta}E[N\mathbb{P}(\delta,\wp)+M\mathbb{P}(\delta,\wp)]. \tag{12}$$

Now by executing the inverse ET to Equation (12),

$$\mathbb{P}(\delta,\wp)=E^{-1}\left[\left\{\sum_{k=0}^{m}s^{2-\eta+k}\mathbb{P}^{k}(\delta,0)+s^{\eta}E[h(\delta,\wp)]\right\}\right]-E^{-1}\left[s^{\eta}E\left[N\mathbb{P}(\delta,\wp)+M\mathbb{P}(\delta,\wp)\right]\right]. \tag{13}$$

By iterative process, we may have

$$\mathbb{P}(\delta,\wp)=\sum_{m=0}^{\infty}\mathbb{P}_{m}(\delta,\wp), \tag{14}$$

$$N\left(\sum_{m=0}^{\infty}\mathbb{P}_{m}(\delta,\wp)\right)=\sum_{m=0}^{\infty}N[\mathbb{P}_{m}(\delta,\wp)], \tag{15}$$

the nonlinear term N is decomposed as

$$N\left(\sum_{m=0}^{\infty}\mathbb{P}_{m}(\delta,\wp)\right)=\mathbb{P}_{0}(\delta,\wp)+N\left(\sum_{k=0}^{m}\mathbb{P}_{k}(\delta,\wp)\right)-M\left(\sum_{k=0}^{m}\mathbb{P}_{k}(\delta,\wp)\right). \tag{16}$$

On utilizing Equations (14)–(16) into Equation (13), we may have

$$\begin{aligned}\sum_{m=0}^{\infty}\mathbb{P}_m(\delta,\wp) &= E^{-1}\left[s^{\eta}\left(\sum_{k=0}^{m}s^{2-\delta+k}\mathbb{P}^{k}(\delta,0)+E[h(\delta,\wp)]\right)\right]\\ &-E^{-1}\left[s^{\eta}E\left[N\left(\sum_{k=0}^{m}\mathbb{P}_k(\delta,\wp)\right)-M\left(\sum_{k=0}^{m}\mathbb{P}_k(\delta,\wp)\right)\right]\right].\end{aligned} \quad (17)$$

By using iterative formula, we may have

$$\mathbb{P}_0(\delta,\wp) = E^{-1}\left[s^{\eta}\left(\sum_{k=0}^{m}s^{2-\delta+k}\mathbb{P}^{k}(\delta,0)+s^{\eta}E(g(\delta,\wp))\right)\right], \quad (18)$$

$$\mathbb{P}_1(\delta,\wp) = -E^{-1}[s^{\eta}E[N[\mathbb{P}_0(\delta,\wp)]+M[\mathbb{P}_0(\delta,\wp)]], \quad (19)$$

$$\mathbb{P}_{m+1}(\delta,\wp) = -E^{-1}\left[s^{\eta}E\left[-N\left(\sum_{k=0}^{m}\mathbb{P}_k(\delta,\wp)\right)-M\left(\sum_{k=0}^{m}\mathbb{P}_k(\delta,\wp)\right)\right]\right],\quad m\geq 1. \quad (20)$$

Lastly, the approximate solution to Equation (9) is taken as

$$\mathbb{P}(\delta,\wp)\cong\mathbb{P}_0(\delta,\wp)+\mathbb{P}_1(\delta,\wp)+\mathbb{P}_2(\delta,\wp)+\cdots,\quad m=1,2,\cdots. \quad (21)$$

4. General Procedure of HPTM

Here, we illustrated the general analysis of the offered approach as given.

$$\begin{aligned}&D_{\wp}^{\eta}\mathbb{P}(\delta,\wp)+M\mathbb{P}(\delta,\wp)+N\mathbb{P}(\delta,\wp)=h(\delta,\wp),\quad \wp>0,\quad 0<\eta\leq 1,\\ &\mathbb{P}(\delta,0)=f(\delta).\end{aligned} \quad (22)$$

By executing the ET to Equation (22), we may have

$$\begin{aligned}&E[D_{\wp}^{\eta}\mathbb{P}(\delta,\wp)+M\mathbb{P}(\delta,\wp)+N\mathbb{P}(\delta,\wp)]=E[h(\delta,\wp)],\quad \wp>0,0<\eta\leq 1,\\ &\mathbb{P}(\delta,\wp)=s^2g(\delta)+s^{\eta}E[h(\delta,\wp)]-s^{\eta}E[M\mathbb{P}(\delta,\wp)+N\mathbb{P}(\delta,\wp)].\end{aligned} \quad (23)$$

Now by employing the inverse ET, we may have

$$\mathbb{P}(\delta,\wp)=F(x,\wp)-E^{-1}[s^{\eta}E\{M\mathbb{P}(\delta,\wp)+N\mathbb{P}(\delta,\wp)\}], \quad (24)$$

where

$$F(\delta,\wp)=E^{-1}\left[s^2g(\delta)+s^{\eta}E[h(\delta,\wp)]\right]=g(v)+E^{-1}[s^{\eta}E[h(\delta,\wp)]]. \quad (25)$$

In terms of the HPM

$$\mathbb{P}(\delta,\wp)=\sum_{k=0}^{\infty}\epsilon^k\mathbb{P}_k(\delta,\wp), \quad (26)$$

with $\epsilon\in[0,1]$ indicates the perturbation parameter.

The nonlinear terms are decomposed as

$$N\mathbb{P}(\delta,\wp)=\sum_{k=0}^{\infty}\epsilon^kH_k(\mathbb{P}_k), \quad (27)$$

with H_n indicates He's polynomials $\mathbb{P}_0,\mathbb{P}_1,\mathbb{P}_2,\ldots,\mathbb{P}_n$, and is demonstrated as

$$H_n(\mathbb{P}_0,\mathbb{P}_1,\cdots,\mathbb{P}_n)=\frac{1}{\eta(n+1)}D_{\epsilon}^{k}\left[N\left(\sum_{k=0}^{\infty}\epsilon^k\mathbb{P}_k\right)\right]_{\epsilon=0}, \quad (28)$$

where $D_{\epsilon}^{k}=\frac{\partial^k}{\partial\epsilon^k}$.

On utilizing Equations (26) and (27) into Equation (24), we may have

$$\sum_{k=0}^{\infty}\epsilon^k\mathbb{P}_k(\delta,\wp)=F(\delta,\wp)-\epsilon\times\left[E^{-1}\left\{s^{\eta}E\{M\sum_{k=0}^{\infty}p^k\mathbb{P}_k(\delta,\wp)+\sum_{k=0}^{\infty}\epsilon^kH_k(\mathbb{P}_k)\}\right\}\right]. \tag{29}$$

On comparing the ϵ coefficients, we may have

$$\begin{aligned}
&\epsilon^0:\mathbb{P}_0(\delta,\wp)=F(\delta,\wp),\\
&\epsilon^1:\mathbb{P}_1(\delta,\wp)=E^{-1}[s^{\eta}E(M\mathbb{P}_0(\delta,\wp)+H_0(\mathbb{P}))],\\
&\epsilon^2:\mathbb{P}_2(\delta,\wp)=E^{-1}[s^{\eta}E(M\mathbb{P}_1(\delta,\wp)+H_1(\mathbb{P}))],\\
&\vdots\\
&\epsilon^k:\mathbb{P}_k(\delta,\wp)=E^{-1}[s^{\eta}E(M\mathbb{P}_{k-1}(\delta,\wp)+H_{k-1}(\mathbb{P}))],\quad k>0,k\in N.
\end{aligned} \tag{30}$$

Lastly, the approximate solution to Equation (22) is taken as

$$\mathbb{P}(\delta,\wp)=\lim_{M\to\infty}\sum_{k=1}^{M}\mathbb{P}_k(\delta,\wp). \tag{31}$$

5. Convergence Analysis

The convergence analysis of the applied approaches are stated as below.

Theorem 1. *Considering that $\wp$ is analytic in a neighborhood of $\mathbb{P}$ and $||\wp^m(\mathbb{P}_0)||=\sup\{||\wp^m(\mathbb{P}_0)(b_0,b_0,\cdots b_n)/||b_k||\leq 1,1\leq k\leq m\}\leq l$, for some real number $l>0$ and for every number m and $||\mathbb{P}_k||\leq M<\frac{1}{e},k=1,2,\cdots$ thus the series $\sum_{m=0}^{\infty}\zeta_m$ is convergent and also*

$$||\zeta_m||\leq lM^me^{m-1}(e-1),\ \ m=1,2,\cdots.$$

Now to define boundedness of $||\mathbb{P}_k||$, for each k the conditions on $\wp^j(\mathbb{P}_0)$ are assumed and is enough to assurance series convergence.

Theorem 2. *If $\wp$ is C^{∞} and $||\wp^m(\mathbb{P}_0)||\leq M\leq e^{-1}$ for all m hence the series $\sum_{m=0}^{\infty}\zeta_m$ is convergent. These are the conditions for series $\sum_{j=0}^{\infty}\mathbb{P}_j$ to be convergent.*

For proof check [63].

Theorem 3. *Considering the precise solution of (22) is $\zeta(\delta,\wp)$ and assume $\zeta(\delta,\wp),\zeta_n(\delta,\wp)\in H$ and $\alpha\in(0,1)$, with H specifies the Hilbert space. The results achieved $\sum_{q=0}^{\infty}\zeta_q(\delta,\wp)$ will converge $\zeta(\delta,\wp)$ if $\zeta_q(\delta,\wp)\leq\zeta_{q-1}(\delta,\wp)\ \forall q>A$, i.e., for each $\Omega>0\exists A>0$, such that $||\zeta_{q+n}(\delta,\wp)||\leq\beta,\forall m,n\in N$.*

Proof. Considering a sequence of $\sum_{q=0}^{\infty}\zeta_q(\delta,\wp)$.

$$\begin{aligned}
\Omega_0(\delta,\wp)=&\zeta_0(\delta,\wp),\\
\Omega_1(\delta,\wp)=&\zeta_0(\delta,\wp)+\zeta_1(\delta,\wp),\\
\Omega_2(\delta,\wp)=&\zeta_0(\delta,\wp)+\zeta_1(\delta,\wp)+\zeta_2(\delta,\wp),\\
\Omega_3(\delta,\wp)=&\zeta_0(\delta,\wp)+\zeta_1(\delta,\wp)+\zeta_2(\delta,\wp)+\zeta_3(\delta,\wp),\\
&\vdots\\
\Omega_q(\delta,\wp)=&\zeta_0(\delta,\wp)+\zeta_1(\delta,\wp)+\zeta_2(\delta,\wp)+\cdots+\zeta_q(\delta,\wp).
\end{aligned} \tag{32}$$

We must specify that $\Omega_q(\delta, \wp)$ forms a "Cauchy sequence". Additionally, let's take

$$
\begin{aligned}
||\Omega_{q+1}(\delta,\wp) - \Omega_q(\delta,\wp)|| = ||\zeta_{q+1}(\delta,\wp)|| \leq \alpha||\zeta_q(\delta,\wp)|| \leq \alpha^2||\zeta_{q-1}(\delta,\wp)|| \leq \alpha^3||\zeta_{q-2}(\delta,\wp)|| \cdots \\
\leq \alpha_{q+1}||\zeta_0(\delta,\wp)||.
\end{aligned} \tag{33}
$$

For $q, n \in N$, we may have

$$
\begin{aligned}
||\Omega_q(\delta,\wp) - \Omega_n(\delta,\wp)|| =& ||\zeta_{q+n}(\delta,\wp)|| = ||\Omega_q(\delta,\wp) - \Omega_{q-1}(\delta,\wp) + (\Omega_{q-1}(\delta,\wp) - \Omega_{q-2}(\delta,\wp)) \\
& + (\Omega_{q-2}(\delta,\wp) - \Omega_{q-3}(\delta,\wp)) + \cdots + (\Omega_{n+1}(\delta,\wp) - \Omega_n(\delta,\wp))|| \\
\leq& ||\Omega_q(\delta,\wp) - \Omega_{q-1}(\delta,\wp)|| + ||(\Omega_{q-1}(\delta,\wp) - \Omega_{q-2}(\delta,\wp))|| \\
& + ||(\Omega_{q-2}(\delta,\wp) - \Omega_{q-3}(\delta,\wp))|| + \cdots + ||(\Omega_{n+1}(\delta,\wp) - \Omega_n(\delta,\wp))|| \\
\leq& \alpha^q||\zeta_0(\delta,\wp)|| + \alpha^{q-1}||\zeta_0(\delta,\wp)|| + \cdots + \alpha^{q+1}||\zeta_0(\delta,\wp)|| \\
=& ||\zeta_0(\delta,\wp)||(\alpha^q + \alpha^{q-1} + \alpha^{q+1}) \\
=& ||\zeta_0(\delta,\wp)||\frac{1-\alpha^{q-n}}{1-\alpha^{q+1}}\alpha^{n+1}.
\end{aligned} \tag{34}
$$

As $0 < \alpha < 1$, and $\zeta_0(\delta, \wp)$ are bound, so assume $\beta = 1 - \alpha/(1 - \alpha_{q-n})\alpha^{n+1}||\zeta_0(\delta, \wp)||$, and we may have

$$
||\zeta_{q+n}(\delta,\wp)|| \leq \beta, \forall q, n \in N. \tag{35}
$$

Therefore, $\{\zeta_q(\delta, \wp)\}_{q=0}^{\infty}$ forms a "Cauchy sequence" in H. It illustrate that the sequence $\{\zeta_q(\delta, \wp)\}_{q=0}^{\infty}$ is a convergent sequence taking limit $\lim_{q\to\infty} \zeta_q(\delta, \wp) = \zeta(\delta, \wp)$ for $\exists\zeta(\delta, \wp) \in \mathcal{H}$ which verified the theorem. □

Theorem 4. *Considering that $\zeta(\delta, \wp)$ reveals the acquired series solution and $\sum_{h=0}^{k} \zeta_h(\delta, \wp)$ is finite. The relation that follows signifies the maximum absolute error, assuming $\alpha > 0$ with $||\zeta_{h+1}(\delta, \wp)|| \leq ||\zeta_h(\delta, \wp)||$.*

$$
||\zeta(\delta,\wp) - \sum_{h=0}^{k} \zeta_h(\delta,\wp)|| < \frac{\alpha^{k+1}}{1-\alpha}||\zeta_0(\delta,\wp)||. \tag{36}
$$

Proof. Assume $\sum_{h=0}^{k} \zeta_h(\delta, \wp)$ is finite which indicates that $\sum_{h=0}^{k} \zeta_h(\delta, \wp) < \infty$.
Considering

$$
\begin{aligned}
||\zeta(\delta,\wp) - \sum_{h=0}^{k} \zeta_h(\delta,\wp)|| =& ||\sum_{h=k+1}^{\infty} \zeta_h(\delta,\wp)|| \\
\leq& \sum_{h=k+1}^{\infty} ||\zeta_h(\delta,\wp)|| \\
\leq& \sum_{h=k+1}^{\infty} \alpha^h||\zeta_0(\delta,\wp)|| \\
\leq& \alpha^{k+1}(1 + \alpha + \alpha^2 + \cdots)||\zeta_0(\delta,\wp)|| \\
\leq& \frac{\alpha^{k+1}}{1-\alpha}||\zeta_0(\delta,\wp)||.
\end{aligned} \tag{37}
$$

which verified the theorem. □

6. Error Estimation

In this section, we introduce error functions to analyse the accuracy and performance of the proposed methods. The absolute error (E_n) in the nth-order approximation is as follows, assuming that $\mathbb{P}(\wp)$ is the accurate solution and $\mathbb{P}_n(\wp)$ is the nth-order approximation of $\mathbb{P}(\wp)$ obtained through the proposed methods.

$$E_n(\wp) = |\mathbb{P}(\wp) - \mathbb{P}_n(\wp)|, \tag{38}$$

then maximum absolute error (ME_n) by

$$ME_n = max_{\wp\in[0,1]}|\mathbb{P}(\wp) - \mathbb{P}_n(\wp)|. \tag{39}$$

The authors of [64–66] discussed the error bound for their numerical approaches using well-known lemmas and theorems. We provide an upper bound on absolute error for the proposed approaches using the following theorem.

Theorem 5 (Error bound). *Assume $\mathbb{P}(\wp) \in C^{(n+1)}[0,1]$ and $\mathbb{P}_n(\wp) = \sum_{i=0}^{n} c_i\wp^i$ demonstrate the precise and nth-order achieved solution of (9) and (22), thus upper bound of the absolute error is as*

$$||\mathbb{P}(\wp) - \mathbb{P}_n(\wp)||_\infty \leq \frac{M}{(n+1)!} + max_{0\leq i\leq n}|a_i|, \tag{40}$$

where $M = max_{0\leq t\leq 1}|\mathbb{P}^{n+1}(\wp)|, \quad a_i = \sum_{i=0}^{n}\left(\frac{\mathbb{P}^i(0)}{i!} - c_i\right).$

Proof. Assume $\mathbb{P}$ to be a continuous function on $[0,1]$; the upper bound of $|\mathbb{P}|$ is taken as

$$||\mathbb{P}||_\infty = \sup_{\wp\in[0,1]} |\mathbb{P}(\wp)|. \tag{41}$$

Employing norm property, we may have

$$||\mathbb{P}(\wp) - \mathbb{P}_n(\wp)||_\infty \leq ||\mathbb{P}(\wp) - \mathbb{P}_n^*(\wp)||_\infty + ||\mathbb{P}_n^*(\wp) - \mathbb{P}(\wp)||_\infty \tag{42}$$

Since $\mathbb{P}(\wp) \in C^{(n+1)}[0,1]$ so by Taylor expansion, we get

$$\mathbb{P}(\wp) = \mathbb{P}_n^*(\wp) + \frac{\mathbb{P}^{n+1}(\wp_0)}{(n+1)!}\wp^{n+1}, \quad \wp_0 \in (0,1), \tag{43}$$

with $\mathbb{P}_n^*(\wp) = \sum_{i=0}^{n} \frac{\mathbb{P}^i(0)}{i!}\wp^i$.

From (43), we may have

$$\begin{aligned} ||\mathbb{P}(\wp) - \mathbb{P}_n^*(\wp)||_\infty &= \max_{0\leq\wp\leq 1} |\frac{\mathbb{P}^{n+1}(\wp)}{(n+1)!}\wp^{n+1}| \\ &\leq \frac{1}{(n+1)!}\max_{0\leq\wp\leq 1}|\mathbb{P}^{n+1}(\wp)|. \end{aligned} \tag{44}$$

Now we find the value of $||\mathbb{P}(\wp) - \mathbb{P}_n^*(\wp)||_\infty$.

Let $A = (a_0, a_1, \cdots, a_n), T = (t_0, t_1, \cdots, t_n)^T$,

with $a_i = \frac{\mathbb{P}^i(0)}{i!} - c_i, i = 0, 1, \cdots, n$ thus

$$\begin{aligned} &||\mathbb{P}_n^*(\wp) - \mathbb{P}_n(\wp)|| = \left\|\sum_{i=0}^{n}\frac{\mathbb{P}^i(0)}{i!}\wp^i - \sum_{i=0}^{n}c_i\wp^i\right\| = \left\|\sum_{i=0}^{n}\left(\frac{\mathbb{P}^i(0)}{i!} - c_i\right)\wp^i\right\| \\ &\|A\|_\infty.\|T\|_\infty, \\ &||\mathbb{P}_n^*(\wp) - \mathbb{P}_n(\wp)|| = \|A\|_\infty.\|T\|_\infty. \end{aligned} \tag{45}$$

From (44), (45) and (42) we may have

$$\begin{aligned}
\|\mathbb{P}(\wp)-\mathbb{P}_n(\wp)\| &\leq\leq \frac{1}{(n+1)!}\max_{0\leq\wp\leq 1}|\mathbb{P}^{n+1}(\wp)|+\|A\|_{\infty}.\|T\|_{\infty},\\
\|\mathbb{P}(\wp)-\mathbb{P}_n(\wp)\| &\leq\leq \frac{M}{(n+1)!}+\max_{0\leq i\leq n}|a_i|.
\end{aligned} \tag{46}$$

which complete the proof. □

7. Applications

7.1. Example

Consider the one-dimensional TF-GBFE

$$\frac{\partial^{\eta}\mathbb{P}(\delta,\wp)}{\partial\wp^{\eta}}=\frac{\partial^2\mathbb{P}}{\partial\wp^2}-\varrho\mathbb{P}\frac{\partial\mathbb{P}}{\partial\wp}-\varrho\mathbb{P}^2+\varrho\mathbb{P},\quad 0<\eta\leq 1, \tag{47}$$

with initial guess

$$\mathbb{P}(\delta,0)=\frac{1}{2}-\frac{1}{2}\tanh\left(\frac{\varrho\delta}{4}\right). \tag{48}$$

By executing the ET to Equation (47), we may have

$$E[\mathbb{P}(\delta,\wp)]=s^2\left(\frac{1}{2}-\frac{1}{2}\tanh\left(\frac{\varrho\delta}{4}\right)\right)+s^{\eta}E\left[\frac{\partial^2\mathbb{P}}{\partial\wp^2}-\varrho\mathbb{P}\frac{\partial\mathbb{P}}{\partial\wp}-\varrho\mathbb{P}^2+\varrho\mathbb{P}\right], \tag{49}$$

Now by employing the inverse ET, we may have

$$\mathbb{P}(\delta,\wp)=\frac{1}{2}-\frac{1}{2}\tanh\left(\frac{\varrho\delta}{4}\right)+E^{-1}\left[s^{\eta}E\left[\frac{\partial^2\mathbb{P}}{\partial\wp^2}-\varrho\mathbb{P}\frac{\partial\mathbb{P}}{\partial\wp}-\varrho\mathbb{P}^2+\varrho\mathbb{P}\right]\right], \tag{50}$$

By NITM, we may have

$$\mathbb{P}_0(\delta,\wp)=\frac{1}{2}-\frac{1}{2}\tanh\left(\frac{\varrho\delta}{4}\right),$$

$$\mathbb{P}_1(\delta,\wp)=E^{-1}\left[s^{\eta}E\left\{\frac{\partial^2\mathbb{P}_0}{\partial\wp^2}-\varrho\mathbb{P}_0\frac{\partial\mathbb{P}_0}{\partial\wp}-\varrho\mathbb{P}_0^2+\varrho\mathbb{P}_0\right\}\right]=$$

$$\frac{1}{16}\frac{\varrho(\varrho+4)}{\cosh\left(\frac{1}{4}\varrho\delta\right)^2}\frac{\wp^{\eta}}{\Gamma(\eta+1)},$$

$$\mathbb{P}_2(\delta,\wp)=E^{-1}\left[s^{\eta}E\left\{\frac{\partial^2(\mathbb{P}_0+\mathbb{P}_1)}{\partial\wp^2}-\varrho(\mathbb{P}_0+\mathbb{P}_1)\frac{\partial(\mathbb{P}_0+\mathbb{P}_1)}{\partial\wp}-\varrho(\mathbb{P}_0+\mathbb{P}_1)^2+\varrho(\mathbb{P}_0+\mathbb{P}_0)\right\}\right]-$$

$$E^{-1}\left[s^{\eta}E\left\{\frac{\partial^2\mathbb{P}_0}{\partial\wp^2}-\varrho\mathbb{P}_0\frac{\partial\mathbb{P}_0}{\partial\wp}-\varrho\mathbb{P}_0^2+\varrho\mathbb{P}_0\right\}\right]=\frac{1}{64}\frac{\varrho^2(\varrho+4)^2\sinh\left(\frac{1}{4}\varrho\delta\right)}{\cosh\left(\frac{1}{4}\varrho\delta\right)^3}\frac{\wp^{2\eta}}{\Gamma(2\eta+1)}-$$

$$\frac{1}{512}\frac{\varrho^3(\varrho+4)^2\left(-\varrho\sinh\left(\frac{1}{4}\varrho\delta\right)+2\cosh\left(\frac{1}{4}\varrho\delta\right)\right)\Gamma(2\eta+1)}{\cosh\left(\frac{1}{4}\varrho\delta\right)^5\Gamma(\eta+1)^2}\frac{\wp^{3\eta}}{\Gamma(3\eta+1)},$$

$$\vdots$$

Lastly, the series solution is taken as

$$\mathbb{P}(\delta,\wp)=\mathbb{P}_0(\delta,\wp)+\mathbb{P}_1(\delta,\wp)+\mathbb{P}_2(\delta,\wp)+\cdots,$$

$$\begin{aligned}\mathbb{P}(\delta,\wp)=&\frac{1}{2}-\frac{1}{2}\tanh\left(\frac{\varrho\delta}{4}\right)+\frac{1}{16}\frac{\varrho(\varrho+4)}{\cosh\left(\frac{1}{4}\varrho\delta\right)^2}\frac{\wp^\eta}{\Gamma(\eta+1)}+\frac{1}{64}\frac{\varrho^2(\varrho+4)^2\sinh\left(\frac{1}{4}\varrho\delta\right)}{\cosh\left(\frac{1}{4}\varrho\delta\right)^3}\frac{\wp^{2\eta}}{\Gamma(2\eta+1)}-\\&\frac{1}{512}\frac{\varrho^3(\varrho+4)^2\left(-\varrho\sinh\left(\frac{1}{4}\varrho\delta\right)+2\cosh\left(\frac{1}{4}\varrho\delta\right)\right)\Gamma(2\eta+1)}{\cosh\left(\frac{1}{4}\varrho\delta\right)^5\Gamma(\eta+1)^2}\frac{\wp^{3\eta}}{\Gamma(3\eta+1)}+\cdots,\end{aligned}\tag{51}$$

By employing the HPTM, we may have

$$\begin{aligned}\sum_{n=0}^{\infty}\epsilon^n\mathbb{P}^n(\delta,\wp)=&\frac{1}{2}-\frac{1}{2}\tanh\left(\frac{\varrho\delta}{4}\right)+\epsilon\left\{E^{-1}\left(s^\eta E\left[\left(\sum_{n=0}^{\infty}\epsilon^n\mathbb{P}_n(\delta,\wp)\right)_{\delta\delta}-\left(\sum_{n=0}^{\infty}\epsilon^nH_n^1(\delta,\wp)\right)-\right.\right.\right.\\&\left.\left.\left.\varrho\left(\sum_{n=0}^{\infty}\epsilon^nH_n^2(\delta,\wp)\right)+\varrho\left(\sum_{n=0}^{\infty}\epsilon^n\mathbb{P}_n(\delta,\wp)\right)\right]\right)\right\},\end{aligned}\tag{52}$$

with He's polynomials $H_k(\delta)$ represent the nonlinear terms and is stated as

$$\begin{aligned}&H_0^1(\delta)=\mathbb{P}_0(\mathbb{P}_0)_\delta\\&H_1^1(\delta)=\mathbb{P}_0(\mathbb{P}_1)_\delta+\mathbb{P}_1(\mathbb{P}_0)_\delta\\&H_2^1(\delta)=\mathbb{P}_2(\mathbb{P}_0)_\delta+\mathbb{P}_1(\mathbb{P}_1)_\delta+\mathbb{P}_0(\mathbb{P}_2)_\delta\\&\vdots\\&H_0^2(\delta)=(\mathbb{P}_0)^2\\&H_1^2(\delta)=2\mathbb{P}_0\mathbb{P}_1\\&H_2^2(\delta)=2\mathbb{P}_0\mathbb{P}_1+(\mathbb{P}_0)^2\end{aligned}$$

On comparing the ϵ coefficients, we may have

$$\begin{aligned}&\epsilon^0:\mathbb{P}_0(\delta,\wp)=\frac{1}{2}-\frac{1}{2}\tanh\left(\frac{\varrho\delta}{4}\right),\\&\epsilon^1:\mathbb{P}_1(\delta,\wp)=\frac{1}{16}\frac{\varrho(\varrho+4)}{\cosh\left(\frac{1}{4}\varrho\delta\right)^2}\frac{\wp^\eta}{\Gamma(\eta+1)},\\&\epsilon^2:\mathbb{P}_2(\delta,\wp)=\frac{1}{64}\frac{\varrho^2(\varrho+4)^2\sinh\left(\frac{1}{4}\varrho\delta\right)}{\cosh\left(\frac{1}{4}\varrho\delta\right)^3}\frac{\wp^{2\eta}}{\Gamma(2\eta+1)},\\&\epsilon^3:\mathbb{P}_3(\delta,\wp)=-\frac{\varrho^3(\varrho+4)^2}{512\cosh\left(\frac{1}{4}\varrho\delta\right)^5}\left(-2\varrho\cosh\left(\frac{1}{4}\varrho\delta\right)^3-8\cosh\left(\frac{1}{4}\varrho\delta\right)^3+2\varrho\sinh\left(\frac{1}{4}\varrho\delta\right)+\right.\\&\qquad\left.3\varrho\cosh\left(\frac{1}{4}\varrho\delta\right)+8\cosh\left(\frac{1}{4}\varrho\delta\right)\right)\frac{\wp^{3\eta}}{\Gamma(3\eta+1)}+\frac{\varrho^3(\varrho+4)^2}{512\cosh\left(\frac{1}{4}\varrho\delta\right)^5\Gamma(\eta+1)^2}\left(\varrho\sinh\left(\frac{1}{4}\varrho\delta\right)\right.\\&\qquad\left.-2\cosh\left(\frac{1}{4}\varrho\delta\right)\right)\Gamma(2\eta+1)\frac{\wp^{3\eta}}{\Gamma(3\eta+1)}\\&\quad\vdots\end{aligned}\tag{53}$$

Lastly, the series solution is taken as

$$\mathbb{P}(\delta,\wp)=\sum_{n=0}^{\infty}\epsilon^n\mathbb{P}_n(\delta,\wp).\tag{54}$$

Hence

$$\mathbb{P}(\delta,\wp)=\mathbb{P}_0(\delta,\wp)+\mathbb{P}_1(\delta,\wp)+\mathbb{P}_2(\delta,\wp)+\cdots,$$

$$\mathbb{P}(\delta,\wp)=\frac{1}{2}-\frac{1}{2}\tanh\left(\frac{\varrho\delta}{4}\right)+\frac{1}{16}\frac{\varrho(\varrho+4)}{\cosh\left(\frac{1}{4}\varrho\delta\right)^2}\frac{\wp^{\eta}}{\Gamma(\eta+1)}+\frac{1}{64}\frac{\varrho^2(\varrho+4)^2\sinh\left(\frac{1}{4}\varrho\delta\right)}{\cosh\left(\frac{1}{4}\varrho\delta\right)^3}\frac{\wp^{2\eta}}{\Gamma(2\eta+1)}-$$
$$\frac{\varrho^3(\varrho+4)^2}{512\cosh\left(\frac{1}{4}\varrho\delta\right)^5}\left(-2\varrho\cosh\left(\frac{1}{4}\varrho\delta\right)^3-8\cosh\left(\frac{1}{4}\varrho\delta\right)^3+2\varrho\sinh\left(\frac{1}{4}\varrho\delta\right)+3\varrho\cosh\left(\frac{1}{4}\varrho\delta\right)+\right. \tag{55}$$
$$\left.8\cosh\left(\frac{1}{4}\varrho\delta\right)\right)\frac{\wp^{3\eta}}{\Gamma(3\eta+1)}+\frac{\varrho^3(\varrho+4)^2}{512\cosh\left(\frac{1}{4}\varrho\delta\right)^5\Gamma(\eta+1)^2}\left(\varrho\sinh\left(\frac{1}{4}\varrho\delta\right)-2\cosh\left(\frac{1}{4}\varrho\delta\right)\right)$$
$$\Gamma(2\eta+1)\frac{\wp^{3\eta}}{\Gamma(3\eta+1)}+\cdots.$$

At $\eta=1$, we get exact solution as

$$\mathbb{P}(\delta,\wp)=\frac{1}{2}+\frac{1}{2}\tanh\left[\frac{-\varrho}{4}\left(\delta-\left(\frac{\varrho}{2}+\frac{2\varrho}{\varrho}\right)\wp\right)\right] \tag{56}$$

This study's graphical and tabular representations offer a thorough understanding of the precision and dependability of the NITM and HPTM when employed to the TF-GBFE. The HPTM approximation solution and the exact solution at $\eta=1$ are compared in Figure 1. The derived solution of NITM and the accurate solution at $\eta=1$ are compared in Figure 2. Excellent agreement can be seen in the graphical comparisons between the precise solution and the solutions from the suggested methods. The 3D depiction of the solutions derived by HPTM and NITM for the TF-GBFE at $\eta=0.6$ and $\eta=0.8$ is shown in Figures 3 and 4. The 2D plot of the found solution for different fractional orders is shown in Figures 5 and 6, along with a comparison of the generated and precise solution. Figures 5 and 6 illustrate the impact of changing the parameter η on the TF-GBFE solutions. The derived solutions are illustrated in Figures 1–6 for a range of η values with $-5\leq\delta\leq5$ and temporal variable $0\leq\wp\leq0.1$. Tables 1 and 2 present the exact solution for the TF-GBFE while maintaining $\eta=0.97, 0.98, 0.98$ and 1, as well as the comparative numerical solutions derived by HPTM and the NITM. Table 3 provides the absolute differences derived from Haar wavelet, OHAM, q-HATM, HPTM, and NITM. This suggests that the solutions generated by NITM and HPTM are more suitable than those obtained using q-HATM, OHAM, and Haar wavelet. It is also clear from Tables 1–3 that the solution obtained by HPTM after the fourth iteration is obtained by NITM after the third iteration. Hence, the solutions obtained by NITM are more suitable and efficient than those obtained by HPTM. Overall, the tabular and graphical data support the finding that both approaches work well, while NITM provides better accuracy in particular fractional contexts.

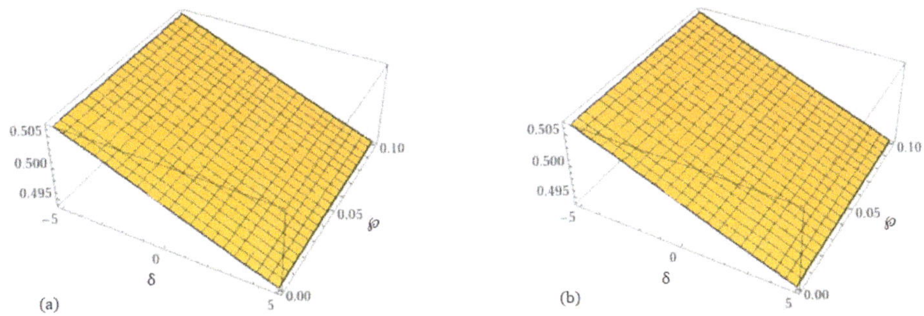

Figure 1. Graphical depict of the (**a**) accurate as well as (**b**) HPTM solution for $\mathbb{P}(\delta, \wp)$.

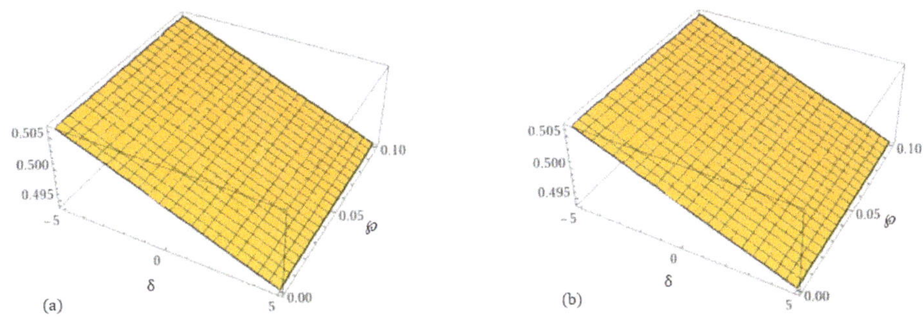

Figure 2. Graphical depict of the (**a**) accurate as well as (**b**) NITM solution for $\mathbb{P}(\delta, \wp)$.

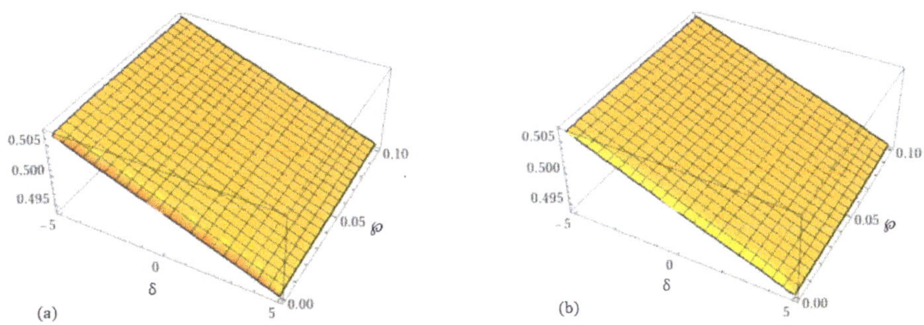

Figure 3. Graphical depict of the HPTM solution at (**a**) $\eta = 0.6$ (**b**) $\eta = 0.8$ for $\mathbb{P}(\delta, \wp)$.

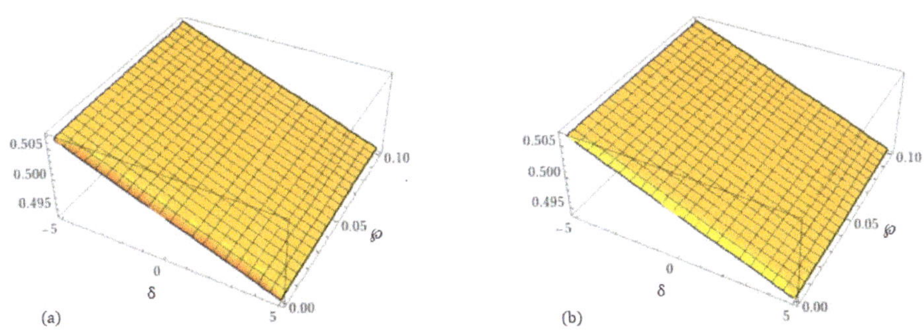

Figure 4. Graphical depict of the NITM solution at (**a**) $\eta = 0.6$ (**b**) $\eta = 0.8$ for $\mathbb{P}(\delta, \wp)$.

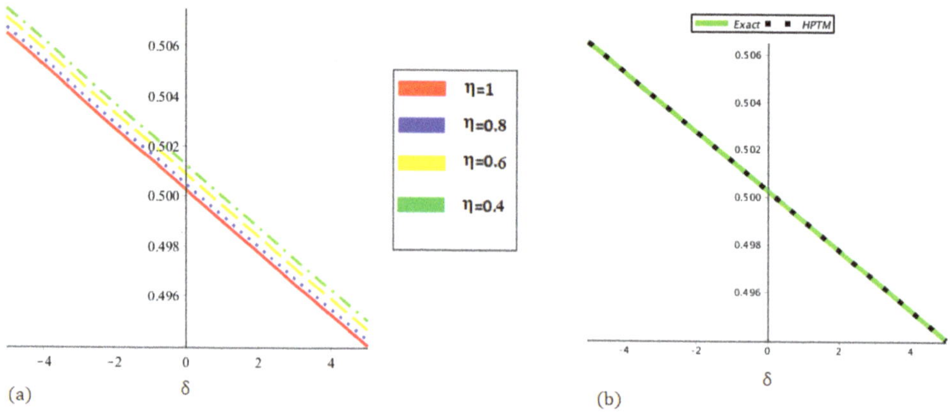

Figure 5. 2D Graphical depict of the HPTM solution at (**a**) several orders of η as well as (**b**) comparison with accurate solution.

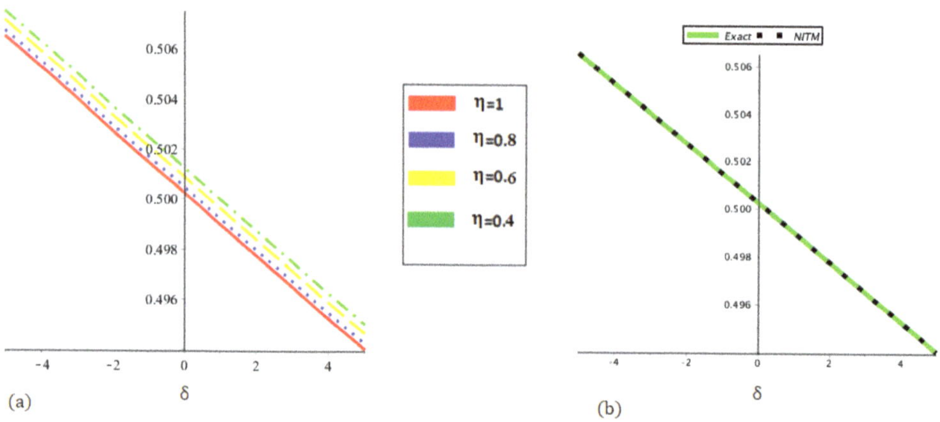

Figure 6. 2D Graphical depict of the NITM solution at (**a**) several orders of η as well as (**b**) comparison with accurate solution.

Table 1. Behavior of the accurate as well as HPTM solution at several η for $\mathbb{P}(\delta, \wp)$.

δ	$\eta = 0.97$	$\eta = 0.98$	$\eta = 0.99$	$\eta = 1\,(HPTM)$	$\eta = 1\,(Aacurate)$
0.0	0.5002718980	0.5002646308	0.5002575411	0.5002506250	0.5002506250
0.1	0.5001468979	0.5001396308	0.5001325410	0.5001256250	0.5001256250
0.2	0.5000218980	0.5000146308	0.5000075411	0.5000006250	0.5000006250
0.3	0.4998968980	0.4998896309	0.4998825411	0.4998756251	0.4998756250
0.4	0.4997718981	0.4997646308	0.4997575411	0.4997506250	0.4997506250
0.5	0.4996468980	0.4996396309	0.4996325412	0.4996256251	0.4996256251
0.6	0.4995218981	0.4995146310	0.4995075413	0.4995006252	0.4995006252
0.7	0.4993968983	0.4993896312	0.4993825414	0.4993756253	0.4993756253
0.8	0.4992718985	0.4992646313	0.4992575416	0.4992506256	0.4992506256
0.9	0.4991468988	0.4991396317	0.4991325420	0.4991256259	0.4991256259
1.0	0.4990218993	0.4990146321	0.4990075424	0.4990006263	0.4990006263

Table 2. Behavior of the accurate as well as NITM solution at several η for $\mathbb{P}(\delta, \wp)$.

δ	$\eta = 0.97$	$\eta = 0.98$	$\eta = 0.99$	$\eta = 1\,(NITM)$	$\eta = 1\,(Accurate)$
0.0	0.5002718980	0.5002646308	0.5002575411	0.5002506250	0.5002506250
0.1	0.5001468979	0.5001396308	0.5001325410	0.5001256250	0.5001256250
0.2	0.5000218980	0.5000146308	0.5000075411	0.5000006250	0.5000006250
0.3	0.4998968980	0.4998896309	0.4998825411	0.4998756251	0.4998756250
0.4	0.4997718981	0.4997646308	0.4997575411	0.4997506250	0.4997506250
0.5	0.4996468980	0.4996396309	0.4996325412	0.4996256251	0.4996256251
0.6	0.4995218981	0.4995146310	0.4995075413	0.4995006252	0.4995006252
0.7	0.4993968983	0.4993896312	0.4993825414	0.4993756253	0.4993756253
0.8	0.4992718985	0.4992646313	0.4992575416	0.4992506256	0.4992506256
0.9	0.4991468988	0.4991396317	0.4991325420	0.4991256259	0.4991256259
1.0	0.4990218993	0.4990146321	0.4990075424	0.4990006263	0.4990006263

Table 3. Comparative analysis of the analytical solution with Haar wavelet, OHAM, and q-HATM.

δ	$\wp$	Haar Wavelet Error [67]	OHAM Error [67]	q-HATM Error [68]	HPTM Error	NITM Error
0.1	0.2	5.4804×10^{-5}	4.2290×10^{-11}	1.1102×10^{-16}	0	0
	0.4	2.3476×10^{-5}	8.4080×10^{-10}	8.8818×10^{-16}	0	0
	0.6	7.8526×10^{-6}	3.4030×10^{-9}	9.6589×10^{-15}	0	0
	0.8	3.9181×10^{-5}	8.7368×10^{-9}	4.7517×10^{-14}	1.0×10^{-10}	1.0×10^{-10}
0.2	0.2	2.3553×10^{-5}	8.3330×10^{-11}	1.1102×10^{-16}	0	0
	0.4	7.7785×10^{-6}	3.3840×10^{-10}	4.4409×10^{-16}	1.0×10^{-10}	1.0×10^{-10}
	0.6	3.9108×10^{-5}	2.2730×10^{-9}	2.7756×10^{-15}	0	0
	0.8	7.0440×10^{-5}	6.7268×10^{-9}	2.6090×10^{-14}	0	0
0.3	0.2	7.0426×10^{-5}	2.0890×10^{-10}	1.1102×10^{-16}	0	0
	0.4	3.9091×10^{-5}	1.6420×10^{-10}	1.7764×10^{-15}	0	0
	0.6	7.7594×10^{-6}	1.1420×10^{-9}	3.9968×10^{-15}	1.0×10^{-10}	1.0×10^{-10}
	0.8	2.3578×10^{-5}	4.7168×10^{-9}	4.5519×10^{-15}	1.0×10^{-10}	1.0×10^{-10}
0.4	0.2	3.9169×10^{-6}	3.3460×10^{-10}	3.3307×10^{-16}	0	0
	0.4	7.8222×10^{-5}	6.6670×10^{-10}	3.3305×10^{-15}	1.0×10^{-10}	1.0×10^{-10}
	0.6	2.3516×10^{-5}	1.1300×10^{-11}	1.088×10^{-14}	0	0
	0.8	5.4870×10^{-5}	2.7068×10^{-9}	1.7097×10^{-14}	0	0
0.5	0.2	7.9054×10^{-6}	4.6020×10^{-10}	3.3307×10^{-16}	1.0×10^{-10}	1.0×10^{-10}
	0.4	2.3463×10^{-5}	1.1692×10^{-9}	4.5519×10^{-15}	0	0
	0.6	5.4812×10^{-5}	1.1190×10^{-9}	1.7652×10^{-14}	1.0×10^{-10}	1.0×10^{-10}
	0.8	8.6199×10^{-6}	6.9680×10^{-10}	3.8636×10^{-14}	1.0×10^{-10}	1.0×10^{-10}
0.6	0.2	5.4768×10^{-5}	5.8580×10^{-10}	4.9960×10^{-16}	1.0×10^{-10}	1.0×10^{-10}
	0.4	2.3384×10^{-5}	1.6717×10^{-9}	5.9952×10^{-15}	0	0
	0.6	7.9731×10^{-6}	2.2490×10^{-9}	2.4536×10^{-14}	1.0×10^{-10}	1.0×10^{-10}
	0.8	3.9384×10^{-5}	1.3132×10^{-9}	6.0174×10^{-14}	1.0×10^{-10}	1.0×10^{-10}
0.7	0.2	2.3489×10^{-5}	7.1150×10^{-10}	4.9960×10^{-16}	0	0
	0.4	7.9370×10^{-6}	2.1742×10^{-9}	7.2164×10^{-15}	0	0
	0.6	3.9317×10^{-5}	3.3810×10^{-9}	3.1419×10^{-14}	0	0
	0.8	7.0791×10^{-5}	3.3232×10^{-9}	8.1712×10^{-14}	1.0×10^{-10}	1.0×10^{-10}

Table 3. *Cont.*

δ	$\wp$	Haar Wavelet Error [67]	OHAM Error [67]	q-HATM Error [68]	HPTM Error	NITM Error
0.8	0.2	7.0337×10^{-5}	8.3710×10^{-10}	6.1062×10^{-16}	1.0×10^{-10}	1.0×10^{-10}
	0.4	3.8884×10^{-6}	2.6767×10^{-9}	8.5487×10^{-15}	0	0
	0.6	7.4894×10^{-5}	4.5110×10^{-9}	3.8192×10^{-14}	0	0
	0.8	2.4026×10^{-5}	5.3332×10^{-9}	1.0325×10^{-13}	1.0×10^{-10}	1.0×10^{-10}
0.9	0.2	3.9031×10^{-5}	9.6270×10^{-10}	7.2164×10^{-16}	0	0
	0.4	7.5074×10^{-6}	3.1792×10^{-9}	9.9365×10^{-15}	0	0
	0.6	2.3923×10^{-5}	5.6420×10^{-9}	4.4964×10^{-14}	1.0×10^{-10}	1.0×10^{-10}
	0.8	5.5543×10^{-5}	7.3432×10^{-9}	1.2479×10^{-13}	1.0×10^{-10}	1.0×10^{-10}
1.0	0.2	8.5852×10^{-5}	1.0883×10^{-9}	7.7716×10^{-16}	0	0
	0.4	5.4286×10^{-5}	3.6817×10^{-9}	1.1269×10^{-14}	0	0
	0.6	2.2833×10^{-5}	6.7720×10^{-9}	5.1736×10^{-14}	0	0
	0.8	8.8514×10^{-6}	9.3532×10^{-9}	1.4622×10^{-13}	1.0×10^{-10}	1.0×10^{-10}

7.2. Example

Consider the one-dimensional TF-GBFE

$$\frac{\partial^\eta \mathbb{P}(\delta,\wp)}{\partial \wp^\eta} = \frac{\partial^2 \mathbb{P}}{\partial \wp^2} + \mathbb{P}^2 \frac{\partial \mathbb{P}}{\partial \wp} - \mathbb{P}^3 + \mathbb{P}, \quad 0 < \eta \le 1, \tag{57}$$

with initial guess

$$\mathbb{P}(\delta,0) = \sqrt{\frac{1}{2}\left(1 + \tanh\left(\frac{\delta}{3}\right)\right)}. \tag{58}$$

By executing the ET to Equation (57), we may have

$$E[\mathbb{P}(\delta,\wp)] = s^2\left(\sqrt{\frac{1}{2}\left(1 + \tanh\left(\frac{\delta}{3}\right)\right)}\right) + s^\eta E\left[\frac{\partial^2 \mathbb{P}}{\partial \wp^2} + \mathbb{P}^2 \frac{\partial \mathbb{P}}{\partial \wp} - \mathbb{P}^3 + \mathbb{P}\right], \tag{59}$$

Now by employing the inverse ET, we may have

$$\mathbb{P}(\delta,\wp) = \sqrt{\frac{1}{2}\left(1 + \tanh\left(\frac{\delta}{3}\right)\right)} + E^{-1}\left[s^\eta E\left[\frac{\partial^2 \mathbb{P}}{\partial \wp^2} + \mathbb{P}^2 \frac{\partial \mathbb{P}}{\partial \wp} - \mathbb{P}^3 + \mathbb{P}\right]\right], \tag{60}$$

By NITM, we may have

$$\mathbb{P}_0(\delta,\wp) = \sqrt{\frac{1}{2}\left(1 + \tanh\left(\frac{\delta}{3}\right)\right)},$$

$$\mathbb{P}_1(\delta,\wp) = E^{-1}\left[s^\eta E\left\{\frac{\partial^2 \mathbb{P}_0}{\partial \wp^2} + \mathbb{P}_0^2 \frac{\partial \mathbb{P}_0}{\partial \wp} - \mathbb{P}_0^3 + \mathbb{P}_0\right\}\right] =$$

$$\frac{5}{18} \frac{\sqrt{2}}{\cosh\left(\frac{\delta}{3}\right)^2 \sqrt{\frac{\cosh\left(\frac{\delta}{3}\right) + \sinh\left(\frac{\delta}{3}\right)}{\cosh\left(\frac{\delta}{3}\right)}}} \frac{\wp^\eta}{\Gamma(\eta+1)},$$

$$\mathbb{P}_2(\delta,\wp) = E^{-1}\left[s^{\eta}E\left\{\frac{\partial^2(\mathbb{P}_0+\mathbb{P}_1)}{\partial\wp^2} + (\mathbb{P}_0+\mathbb{P}_1)^2\frac{\partial(\mathbb{P}_0+\mathbb{P}_1)}{\partial\wp} - (\mathbb{P}_0+\mathbb{P}_1)^3 + (\mathbb{P}_0+\mathbb{P}_1)\right\}\right] -$$
$$E^{-1}\left[s^{\eta}E\left\{\frac{\partial^2\mathbb{P}_0}{\partial\wp^2} + \mathbb{P}_0^2\frac{\partial\mathbb{P}_0}{\partial\wp} - \mathbb{P}_0^3 + \mathbb{P}_0\right\}\right] =$$
$$-\frac{25}{162}\frac{\sqrt{2}\left(8\sinh\left(\frac{\delta}{3}\right)\cosh\left(\frac{\delta}{3}\right)^2 + 8\cosh\left(\frac{\delta}{3}\right)^3 - 3\sinh\left(\frac{\delta}{3}\right) - 7\cosh\left(\frac{\delta}{3}\right)\right)}{\cosh\left(\frac{\delta}{3}\right)^3\left(\cosh\left(\frac{\delta}{3}\right)+\sinh\left(\frac{\delta}{3}\right)\right)^2\sqrt{\frac{\cosh\left(\frac{\delta}{3}\right)+\sinh\left(\frac{\delta}{3}\right)}{\cosh\left(\frac{\delta}{3}\right)}}}\frac{\wp^{2\eta}}{\Gamma(2\eta+1)}$$
$$-\frac{25}{1944}\frac{\sqrt{2}\left(52\sinh\left(\frac{\delta}{3}\right)\cosh\left(\frac{\delta}{3}\right)^2 + 52\cosh\left(\frac{\delta}{3}\right)^3 - 7\sinh\left(\frac{\delta}{3}\right) - 33\cosh\left(\frac{\delta}{3}\right)\right)\Gamma(2q+1)}{\cosh\left(\frac{\delta}{3}\right)^5\left(\cosh\left(\frac{\delta}{3}\right)+\sinh\left(\frac{\delta}{3}\right)\right)^2\sqrt{\frac{\cosh\left(\frac{\delta}{3}\right)+\sinh\left(\frac{\delta}{3}\right)}{\cosh\left(\frac{\delta}{3}\right)}}\Gamma(\eta+1)^2}\frac{\wp^{3\eta}}{\Gamma(3\eta+1)}$$
$$-\frac{125}{17496}\frac{\sqrt{2}\left(10\cosh\left(\frac{\delta}{3}\right)^2 + 10\cosh\left(\frac{\delta}{3}\right)\sinh\left(\frac{\delta}{3}\right) - 3\right)\Gamma(3q+1)}{\cosh\left(\frac{\delta}{3}\right)^6\left(\cosh\left(\frac{\delta}{3}\right)+\sinh\left(\frac{\delta}{3}\right)\right)^2\sqrt{\frac{\cosh\left(\frac{\delta}{3}\right)+\sinh\left(\frac{\delta}{3}\right)}{\cosh\left(\frac{\delta}{3}\right)}}\Gamma(\eta+1)^3}\frac{\wp^{4\eta}}{\Gamma(4\eta+1)}$$
$$\vdots$$

Lastly, the series solution is taken as

$$\begin{aligned}
&\mathbb{P}(\delta,\wp) = \mathbb{P}_0(\delta,\wp) + \mathbb{P}_1(\delta,\wp) + \mathbb{P}_2(\delta,\wp) + \cdots, \\
&\mathbb{P}(\delta,\wp) = \sqrt{\frac{1}{2}\left(1+\tanh\left(\frac{\delta}{3}\right)\right)} + \frac{5}{18}\frac{\sqrt{2}}{\cosh\left(\frac{\delta}{3}\right)^2\sqrt{\frac{\cosh\left(\frac{\delta}{3}\right)+\sinh\left(\frac{\delta}{3}\right)}{\cosh\left(\frac{\delta}{3}\right)}}}\frac{\wp^{\eta}}{\Gamma(\eta+1)} \\
&-\frac{25}{162}\frac{\sqrt{2}\left(8\sinh\left(\frac{\delta}{3}\right)\cosh\left(\frac{\delta}{3}\right)^2 + 8\cosh\left(\frac{\delta}{3}\right)^3 - 3\sinh\left(\frac{\delta}{3}\right) - 7\cosh\left(\frac{\delta}{3}\right)\right)}{\cosh\left(\frac{\delta}{3}\right)^3\left(\cosh\left(\frac{\delta}{3}\right)+\sinh\left(\frac{\delta}{3}\right)\right)^2\sqrt{\frac{\cosh\left(\frac{\delta}{3}\right)+\sinh\left(\frac{\delta}{3}\right)}{\cosh\left(\frac{\delta}{3}\right)}}}\frac{\wp^{2\eta}}{\Gamma(2\eta+1)} \\
&-\frac{25}{1944}\frac{\sqrt{2}\left(52\sinh\left(\frac{\delta}{3}\right)\cosh\left(\frac{\delta}{3}\right)^2 + 52\cosh\left(\frac{\delta}{3}\right)^3 - 7\sinh\left(\frac{\delta}{3}\right) - 33\cosh\left(\frac{\delta}{3}\right)\right)\Gamma(2\eta+1)}{\cosh\left(\frac{\delta}{3}\right)^5\left(\cosh\left(\frac{\delta}{3}\right)+\sinh\left(\frac{\delta}{3}\right)\right)^2\sqrt{\frac{\cosh\left(\frac{\delta}{3}\right)+\sinh\left(\frac{\delta}{3}\right)}{\cosh\left(\frac{\delta}{3}\right)}}\Gamma(\eta+1)^2}\frac{\wp^{3\eta}}{\Gamma(3\eta+1)} \\
&-\frac{125}{17496}\frac{\sqrt{2}\left(10\cosh\left(\frac{\delta}{3}\right)^2 + 10\cosh\left(\frac{\delta}{3}\right)\sinh\left(\frac{\delta}{3}\right) - 3\right)\Gamma(3\eta+1)}{\cosh\left(\frac{\delta}{3}\right)^6\left(\cosh\left(\frac{\delta}{3}\right)+\sinh\left(\frac{\delta}{3}\right)\right)^2\sqrt{\frac{\cosh\left(\frac{\delta}{3}\right)+\sinh\left(\frac{\delta}{3}\right)}{\cosh\left(\frac{\delta}{3}\right)}}\Gamma(\eta+1)^3}\frac{\wp^{4\eta}}{\Gamma(4\eta+1)} + \cdots,
\end{aligned} \tag{61}$$

By employing the HPTM, we may have

$$\sum_{n=0}^{\infty}\epsilon^n\mathbb{P}^n(\delta,\wp)=\sqrt{\frac{1}{2}\left(1+\tanh\left(\frac{\delta}{3}\right)\right)}+\epsilon\left\{E^{-1}\left(s^{\eta}E\left[\left(\sum_{n=0}^{\infty}\epsilon^n\mathbb{P}_n(\delta,\wp)\right)_{\delta\delta}+\left(\sum_{n=0}^{\infty}\epsilon^n H_n^1(\delta,\wp)\right)-\left(\sum_{n=0}^{\infty}\epsilon^n H_n^2(\delta,\wp)\right)+\left(\sum_{n=0}^{\infty}\epsilon^n\mathbb{P}_n(\delta,\wp)\right)\right]\right)\right\}, \tag{62}$$

with He's polynomials $H_k(\delta)$ represent the nonlinear terms and is stated as

$$\begin{aligned}
&H_0^1(\delta)=\mathbb{P}_0^2(\mathbb{P}_0)_\delta\\
&H_1^1(\delta)=\mathbb{P}_0^2(\mathbb{P}_1)_\delta+2\mathbb{P}_0\mathbb{P}_1(\mathbb{P}_0)_\delta\\
&\vdots\\
&H_0^2(\delta)=(\mathbb{P}_0)^3\\
&H_1^2(\delta)=3\mathbb{P}_0^2\mathbb{P}_1
\end{aligned}$$

On comparing the ϵ coefficients, we may have

$$\begin{aligned}
&\epsilon^0:\mathbb{P}_0(\delta,\wp)=\sqrt{\frac{1}{2}\left(1+\tanh\left(\frac{\delta}{3}\right)\right)},\\
&\epsilon^1:\mathbb{P}_1(\delta,\wp)=\frac{5}{18}\frac{\sqrt{2}}{\cosh\left(\frac{\delta}{3}\right)^2\sqrt{\frac{\cosh\left(\frac{\delta}{3}\right)+\sinh\left(\frac{\delta}{3}\right)}{\cosh\left(\frac{\delta}{3}\right)}}}\frac{\wp^{\eta}}{\Gamma(\eta+1)},\\
&\epsilon^2:\mathbb{P}_2(\delta,\wp)=-\frac{25}{162}\frac{\sqrt{2}\left(8\sinh\left(\frac{\delta}{3}\right)\cosh\left(\frac{\delta}{3}\right)^2+8\cosh\left(\frac{\delta}{3}\right)^3-3\sinh\left(\frac{\delta}{3}\right)-7\cosh\left(\frac{\delta}{3}\right)\right)}{\cosh\left(\frac{\delta}{3}\right)^3\left(\cosh\left(\frac{\delta}{3}\right)+\sinh\left(\frac{\delta}{3}\right)\right)^2\sqrt{\frac{\cosh\left(\frac{\delta}{3}\right)+\sinh\left(\frac{\delta}{3}\right)}{\cosh\left(\frac{\delta}{3}\right)}}}\frac{\wp^{2\eta}}{\Gamma(2\eta+1)},\\
&\vdots
\end{aligned} \tag{63}$$

Lastly, the series solution is taken as

$$\mathbb{P}(\delta,\wp)=\sum_{n=0}^{\infty}\epsilon^n\mathbb{P}_n(\delta,\wp). \tag{64}$$

Hence

$$\mathbb{P}(\delta,\wp) = \mathbb{P}_0(\delta,\wp) + \mathbb{P}_1(\delta,\wp) + \mathbb{P}_2(\delta,\wp) + \cdots,$$

$$\mathbb{P}(\delta,\wp) = \sqrt{\frac{1}{2}\left(1+\tanh\left(\frac{\delta}{3}\right)\right)} + \frac{5}{18}\frac{\sqrt{2}}{\cosh\left(\frac{\delta}{3}\right)^2\sqrt{\frac{\cosh\left(\frac{\delta}{3}\right)+\sinh\left(\frac{\delta}{3}\right)}{\cosh\left(\frac{\delta}{3}\right)}}}\frac{\wp^{\eta}}{\Gamma(\eta+1)} + \tag{65}$$

$$-\frac{25}{162}\frac{\sqrt{2}\left(8\sinh\left(\frac{\delta}{3}\right)\cosh\left(\frac{\delta}{3}\right)^2 + 8\cosh\left(\frac{\delta}{3}\right)^3 - 3\sinh\left(\frac{\delta}{3}\right) - 7\cosh\left(\frac{\delta}{3}\right)\right)}{\cosh\left(\frac{\delta}{3}\right)^3\left(\cosh\left(\frac{\delta}{3}\right)+\sinh\left(\frac{\delta}{3}\right)\right)^2\sqrt{\frac{\cosh\left(\frac{\delta}{3}\right)+\sinh\left(\frac{\delta}{3}\right)}{\cosh\left(\frac{\delta}{3}\right)}}}\frac{\wp^{2\eta}}{\Gamma(2\eta+1)} + \cdots.$$

At $\eta = 1$, we get exact solution as

$$\mathbb{P}(\delta,\wp) = \sqrt{\frac{1}{2}\left(1+\tanh\left(\frac{\delta}{3}+\frac{10\wp}{9}\right)\right)} \tag{66}$$

The HPTM approximation solution and the accurate solution at $\eta = 1$ are compared in Figure 7. The derived solution of NITM and the accurate solution at $\eta = 1$ are compared in Figure 8. Excellent agreement can be seen in the graphical comparisons between the precise solution and the solutions from the suggested methods. The 3D depiction of the solutions derived by HPTM and NITM for the TF-GBFE at $\eta = 0.6$ and $\eta = 0.8$ is shown in Figures 9 and 10. The 2D plot of the found solution for different fractional orders is shown in Figures 11 and 12, along with a comparison of the generated and precise solution. Figures 11 and 12 illustrate the impact of changing the parameter η on the TF-GBFE solutions. The derived solutions are illustrated in Figures 7–12 for a range of η values with $-5 \leq \delta \leq 5$ and temporal variable $0 \leq \wp \leq 0.1$. Tables 4 and 5 present the exact solution for the TF-GBFE while maintaining $\eta = 0.97, 0.98, 0.98$ and 1, as well as the comparative numerical solutions derived by HPTM and the NITM.

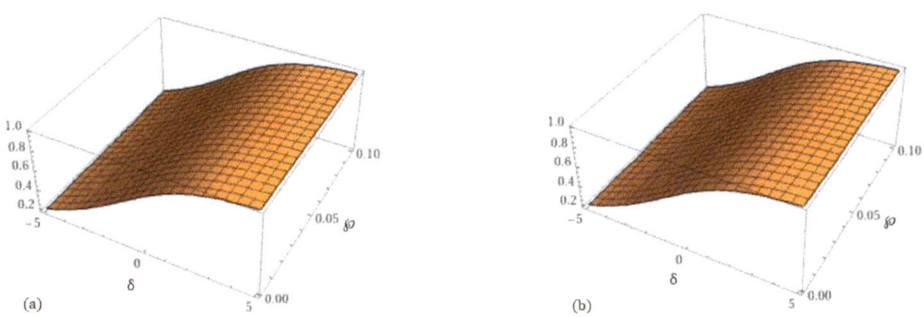

Figure 7. Graphical depict of the (**a**) accurate as well as (**b**) HPTM solution for $\mathbb{P}(\delta,\wp)$.

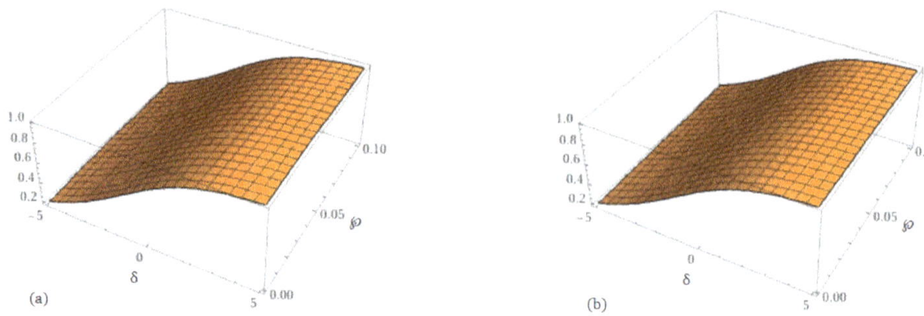

Figure 8. Graphical depict of the (**a**) accurate as well as (**b**) NITM solution for $\mathbb{P}(\delta, \wp)$.

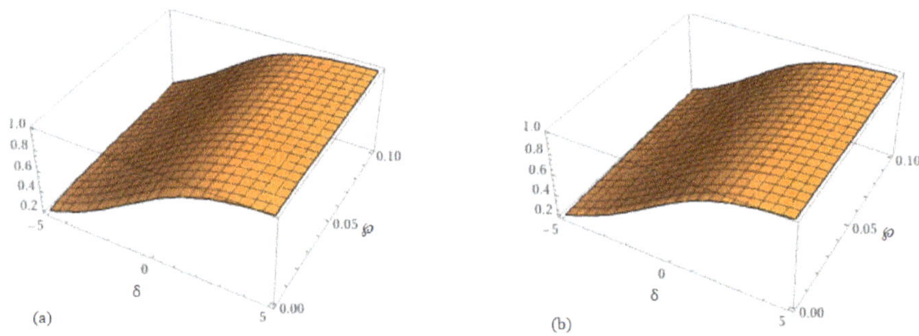

Figure 9. Graphical depict of the HPTM solution at (**a**) $\eta = 0.6$ (**b**) $\eta = 0.8$ for $\mathbb{P}(\delta, \wp)$.

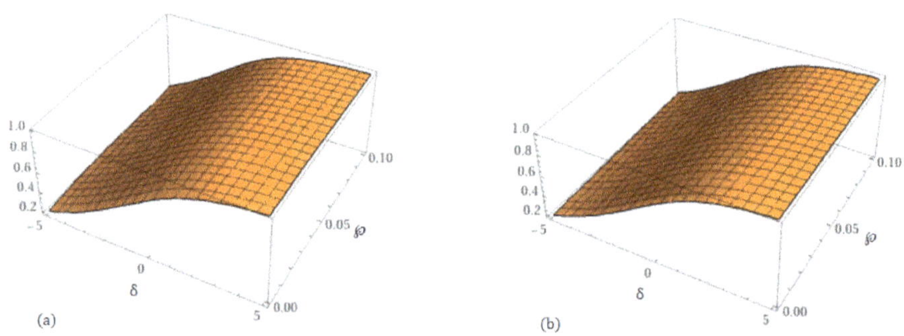

Figure 10. Graphical depict of the NITM solution at (**a**) $\eta = 0.6$ (**b**) $\eta = 0.8$ for $\mathbb{P}(\delta, \wp)$.

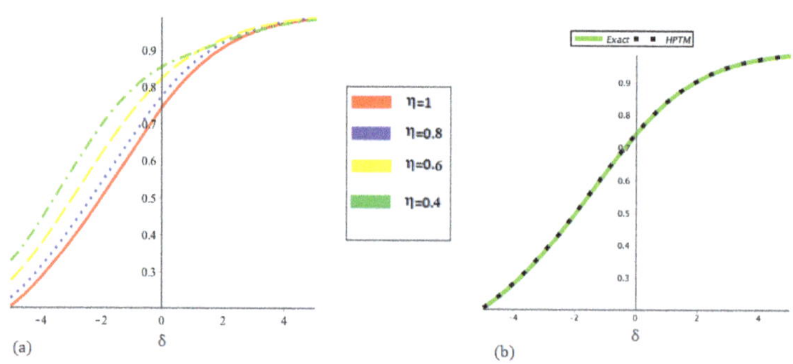

Figure 11. 2D Graphical depict of the HPTM solution at (**a**) several orders of η as well as (**b**) comparison with accurate solution.

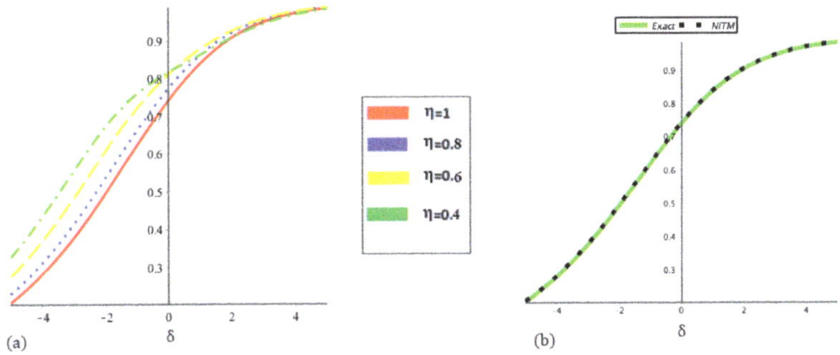

Figure 12. 2D Graphical depict of the HPTM solution at (**a**) several orders of η as well as (**b**) comparison with accurate solution.

Table 4. Behavior of the accurate as well as HPTM solution at several of η for $\mathbb{P}(\delta, \wp)$.

δ	$\eta = 0.97$	$\eta = 0.98$	$\eta = 0.99$	$\eta = 1\,(HPTM)$	$\eta = 1\,(Accurate)$
0.0	0.7116581992	0.7114365594	0.7112253981	0.7110242400	0.7110241395
0.1	0.7232619661	0.7230443269	0.7228369684	0.7226394249	0.7226393305
0.2	0.7346476339	0.7344342783	0.7342309925	0.7340373213	0.7340372335
0.3	0.7458007792	0.7455919690	0.7453930058	0.7452034453	0.7452033650
0.4	0.7567081326	0.7565041070	0.7563096947	0.7561244628	0.7561243895
0.5	0.7673576479	0.7671586222	0.7669689664	0.7667882594	0.7667881945
0.6	0.7777385630	0.7775447277	0.7773600105	0.7771840022	0.7771839460
0.7	0.7878414402	0.7876529605	0.7874733396	0.7873021809	0.7873021325
0.8	0.7976581905	0.7974752057	0.7973008145	0.7971346329	0.7971345930
0.9	0.8071820859	0.8070047096	0.8068356568	0.8066745564	0.8066745250
1.0	0.8164077556	0.8162360756	0.8160724457	0.8159165074	0.8159164840

Table 5. Behavior of the accurate as well as NITM solution at several η for $\mathbb{P}(\delta, \wp)$.

δ	$\eta = 0.97$	$\eta = 0.98$	$\eta = 0.99$	$\eta = 1(NITM)$	$\eta = 1(Accurate)$
0.0	0.7116580097	0.7114363988	0.7112252619	0.7110241247	0.7110241395
0.1	0.7232617778	0.7230441673	0.7228368331	0.7226393103	0.7226393305
0.2	0.7346474475	0.7344341203	0.7342308586	0.7340372079	0.7340372335
0.3	0.7458005955	0.7455918133	0.7453928739	0.7452033335	0.7452033650
0.4	0.7567079523	0.7565039542	0.7563095652	0.7561243531	0.7561243895
0.5	0.7673574716	0.7671584728	0.7669688398	0.7667881521	0.7667881945
0.6	0.7777383914	0.7775445823	0.7773598872	0.7771838978	0.7771839460
0.7	0.7878412738	0.7876528195	0.7874732201	0.7873020797	0.7873021325
0.8	0.7976580298	0.7974750695	0.7973006991	0.7971345351	0.7971345930
0.9	0.8071819313	0.8070045785	0.8068355457	0.8066744623	0.8066745250
1.0	0.8164076073	0.8162359500	0.8160723393	0.8159164172	0.8159164840

8. Conclusions

In this work, we offer the HPTM and NITM for nonlinear TF-GBFE solutions. The derivative is considered in the Caputo sense. The solution derived from the methods presented shows that our findings strongly match the precise solution. We have compared the solutions we found with some of the solutions provided in the literature to demonstrate the effectiveness of the existing methodologies. A comparison with the other three approaches validates the accuracy and convergence of our offered strategies. Finding the solution to fractional problems is made more straightforward by the hybrid techniques that have been offered. The results acquired are plotted in their graphical form. Graphs and tables are used to show a very strong correlation between the actual and suggested technique solutions. The fractional solutions are used to illustrate the behaviour of different dynamics of the specified physical phenomena. The aforementioned issues can be seen in tabular and graphical form with Maple's assistance.

In conclusion, the suggested methods were found to be quite precise, efficient, and simple to use. It provides a practical tool for solving nonlinear fractional equations in a variety of academic fields and creates new opportunities for fractional differential equation research. Thus, we can say that the methods presented are sufficiently consistent and applicable to the analysis of a wide range of fractional-order nonlinear mathematical models that aid in explaining the behaviour of complex, highly nonlinear phenomena in significant scientific and engineering domains.

Future Work

In future work, these techniques are expected to be considered for fractional problems in the sense of Atangana–Baleanu derivatives and other partial differential equations employing fractional calculus and fractal theory. We expect that these methods will be used in the future to swiftly and efficiently tackle other fractional differential problems in scientific domains.

Funding: This study is funded by Prince Sattam bin Abdulaziz University under project number PSAU/2025/R/1446.

Data Availability Statement: The numerical data used to support the findings of this study are included within the article.

Acknowledgments: The author extends her appreciation to Prince Sattam bin Abdulaziz University for funding this research work through project number PSAU/2025/R/1446.

Conflicts of Interest: The author declares no conflict of interest.

Abbreviations

The following abbreviations are used in this manuscript:

TF-GBFE	time-fractional generalized Burger-Fisher equation
HPTM	homotopy perturbation transform method
YTDM	yang transform decomposition method
OHAM	optimal homotopy asymptotic method
q-HATM	q-homotopy analysis transform method
PDE	partial differential equation
FPDEs	Fractional partial differential equations
ET	Elzaki transform
δ	Independent variable
$\wp$	Time
$\mathbb{P}(\delta, \wp)$	Dependent function representing the physical quantity
η	Fractional order
ϵ	Perturbation parameter

References

1. Rezapour, S.; Liaqat, M.I.; Etemad, S. An effective new iterative method to solve conformable cauchy reaction-diffusion equation via the Shehu transform. *J. Math.* **2022**, *12*, 4172218. [CrossRef]
2. Bas, E.; Ozarslan, R. Real world applications of fractional models by Atangana-Baleanu fractional derivative. *Chaos Solitons Fractals* **2018**, *116*, 121–125. [CrossRef]
3. Liaqat, M.I.; Khan, A.; Akgül, A.; Ali, M. A novel numerical technique for fractional ordinary differential equations with proportional delay. *J. Funct. Spaces* **2022**, *21*, 6333084. [CrossRef]
4. Traore, A.; Sene, N. Model of economic growth in the context of fractional derivative. *Alex. Eng. J.* **2020**, *59*, 4843–4850. [CrossRef]
5. Khan, A.; Liaqat, M.I.; Younis, M.; Alam, A. Approximate and exact solutions to fractional order Cauchy reaction-diffusion equations by new combine techniques. *J. Math.* **2021**, *12*, 5337255. [CrossRef]
6. AlBaidani, M.M.; Ganie, A.H.; Khan, A.; Aljuaydi, F. An Approximate Analytical View of Fractional Physical Models in the Frame of the Caputo Operator. *Fractal Fract.* **2025**, *9*, 199. [CrossRef]
7. Shah, N.A.; El-Zahar, E.R.; Akgül, A.; Khan, A.; Kafle, J. Analysis of Fractional-Order Regularized Long-Wave Models via a Novel Transform. *J. Funct. Spaces* **2022**, *2022*, 2754507. [CrossRef]
8. Hilfer, R.; Luchko, Y.; Tomovski, Z. Operational method for the solution of fractional differential equations with generalized Riemann-Liouville fractional derivatives. *Fract. Calc. Appl. Anal.* **2009**, *12*, 299–318.
9. AlBaidani, M.M. Analytical Insight into Some Fractional Nonlinear Dynamical Systems Involving the Caputo Fractional Derivative Operator. *Fractal Fract.* **2025**, *9*, 320. [CrossRef]
10. Ali, L.; Zou, G.; Li, N.; Mehmood, K.; Fang, P.; Khan, A. Analytical treatments of time-fractional seventh-order nonlinear equations via Elzaki transform. *J. Eng. Math.* **2024**, *145*, 1. [CrossRef]
11. Jia, H.; Guo, Z.; Qi, G.; Chen, Z. Analysis of a four-wing fractional-order chaotic system via frequency-domain and time-domain approaches and circuit implementation for secure communication. *Optik* **2018**, *155*, 233–241. [CrossRef]
12. He, S.; Sun, K.; Wang, H. Complexity analysis and DSP implementation of the fractional-order Lorenz hyperchaotic system. *Entropy* **2015**, *17*, 8299–8311. [CrossRef]
13. Wang, Y.; Sun, K.; He, S.; Wang, H. Dynamics of fractional-order sinusoidally forced simplified Lorenz system and its synchronization. *Eur. Phys. J. Spec. Top.* **2014**, *223*, 1591–1600. [CrossRef]
14. He, S.; Sun, K.; Wang, H.; Mei, X.; Sun, Y. Generalized synchronization of fractional-order hyperchaotic systems and its DSP implementation. *Nonlinear Dyn.* **2018**, *92*, 85–96. [CrossRef]
15. Li, C.; Su, K.; Tong, Y.; Li, H. Robust synchronization for a class of fractional-order chaotic and hyperchaotic systems. *Opt.-Int. J. Light Electron Opt.* **2013**, *124*, 3242–3245. [CrossRef]
16. Adomian, G. A review of the decomposition method and some recent results for nonlinear equations. *Math. Comput. Model.* **1990**, *13*, 17–43. [CrossRef]
17. Deng, W. Short memory principle and a predictor-corrector approach for fractional differential equations. *J. Comput. Appl. Math.* **2007**, *206*, 174–188. [CrossRef]
18. He, S.; Banerjee, S.; Yan, B. Chaos and symbol complexity in a conformable fractional-order memcapacitor system. *Complexity* **2018**, *2018*, 4140762. [CrossRef]
19. Diethelm, K.; Ford, N.J.; Freed, A.D. A predictor-corrector approach for the numerical solution of fractional differential equations. *Nonlinear Dyn.* **2002**, *29*, 3–22. [CrossRef]
20. Tavazoei, M.S.; Haeri, M. Unreliability of frequency-domain approximation in recognising chaos in fractional-order systems. *IET Signal Process.* **2007**, *1*, 171–181. [CrossRef]
21. He, S.B.; Sun, K.H.; Wang, H.H. Solution of the fractional-order chaotic system based on Adomian decomposition algorithm and its complexity analysis. *Acta Phys. Sin.* **2014**, *63*, 030502.
22. He, K.; Zhang, X.; Ren, S.; Sun, J. Deep residual learning for image recognition. In Proceedings of the IEEE Conference on Computer Vision and Pattern Recognition, Las Vegas, NV, USA, 27–30 June 2016; pp. 770–778.
23. Wu, Z.; Shen, C.; Van Den Hengel, A. Wider or deeper: Revisiting the resnet model for visual recognition. *Pattern Recognit.* **2019**, *90*, 119–133. [CrossRef]
24. Xu, W.; Fu, Y.L.; Zhu, D. ResNet and its application to medical image processing: Research progress and challenges. *Comput. Methods Programs Biomed.* **2023**, *240*, 107660. [CrossRef] [PubMed]
25. Yan, H.; Du, J.; Tan, V.Y.; Feng, J. On robustness of neural ordinary differential equations. *arXiv* **2019**, arXiv:1910.05513.
26. Poli, M.; Massaroli, S.; Park, J.; Yamashita, A.; Asama, H.; Park, J. Graph neural ordinary differential equations. *arXiv* **2019**, arXiv:1911.07532.
27. Zhu, A.; Jin, P.; Zhu, B.; Tang, Y. On numerical integration in neural ordinary differential equations. In Proceedings of the International Conference on Machine Learning, Baltimore, MD, USA, 17–23 July 2022; pp. 27527–27547.
28. Yang, Y.; Li, H. Neural ordinary differential equations for robust parameter estimation in dynamic systems with physical priors. *Appl. Soft Comput.* **2025**, *169*, 112649. [CrossRef]

29. Yue, P. Uncertain Numbers. *Mathematics* **2025**, *13*, 496. [CrossRef]
30. Yao, K.; Liu, B. Parameter estimation in uncertain differential equations. *Fuzzy Optim. Decis. Mak.* **2020**, *19*, 1–12. [CrossRef]
31. Liu, Z.; Jia, L. Moment estimations for parameters in uncertain delay differential equations. *J. Intell. Fuzzy Syst.* **2020**, *39*, 841–849. [CrossRef]
32. Wu, G.C.; Wei, J.L.; Luo, C.; Huang, L.L. Parameter estimation of fractional uncertain differential equations via Adams method. *Nonlinear Anal. Model. Control* **2022**, *27*, 413–427. [CrossRef]
33. Ning, J.; Li, Z.; Xu, L. Parameter Estimation of Fractional Uncertain Differential Equations. *Fractal Fract.* **2025**, *9*, 138. [CrossRef]
34. Rosales-García, J.; Andrade-Lucio, J.A.; Shulika, O. Conformable derivative applied to experimental Newtonas law of cooling. *Rev. Mex. Fís.* **2020**, *66*, 224–227. [CrossRef]
35. Ionescu, C.; Lopes, A.; Copot, D.; Machado, J.T.; Bates, J.H. The role of fractional calculus in modeling biological phenomena: A review. *Commun. Nonlinear Sci. Numer. Simul.* **2017**, *51*, 141–159. [CrossRef]
36. Rabtah, A.A.; Erturk, R.S.; Momani, S. Solution of fractional oscillator by using differential transformation method. *Comput. Math. Appl.* **2010**, *59*, 1356–1362. [CrossRef]
37. Archibald, A.M.; Gusinskaia, N.V.; Hessels, J.W.; Deller, A.T.; Kaplan, D.L.; Lorimer, D.R. Universality of free fall from the orbital motion of a pulsar in a stellar triple system. *Nature* **2018**, *559*, 73–76. [CrossRef]
38. Cresson, J. Fractional embedding of differential operators and Lagrangian systems. *J. Math. Phys.* **2007**, *48*, 033504. [CrossRef]
39. Katugampola, U.N. A New Approach to Generalized Fractional Derivatives. *arXiv* **2011**, arXiv:1106.0965.
40. Klimek, M. Lagrangian fractional mechanics-a noncommutative approach. *Czechoslov. J. Phys.* **2005**, *55*, 1447–1453. [CrossRef]
41. Ray, S.S.; Sahoo, S. New exact solutions of fractional Zakharov-Kuznetsov and modified Zakharov-Kuznetsov equations using fractional sub-equation method. *Commun. Theor. Phys.* **2015**, *63*, 25. [CrossRef]
42. Gepreel, K.A.; Nofal, T.A. Optimal homotopy analysis method for nonlinear partial fractional differential equations. *Math. Sci.* **2015**, *9*, 47–55. [CrossRef]
43. Khirsariya, S.R.; Chauhan, J.P.; Rao, S.B. A robust computational analysis of residual power series involving general transform to solve fractional differential equations. *Math. Comput. Simul.* **2024**, *216*, 168–186. [CrossRef]
44. Zurigat, M.; Momani, S.; Odibat, Z.; Alawneh, A. The homotopy analysis method for handling systems of fractional differential equations. *Appl. Math. Model.* **2010**, *34*, 24–35. [CrossRef]
45. Li, M.; Huang, C.; Wang, P. Galerkin finite element method for nonlinear fractional Schrödinger equations. *Numer. Algorithms* **2017**, *74*, 499–525. [CrossRef]
46. Li, C.; Zeng, F. Finite difference methods for fractional differential equations. *Int. J. Bifurc. Chaos* **2012**, *22*, 1230014. [CrossRef]
47. Kanth, A.R.; Aruna, K.; Raghavendar, K.; Rezazadeh, H.; İnç, M. Numerical solutions of nonlinear time fractional Klein-Gordon equation via natural transform decomposition method and iterative Shehu transform method. *J. Ocean Eng. Sci.* **2021**. [CrossRef]
48. Kumar, R.; Verma, R.S.; Tiwari, A.K. On similarity solutions to (2+ 1)-dispersive long-wave equations. *J. Ocean Eng. Sci.* **2023**, *8*, 11–123. [CrossRef]
49. Ahmad, I.; Ahmad, H.; Inc, M.; Rezazadeh, H.; Akbar, M.A.; Khater, M.M.; Akinyemi, L.; Jhangeer, A. Solution of fractional-order Korteweg-de Vries and Burgers equations utilizing local meshless method. *J. Ocean Eng. Sci.* **2021**. [CrossRef]
50. Tang, S.; Wu, J.; Cui, M. The nonlinear convection-reaction-diffusion equation for modelling El Niño events. *Commun. Nonlinear Sci. Numer. Simul.* **1996**, *1*, 27–31. [CrossRef]
51. Fakhrusy, Q.Z.; Anggraeni, C.P.; Gunawan, P.H. Simulating water and sediment flow using swe-convection diffusion model on openmp platform. In Proceedings of the 2019 7th International Conference on Information and Communication Technology (ICoICT), Kuala Lumpur, Malaysia, 24–26 July 2019; pp. 1–6.
52. Khuri, S.A. A Laplace decomposition algorithm applied to a class of nonlinear differential equations. *J. Appl. Math.* **2001**, *1*, 141–155. [CrossRef]
53. Khan, Y.; Wu, Q. Homotopy perturbation transform method for nonlinear equations using He's polynomials. *Comput. Math. Appl.* **2011**, *61*, 1963–1967. [CrossRef]
54. Khuri, S.A.; Sayfy, A. A Laplace variational iteration strategy for the solution of differential equations. *Appl. Math. Lett.* **2012**, *25*, 2298–2305. [CrossRef]
55. Zurigat, M. Solving fractional oscillators using Laplace homotopy analysis method. *Ann. Univ. -Craiova-Math. Comput. Sci. Ser.* **2011**, *38*, 1–11.
56. Guo, S.; Li, Y.; Wang, D. 2-Term Extended Rota-Baxter Pre-Lie $_\infty$-Algebra and Non-Abelian Extensions of Extended Rota-Baxter Pre-Lie Algebras. *Results Math.* **2025**, *80*, 96. [CrossRef]
57. Ali, N.; Nawaz, R.; Zada, L.; Mouldi, A.; Bouzgarrou, S.M.; Sene, N. Analytical approximate solution of the fractional order biological population model by using natural transform. *J. Nanomater.* **2022**, *2022*, 6703086. [CrossRef]
58. He, J.H. Homotopy perturbation technique. Comput. *Methods Appl. Mech. Eng.* **1999**, *178*, 257–262. [CrossRef]
59. He, J.H. A coupling method of a homotopy technique and a perturbation technique for non-linear problems. *Int. J. Non-Linear Mech.* **2000**, *35*, 37–43. [CrossRef]

60. Neamaty, A.; Agheli, B.; Darzi, R. Applications of homotopy perturbation method and Elzaki transform for solving nonlinear partial differential equations of fractional order. *J. Nonlin. Evolut. Equat. Appl.* **2016**, *2015*, 91–104.
61. Podlubny, I. *Fractional Differential Equations: An Introduction to Fractional Derivatives, Fractional Differential Equations, to Methods of Their Solution and Some of Their Applications*; Academic Press: New York, NY, USA, 1998; 340p.
62. Sedeeg, A.K.H. A coupling Elzaki transform and homotopy perturbation method for solving nonlinear fractional heat-like equations. *Am. J. Math. Comput. Model.* **2016**, *1*, 15–20.
63. Bhalekar, S.; Daftardar-Gejji, V. Convergence of the new iterative method. *Int. J. Differ. Equ.* **2011**, *2011*, 989065. [CrossRef]
64. Cooper, G.J. Error bounds for numerical solutions of ordinary differential equations. *Numer. Math.* **1971**, *18*, 162–170. [CrossRef]
65. Warne, P.G.; Warne, D.P.; Sochacki, J.S.; Parker, G.E.; Carothers, D.C. Explicit a-priori error bounds and adaptive error control for approximation of nonlinear initial value differential systems. *Comput. Math. Appl.* **2006**, *52*, 1695–1710. [CrossRef]
66. Yüzbaşi, Ş. A numerical approach for solving a class of the nonlinear Lane-Emden type equations arising in astrophysics. *Math. Methods Appl. Sci.* **2011**, *34*, 2218–2230. [CrossRef]
67. Gupta, A.K.; Ray, S.S. On the Solutions of Fractional Burgers-Fisher and Generalized Fisher's Equations Using Two Reliable Methods. *Int. J. Math. Math. Sci.* **2014**, *2014*, 682910. [CrossRef]
68. Veeresha, P.; Prakasha, D.G.; Baskonus, H.M. Novel simulations to the time-fractional Fisher's equation. *Math. Sci.* **2019**, *13*, 33–42. [CrossRef]

fractal and fractional

MDPI

Article

A Robust and Versatile Numerical Framework for Modeling Complex Fractional Phenomena: Applications to Riccati and Lorenz Systems

Waleed Mohammed Abdelfattah [1,*], Ola Ragb [2], Mohamed Salah [2] and Mokhtar Mohamed [3,*]

[1] College of Engineering, University of Business and Technology, Jeddah 23435, Saudi Arabia
[2] Department of Engineering Mathematics and Physics, Faculty of Engineering, Zagazig University, Zagazig 44519, Egypt; ormohamed@eng.zu.edu.eg (O.R.); msalaheldin@zu.edu.eg (M.S.)
[3] Basic Science Department, Faculty of Engineering, Delta University for Science and Technology, Gamasa 11152, Egypt
* Correspondence: w.abdelfattah@ubt.edu.sa (W.M.A.); mokhtar.alsaidi@deltauniv.edu.eg (M.M.)

Abstract: The fractional differential quadrature method (FDQM) with generalized Caputo derivatives is used in this paper to show a new numerical way to solve fractional Riccati equations and fractional Lorenz systems. Unlike previous FDQM applications that have primarily focused on linear problems, our work pioneers the use of this method for nonlinear fractional initial value problems. By combining Lagrange interpolation polynomials and discrete singular convolution (DSC) shape functions with the generalized Caputo operator, we effectively transform nonlinear fractional equations into algebraic systems. An iterative method is then utilized to address the nonlinearity. Our numerical results, obtained using MATLAB, demonstrate the exceptional accuracy and efficiency of this approach, with convergence rates reaching 10^{-8}. Comparative analysis with existing methods highlights the superior performance of the DSC shape function in terms of accuracy, convergence speed, and reliability. Our results highlight the versatility of our approach in tackling a wider variety of intricate nonlinear fractional differential equations.

Keywords: fractional derivative; generalized Caputo; differential quadrature technique; discrete singular convolution; fractional Riccati; fractional Lorenz system

1. Introduction

Many phenomena in chemistry, biology, acoustics, psychology, control theory, rheology, damping laws, diffusion processes, and other fields of science have been successfully modeled using fractional-order derivatives in recent years. This is because fractional calculus can be used to successfully model a physical phenomenon that is dependent not only on the time instant but also on the prior time history [1–6]. Hence, numerous physical problems are defined by fractional differential equations (FDEs), and solving these equations has been the focus of several studies in recent years. Several techniques have recently been developed to solve FDEs, including numerical and analytical techniques. Various methods, including homotopy perturbation [7–9], homotopy analysis [10,11], Taylor matrix [12], Adomian decomposition [11], and Haar wavelet [13] methods, have been employed to solve the fractional-order Riccati differential equation. Unfortunately, the convergence region for the corresponding outcomes is relatively limited. The fractional derivative operator's unique properties can make the numerical solution of fractional equations challenging, particularly in high-dimensional spaces. To address this challenge, numerical methods such as the Finite Difference Method (FDM) [14–17], Galerkin [18–21], Collocation [22–25], and finite volume element methods [26–28] have been utilized to tackle such fractional equations.

Liu et al. [29] introduced a radial basis function finite difference approach for studying the time fractional convection equation. Saadeh [30] employed the finite-difference and space finite-volume techniques to solve fractional diffusion equations. To address a two-dimensional space fractional diffusion equation, Tuan et al. [31] employed finite difference discretization with Caputo derivatives. Devshali and Arora [32] proposed differential transform and differential quadrature methods for solving the fractional diffusion equation. Odibat and Momani [9] utilized a modified homotopy perturbation technique to solve fractional Riccati differential equations (FRDEs). Khader [33] applied the fractional Chebyshev FDM to solve FRDEs. Li et al. [34] solved FRDEs via the quasi-linearization method. Sakar et al. [34] explained an iterative reproducing kernel Hilbert space technique to obtain the solutions of FRDEs. Agheli [35] explained an iterative reproducing kernel Hilbert space technique to obtain the solutions of FRDEs. Agheli [36] presented numerical solutions for solving FRDEs using trigonometric basic functions. Liu et al. [37] offered the Laplace transform and quadrature rule with Caputo sense to solve FRDEs.

In the last ten years, chaos has emerged as a popular topic in fractional calculus [38]. The chaotic behavior becomes more complicated because the equation contains fractional orders. Numerical methods were developed to analyze nonlinear dynamics to better understand physical phenomena. To find numerical solutions to various nonlinear fractional differential equations, the predictor–corrector method (P-C) was developed [39–41]. Fuzzy fractional differential and fractional delay equations [42–45] demonstrate the emergence of new trends in fractional differential equations.

Despite yielding fruitful results, finding more general chaotic differential equations remains an intriguing task. A generalized fractional derivative was recently proposed in [46]. Fractional derivatives have demonstrated superior performance compared to regular derivatives in several respects and may have even more real-world applications. One such application is in image encryption, where fractional differential equations have been suggested as a means of introducing chaos [47,48]. This means that image encryption results can be made more secure by using fractional chaotic equations with two parameters. This derivative was recently proposed in quantum mechanics [49]. Furthermore, two-parameter models in control theory and diffusion issues can have degrees of freedom in control and fitting. This derivative and its applications are depicted as a new direction in fractional calculus. Li and Chen [50] demonstrated the chaotic behaviors in the fractional order Chen system. Alomari [51] used the step homotopy analysis technique to solve the fractional chaotic Chen system. Luo and Wang [44] solved chaos in the fractional-order complex Lorenz system and its synchronization. Petráš [2] introduced a new classification of the fractional-order Lorenz-type systems. Erturka and Kumar [52] presented a solution for a COVID-19 model using new generalized Caputo-type fractional derivatives. Xu et al. [53] studied numerical and analytical solutions of a new generalized fractional diffusion equation. Kumar et al. [54] proposed a new technique to solve generalized Caputo-type FDEs with the example of a computer virus model.

The primary goal of this paper is to apply the novel fractional Differential Quadrature Method (FDQM) with generalized Caputo definition fractional to solve nonlinear initial value fractional problems. Two different shape functions, the Lagrange interpolation [55,56] and the regularized Shannon kernel [57–60], have been successfully employed to address initial value problems involving fractional derivatives. To exhibit the efficacy, efficiency, and capabilities of the proposed algorithm, two test problems were investigated, including FRDEs and the fractional Lorenz system. Then, by the proposed methods, the given problems are reduced to a system of nonlinear algebraic equations, and by solving this system via the iterative method, we obtain the solution of FRDEs and the fractional Lorenz system. Furthermore, we create a MATLAB code for each approach to obtain a numerical solution for the two problems under consideration. A comparison between the computed results and previous analytical and numerical [61–65] methodologies is included to demonstrate the validity and applicability of the proposed methods. Furthermore, we conducted some parametric investigations to showcase the reliability of our techniques in the presence of fractional order derivatives.

This paper introduces a novel fractional Differential Quadrature Method (FDQM) to solve nonlinear initial value fractional problems. This method employs the generalized Caputo fractional derivative and utilizes Lagrange interpolation and the Regularized Shannon kernel as shape functions. Numerical simulations demonstrate the method's superior accuracy, efficiency, and versatility in handling fractional Riccati and Lorenz systems. The FDQM's potential applications extend to various fields where it can be used to model complex systems with memory effects and nonlinearities [66].

2. Formulation of the Problem

The following two nonlinear fractional differential equations serve as examples to illustrate the capabilities of our proposed methods:

2.1. Our 1st Example Is the Fractional Riccati Equation

$$\frac{d^{\alpha,\rho}v(t)}{dt} = 2v(t) - v^2(t) + 1, \qquad \text{when } (0 < \text{ t and } 0 < \alpha \leq 1) \tag{1}$$

where $\frac{d^{\alpha,\rho}}{dt}$ is the operator of the generalized Caputo-type fractional derivative [61].

Also, the initial condition for FRDE is:

$$v(0) = 0 \tag{2}$$

In addition, the exact solution of FRDE at $\alpha = 1$, and $\rho = 1$ is given by [67]:

$$v(x,t) = 1 + \sqrt{2}\tanh\left[\sqrt{2}t + \log\sqrt{\frac{\sqrt{2}-1}{\sqrt{2}+1}}\right] \tag{3}$$

2.2. Our 2nd Example Is the Fractional Lorenz System

$$\frac{d^{\alpha,\rho}X(t)}{dt} = \lambda(Y(t) - X(t)) \tag{4}$$

$$\frac{d^{\alpha,\rho}Y(t)}{dt} = (\phi - \lambda)X(t) - X(t)Z(t) + \phi Y(t) \tag{5}$$

$$\frac{d^{\alpha,\rho}Z(t)}{dt} = X(t)Y(t) - \beta\, Z(t) \tag{6}$$

where λ, ϕ, and β are constant parameters $\in \mathbb{R}$ that affect chaotic behavior.

Consequently, the fractional Lorenz system is subject to the following initial condition:

$$X(0) = x_0,\ Y(0) = y_0,\ Z(0) = z_0 \tag{7}$$

3. Method of Solution

This paper introduces a novel application of the FDQM to solve initial value fractional problems. We employ two distinct shape functions, Lagrange interpolation and the regularized Shannon kernel, in conjunction with the generalized Caputo fractional derivative to transform fractional problems into nonlinear algebraic systems.

We begin by defining a fractional derivative, of which several definitions exist. In this work, we utilize the recently proposed generalized Caputo definition.

3.1. Generalized Caputo-Kind Fractional Derivative [63]

The fractional derivative has good memory effects compared to ordinary calculus. FDEs are realized in model problems in fluid flow, viscoelasticity, finance, engineering, and other areas of applications.

Caputo's Fractional Derivative

A concise overview of Caputo's fractional derivative is presented in this section. This definition, which is derived from the Riemann–Liouville Fractional Derivative [68], is explained in greater detail in our prior publication [69].

Suppose $\alpha \in R^{+}$, If $\mathbb{N}$ is a positive integer, and $\mathbb{N}-1<\alpha \leq \mathbb{N}$. According to Riemann–Liouville fractional, which is one of the most researched definitions, the fraction derivative of a function $v(t)$ of order α is defined as follows:

$$D_{c}^{\alpha} v(t)=\frac{1}{\Gamma(\mathbb{N}-\alpha)} \frac{d^{\mathbb{N}}}{dt^{\mathbb{N}}} \int_{c}^{t}(t-x)^{\mathbb{N}-\alpha-1} v^{\mathbb{N}}(x)\, dx \tag{8}$$

Generalized Caputo's Fractional Derivative of operator $D_{c+}^{\alpha,\rho}$ and order α is defined as [52–54]:

$$D_{c+}^{\alpha,\rho} v(t)=\frac{\rho^{\alpha-\mathbb{N}+1}}{\Gamma(\mathbb{N}-\alpha)} \int_{c}^{t} x^{\rho-1}\left(t^{\rho}-x^{\rho}\right)^{\mathbb{N}-\alpha-1}\left(x^{1-\rho} \frac{d}{dx}\right)^{\mathbb{N}} v(x)\, dx, \quad \mathbb{N}-1<\alpha<\mathbb{N},\ \rho>0,\ c \geq 0 \tag{9}$$

where c is the lower limit of integration.

Consequently, the solution to Equation (9) can be written as [52–54]:

$$D_{c+}^{\alpha,\rho}\left(t^{\rho}-x^{\rho}\right)^{\gamma}=\rho^{\alpha} \frac{\Gamma(\gamma+1)}{\Gamma(\gamma-\alpha+1)}\left(t^{\rho}-c^{\rho}\right)^{\gamma-\alpha} \tag{10}$$

Next, we will discuss the differential quadrature technique using the specified shape functions.

3.2. Our First Shape Function Is Lagrange Interpolation Polynomial Based DQM (PDQM)

Within this partition, the functional values of any unknown P at a specific set of N grid points can be represented using this shape function, as described in [55,56]:

$$\mathrm{P}(\mathrm{t_i})=\sum_{\mathrm{j}=1}^{\mathrm{N}} \frac{1}{\mathrm{t_i}-\mathrm{t_j}} \times \frac{\prod_{\mathrm{k}=1}^{\mathrm{N}}(\mathrm{t_i}-\mathrm{t_k})}{\prod_{\mathrm{j}=1, \mathrm{j} \neq \mathrm{k}}^{\mathrm{N}}(\mathrm{t_j}-\mathrm{t_k})} \mathrm{P}(t_j), \quad (\mathrm{i}=1: \mathrm{N}) \tag{11}$$

As a result, the following are the different derivatives of this unknown P:

$$\left.\frac{\partial^{\mathrm{r}} \mathrm{P}}{\partial t^{\mathrm{r}}}\right|_{\mathrm{t}=\mathrm{t_i}}=\sum_{\mathrm{j}=1}^{\mathrm{N}} \mathrm{a_{ij}^{(r)}} \mathrm{P}(\mathrm{t_j}), \quad (\mathrm{i}=1: \mathrm{N}) \tag{12}$$

where $\mathrm{a_{ij}^{(r)}}$ is the rth derivative weighting coefficient. However, determining the weighting coefficients is critical to DQM accuracy. As a result, they differ based on the shape function.

Differentiating Equation (12) results in the calculation of the weighting coefficients $\mathrm{a_{ij}^{(1)}}$ and $\mathrm{a_{ij}^{(2)}}$, representing the first and second derivatives.

$$\mathrm{a_{ij}^{(1)}}=\begin{cases} \dfrac{1}{(\mathrm{t_i}-\mathrm{t_j})} \displaystyle\prod_{\substack{\mathrm{k}=1, \\ \mathrm{k} \neq \mathrm{i,j}}}^{\mathrm{N}} \dfrac{(\mathrm{t_i}-\mathrm{t_k})}{(\mathrm{t_j}-\mathrm{t_k})} & \mathrm{i} \neq \mathrm{j} \\ -\displaystyle\sum_{\substack{\mathrm{j}=1, \\ \mathrm{j} \neq \mathrm{i}}}^{\mathrm{N}} \mathrm{a_{ij}^{(1)}} & \mathrm{i}=\mathrm{j} \end{cases}, \quad \mathrm{a_{ij}^{(2)}}=\left[\mathrm{a_{ij}^{(1)}}\right]\left[\mathrm{a_{ij}^{(1)}}\right] \tag{13}$$

The distribution of grid points N, whether uniform or non-uniform, significantly influences the accuracy of the PDQM results. The non-uniform distribution is defined by the following equation, based on Chebyshev's distribution:

$$x_i = \frac{1}{2} L_x \left(1 - \cos\left(\frac{\pi(i-1)}{N-1}\right)\right), \qquad (i = 1 : N) \tag{14}$$

3.3. Discrete Singular Convolution-Based DQM (DSCDQM)

In this part, according to previous research [59,70,71], singular convolution can be expressed as follows:

$$Y(t) = (F * H)(t) = \int_{-\infty}^{\infty} F(t-s)\, H(s)\, ds \tag{15}$$

$F(t-s)$ and $H(t)$ denote a singular kernel and a test function space element, respectively.

The choice of kernel type determines the shape function used in this technique. Given the variety of available kernels, we have selected the kernel demonstrated to have the highest accuracy [69] to represent the functional values of the unknown P and its derivatives at a specified number of grid points N:

- Our second shape function is the Regularized Shannon kernel (DSCDQM–RSK)

$$P(t_i) = \sum_{j=-M}^{M} \left\langle \frac{\sin\left[\frac{\pi(t_i - t_j)}{\Delta}\right]}{\frac{\pi(t_i - t_j)}{\Delta}} \exp\left(\frac{-(t_i - t_j)^2}{2\sigma^2}\right) \right\rangle P(x_j), \qquad (i = -N : N), \sigma = (h \times \Delta) > 0 \tag{16}$$

The parameters σ, h, and Δ represent the Regularized Shannon factor, the computational parameter, and the mesh size, respectively.

$$\frac{\partial^r P}{\partial t^r}\Big|t = t_i = \sum_{j=1}^{N} a_{ij}^{(r)} P(t_j) \qquad (i = -N : N) \tag{17}$$

Differentiating Equation (15) allows us to determine the coefficients $a_{ij}^{(1)}$ and $a_{ij}^{(2)}$, as described in [72]:

$$a_{ij}^{(1)} = \begin{cases} \frac{(-1)^{i-j}}{\Delta(i-j)} \exp\left(-\Delta^2\left(\frac{(i-j)^2}{2\sigma^2}\right)\right), & i \neq j \\ 0 & i = j \end{cases}, \quad a_{ij}^{(2)} = \begin{cases} \left[2\frac{(-1)^{i-j+1}}{a^2(i-j)^2} + \frac{1}{\sigma^2}\right] \exp\left(-\Delta^2\left(\frac{(i-j)^2}{2\sigma^2}\right)\right), & i \neq j \\ -\frac{1}{\sigma^2} - \frac{\pi^2}{3\Delta^2} & i = j \end{cases} \tag{18}$$

The kernel type, grid points (N), and bandwidth (2K + 1) are all important parameters that affect the convergence and accuracy of the solutions, as our analysis shows.

Now, after mentioning DQM based on two shape functions, we will demonstrate the effect of the generalized Caputo's fractional derivative, which is shown in Equation (9) on the FDQM in Equation (12), to determine the weighting coefficients a_{ij}^{α} for $\alpha \in (0,1]$ and $\rho > 0$, as follows [69]:

$$D_{c+}^{\alpha,\rho} P(t) = \begin{cases} \sum_{j=1}^{N} a_{ij}^{\alpha,\rho}\, P(t_j, x), & 0 < \alpha \leq 1, \ \rho > 0 \\ \sum_{j=1}^{N} a_{ij}^{(1)}\, P(t_j, x) & \alpha = \rho = 1 \end{cases} \tag{19}$$

Hence, the weighting coefficient $a_{ij}^{\alpha,\rho}$ is calculated as:

$$a_{ij}^{\alpha,\rho} = A^{1-\alpha}\rho^{\alpha}\, a_{ij}^{(1)} + \frac{\rho^{\alpha} a_{1,j}^{(1)}}{\Gamma(2-\alpha)}\left(t^{\rho} - c^{\rho}\right)^{1-\alpha}, \quad A_{ij} = a_{ij}^{(1)} - a_{1j}^{(1)} \tag{20}$$

3.4. Algorithm: Fractional Differential Quadrature Method (FDQM) for Nonlinear Initial Value Problems

This pseudo-code (Algorithm 1) outlines the key steps for implementing the proposed numerical framework for solving nonlinear fractional differential equations using the FDQM approach.

Algorithm 1: Fractional Differential Quadrature Method (FDQM) for Nonlinear Initial Value Problems

Input:

- Fractional order, constants in the fractional differential equation
- Nonlinear fractional differential equation.
- Initial conditions.
- Grid points (N)
- Shape functions (Lagrange, Regularized Shannon)
- Tolerance for convergence (ε)

Output:

- The solution of the fractional differential equation numerically.

1. Define the generalized Caputo fractional derivative operator.
2. Initialize grid points $x_1, x_2, \ldots, x_N$ based on Chebyshev distribution or uniform distribution.
3. For each time step "t:
   - Construct the shape functions using Lagrange interpolation and Regularized Shannon kernel.
   - Formulate the algebraic system from the fractional differential equation using FDQM:

   a. Apply shape functions to approximate the unknown function and its derivatives.
   b. Substitute into the original FDE to derive a system of nonlinear algebraic equations.
4. Initialize solution guess for the unknown function.
5. While not converged ($||f_{new} - f_{old}|| > \varepsilon$)
6. Solve the algebraic system iteratively:

   a. Use a numerical method (iterative differential quadrature method) to update the solution.
   b. Update f_{old} with f_{new}
7. End while
8. Return the numerical solution for the fractional differential equation at the specified time steps.

End Algorithm

4. Numerical Results

Now that it is easier to understand FDQM with different shape functions such as PDQM [55,56], and DSCDQM–RSK [59,70,71] based on the generalized Caputo definition fractional derivative, two examples will be given here and then will be discussed. In all these examples, MATLAB software(R2022b) is used for computations and graphs. The primary goal of this article is to learn about the performance, validity, efficiency, and accuracy of developed techniques by comparing the computed results to previous numerical and analytical solutions.

4.1. Problem 4.1

We introduce the first example fractional Riccati equation after substituting the Equations (19) and (20) for the proposed methods in Equation (1) as follows:

$$\sum_{j=1}^{L} a_{ij}^{\alpha,\rho}\, \upsilon(t_j) = 2\sum_{j=1}^{N} \delta_{ij}\, \upsilon(t_j) - \left(\sum_{j=1}^{N} \delta_{ij}\, \upsilon(t_j)\right)^2 + 1 \tag{21}$$

The governing Equation (21) is also used to deal with the initial condition (2). To solve the nonlinear problem, the iterative method is applied [55,72,73]. As a first step, the governing equation is solved as a linear system. Then we solve them iteratively as a nonlinear system until we reach the requisite convergence, which is as follows:

$$\left|\frac{\upsilon_{m+1}}{\upsilon_m}\right| < 1, \qquad \text{where } m = 0, 1, 2, \ldots \tag{22}$$

Also, to assess the convergence and accuracy of the developed methods, we use the error computation method:

$$L_\infty \text{ Error} = \max_{1\le i\le N} |\upsilon_{numerical} - \upsilon_{exact}| \tag{23}$$

Now, the obtained results will be demonstrated as follows:

The effect of applying PDQM with uniform and non-uniform grid distributions on the computation of the fractional Riccati equation with fractions $(\alpha = 1,\ \rho = 1)$ at different grid points (N) and times (T) is shown in Table 1. Hence, it is found that non-uniform grid results are higher and more consistent with earlier solutions than uniform ones with an error $\le 10^{-8}$, and execution time of about (0.024 s). Also, when the grid points increase with time, the accuracy increases; for example, at time (t = 1), we make (N = 13), and at time (t = 2), we make (N = 26) Furthermore, the maximum number of grids we use is significantly less than in previous studies (N = 3200).

Table 2 compares non-uniform PDQM and DSCDQM–RSK for the fractional Riccati equation under various conditions of time (T = 1), fraction $(\alpha = 1,\ \rho = 1)$, different grid points (N), regularized Shannon factor $(\sigma = h \times \Delta)$, and bandwidth (2K + 1). To begin, Table 2 ensures that the best value of the regularized Shannon factor is $\sigma = 0.45 \times \Delta$, with results matching previous studies and PDQM shown in Table 1 at the fewest grid points (N = 9), bandwidth (2K + 1 = 7) and performance time of about (0.018 s). DSCDQM–RSK is the best method overall, based on low grid points and performance time when compared to PDQM (N = 16) and previous studies (N = 640).

The efficiency, validity, and accuracy of the created methodologies are presently being explored by comparing the calculated results to earlier numerical and analytical solutions at various powers of fraction (α, ρ), as shown in Tables 3–6. Tables 3–6 show that increasing the fraction power (α or ρ) decreases the value of $\upsilon(t)$, but increases with time for the fractional Riccati equation. Furthermore, the results show that DSCDQM–RSK outperforms non-uniform PDQM in terms of efficiency, validity, and accuracy.

In addition, the dynamic behaviors of the fractional Riccati equation with respect to the parameters (α and ρ) and against the time variable t are depicted in Figures 1 and 2.

Table 1. Computation of $\upsilon(t)$ via uniform and non-uniform PDQM for fractional Riccati equation with fraction ($\alpha = 1,\ \rho = 1$) at different grid points (N), and times (T).

T	PDQ Solutions							Previous Solutions		
	N	Uniform	CPU (s)	Error	Non-Uniform	CPU (s)	Error	N	Earlier Numerical [64]	Exact [61]
1	4	1.59030488	0.016	0.0971	1.64023865	0.013	0.04721	10	1.68745117	1.68949839
	6	1.68745374	0.018	0.0015	1.67122383	0.017	0.01774	20	1.68896723	
	8	1.68821427	0.018	0.0011	1.68941502	0.017	5.16×10^{-5}	40	1.68936339	
	9	1.68921673	0.019	0.0002	1.68948616	0.018	2.18×10^{-5}	80	1.68946438	
	11	1.68941775	0.020	7.2×10^{-5}	1.68949815	0.018	8.29×10^{-6}	160	1.68948986	
	12	1.68948043	0.021	1.6×10^{-5}	1.68949820	0.020	1.95×10^{-6}	320	1.68949625	
	13	1.68949755	0.021	3.1×10^{-7}	1.68949839	0.020	1.2×10^{-8}	640	1.68949786	
2	8	2.34267643	0.029	0.001168	2.35647559	0.019	0.012631	20	2.35530727	2.35777165
	12	2.35721628	0.031	0.00056	2.35777266	0.020	3.73×10^{-6}	40	2.35721255	
	16	2.35757661	0.032	0.00014	2.35777175	0.021	6.14×10^{-5}	80	2.35763805	
	18	2.35773329	0.033	3.27×10^{-5}	2.35777169	0.021	5.68×10^{-6}	160	2.35773897	
	22	2.35777129	0.034	8.08×10^{-6}	2.35777165	0.022	7.72×10^{-6}	320	2.35776357	
	24	2.35777151	0.035	2.01×10^{-6}	2.35777165	0.023	1.87×10^{-6}	640	2.35776964	
	26	2.35777167	0.036	5×10^{-7}	2.35777165	0.024	2×10^{-8}	1280	2.35777115	
5	20	2.41421578	0.033	1.743×10^{-5}	2.41420169	0.021	3.34×10^{-6}	50	2.41419835	2.41420167
	21	2.41420238	0.033	1.37×10^{-6}	2.41420169	0.021	6.8×10^{-7}	100	2.41420101	
	22	2.41420214	0.034	6.2×10^{-7}	2.41420168	0.022	1.6×10^{-7}	200	2.41420152	
	23	2.41420177	0.034	1.4×10^{-7}	2.41420167	0.022	4×10^{-8}	400	2.41420163	
	24	2.41420175	0.035	9×10^{-8}	2.41420167	0.023	1×10^{-8}	800	2.41420166	
	25	2.41420171	0.035	4×10^{-8}	2.41420167	0.023	1×10^{-8}	1600	2.41420167	
	26	2.41420169	0.036	2×10^{-8}	2.41420167	0.024	1×10^{-8}	3200	2.41420167	

Table 2. Computation of $\upsilon(t)$ via non-uniform PDQM and DSCDQM–RSK for fractional Riccati equation with time (T = 1) and fraction ($\alpha = 1,\ \rho = 1$) at various grid points (N), regularized Shannon factor ($\sigma = h \times \Delta$), and bandwidth (2K + 1).

N	2K + 1	Non-Uniform PDQM	DSCDQM–RSK				
			σ=0.2×Δ	σ=0.4×Δ	σ=0.45×Δ	σ=0.5×Δ	CPU (s)
9	3	1.68948616	1.69745751	1.689880214	1.68950741	1.64023989	0.008
	5	1.68948616	1.69745647	1.689876547	1.68949956	1.64023942	0.01
	7	1.68948616	1.69745559	1.689875120	1.68949839	1.64023865	0.012
	9	1.68948616	1.69745559	1.689875120	1.68949839	1.64023865	0.014
	11	1.68948616	1.69745559	1.689875120	1.68949839	1.64023865	0.016
11	3	1.68949815	1.69745666	1.689877415	1.68949951	1.64023937	0.009
	5	1.68949815	1.69745559	1.689875120	1.68949839	1.64023865	0.01
	7	1.68949815	1.69745559	1.689875120	1.68949839	1.64023865	0.011
	9	1.68949815	1.69745559	1.689875120	1.68949839	1.64023865	0.012
	11	1.68949815	1.69745559	1.689875120	1.68949839	1.64023865	0.014
13	3	1.68949839	1.69745578	1.689876014	1.6894990	1.64023900	0.01
	5	1.68949839	1.69745559	1.689875120	1.68949839	1.64023865	0.012
	7	1.68949839	1.69745559	1.689875120	1.68949839	1.64023865	0.014
	9	1.68949839	1.69745559	1.689875120	1.68949839	1.64023865	0.016
	11	1.68949839	1.69745559	1.689875120	1.68949839	1.64023865	0.018
Earlier numerical solutions [64]				1.68949786 at (N = 640)			
Exact [61]					1.68949839		

Table 3. Computation of $\upsilon(t)$ via non-uniform PDQM and DSCDQM–RSK for fractional Riccati equation at various times (T), fractions (α), and $\rho = 1$.

T	Non-Uniform PDQM		DSCDQM–RSK		Previous Results [61–65]	
	$\alpha = 0.5$	$\alpha = 0.75$	$\alpha = 0.5$	$\alpha = 0.75$	$\alpha = 0.5$	$\alpha = 0.75$
0.1	0.59149371	0.24512554	0.59149373	0.24512556	0.59149373	0.24512556
0.2	0.93141486	0.47450194	0.93141488	0.47450196	0.93141488	0.47450196
0.3	1.171926469	0.709154008	1.171926471	0.709154010	1.171926471	0.709154010
0.4	1.344407759	0.937441050	1.344407761	0.937441052	1.344407761	0.937441052
0.5	1.471501155	1.147807349	1.471501157	1.147807351	1.471501157	1.147807351
0.6	1.568070430	1.332985034	1.568070432	1.332985036	1.568070432	1.332985036
0.7	1.643596282	1.490535187	1.643596284	1.490535189	1.643596284	1.490535189
0.8	1.704182955	1.621592245	1.704182957	1.621592247	1.704182957	1.621592247
0.9	1.753855962	1.729220378	1.753855964	1.729220380	1.753855964	1.729220380
1	1.817133594	1.795344168	1.817133596	1.795344170	1.817133596	1.795344170

Table 4. Computation of $\upsilon(t)$ via non-uniform PDQM and DSCDQM–RSK for fractional Riccati equation with fraction $(\alpha = 1)$ at various times (T), and fractions (ρ).

T	Non-Uniform PDQM		DSCDQM–RSK		Previous Results [61–65]	
	$\rho = 0.8$	$\rho = 1.2$	$\rho = 0.8$	$\rho = 1.2$	$\rho = 0.8$	$\rho = 1.2$
0.1	0.14117992	0.09045268	0.14117994	0.09045271	0.14117994	0.09045271
0.2	0.31592641	0.195667845	0.31592645	0.19566787	0.31592645	0.19566787
0.3	0.52298485	0.315926409	0.52298488	0.315926411	0.52298488	0.315926411
0.4	0.75601439	0.450653813	0.75601442	0.450653816	0.75601442	0.450653816
0.5	1.00354951	0.59824597	1.00354953	0.59824599	1.00354953	0.59824599
0.6	1.25086733	0.75601439	1.25086736	0.75601442	1.25086736	0.75601442
0.7	1.48329584	0.92030072	1.48329586	0.92030075	1.48329586	0.92030075
0.8	1.68949839	1.08677371	1.68949842	1.08677374	1.68949842	1.08677374
0.9	1.86328744	1.25086733	1.86328746	1.25086736	1.86328746	1.25086736
1	2.00353694	1.40827080	2.00353696	1.40827081	2.00353696	1.40827081

Table 5. Computation of $\upsilon(t)$ via non-uniform PDQM for fractional Riccati equation at different grid points (N), and fractions $(\alpha,\ \rho)$.

T	Non-Uniform				Earlier Numerical Solutions [62]			
	N	$\alpha = 1$, $\rho = 0.9$	$\alpha = 0.95$, $\rho = 0.75$	$\alpha = 0.9$, $\rho = 1.2$	N	$\alpha = 1$, $\rho = 0.9$	$\alpha = 0.95$, $\rho = 0.75$	$\alpha = 0.9$, $\rho = 1.2$
1	4	1.80602802	1.96263496	1.39368786	10	1.84281224	2.06729863	1.52944766
	6	1.84319793	2.04896144	1.49050147	20	1.84491385	2.07202706	1.53119172
	8	1.84556010	2.06510470	1.51019655	40	1.84546411	2.07322261	1.53167452
	9	1.84561319	2.06904164	1.52085146	80	1.84560424	2.07352741	1.53180584
	11	1.84565025	2.07362649	1.52696219	160	1.84563955	2.07360571	1.53184129
	12	1.84565137	2.07363589	1.52945738	320	1.84564841	2.07362592	1.53185082
	13	1.84565137	2.07363256	1.53185408	640	1.84565063	2.07363115	1.53185339
	14	1.84565137	2.07363256	1.53185408	1280	1.84565119	2.07363250	1.53185407
2	8	2.28430436	2.32839830	2.20693947	20	2.36576348	2.34646084	2.26631061
	12	2.32381757	2.33437164	2.21000463	40	2.36763874	2.34834846	2.26840179
	16	2.34381756	2.34307946	2.22083045	80	2.36805246	2.34876916	2.26890814
	18	2.36382620	2.34836151	2.23103727	160	2.36815011	2.34887135	2.26903810
	22	2.36832617	2.34863032	2.24089052	320	2.36817385	2.34889710	2.26907235
	24	2.36818255	2.34889017	2.26879047	640	2.36817971	2.34890369	2.26908148
	26	2.36818153	2.34890584	2.26908459	1280	2.36818116	2.34890540	2.26908393
	27	2.36818153	2.34890584	2.26908459	2560	2.36818153	2.34890584	2.26908459

Table 6. Computation of $\upsilon(t)$ via DSCDQM–RSK for fractional Riccati equation at different values of (α, ρ) and times.

α	ρ	T = 0.5	T = 1	T = 2	T = 2.5	T = 3
0.4	1	1.58967600	1.77525996	2.09537035	2.21247852	2.22642314
	1.1	1.54739283	1.74403298	2.07553739	2.19214756	2.20554878
	1.2	1.50756398	1.71405017	2.05317313	2.17021456	2.18875143
	1.4	1.43438179	1.65736347	2.02666948	2.14654879	2.16214787
	1.9	1.28182554	1.53134020	2.01520768	2.12958092	2.13478462
0.5	1	1.68300421	1.79935747	2.12065899	2.25983372	2.27664509
	1.1	1.66554391	1.75798866	2.10285480	2.23984120	2.25471201
	1.2	1.65154233	1.71762640	2.09852919	2.21874621	2.23789123
	1.4	1.62320069	1.66991063	2.07719592	2.20997411	2.21987423
	1.9	1.58526142	1.56342314	2.05661402	2.20278414	2.17645789
0.7	1	1.71613371	1.82286926	2.14596688	2.29139917	2.31617003
	1.1	1.69532577	1.79031758	2.12529159	2.27075056	2.29157030
	1.2	1.67462609	1.77811144	2.10299487	2.25941935	2.26895529
	1.4	0.65934200	1.73806497	2.08048316	2.22364828	2.24318890
	1.9	0.60930946	1.65504250	2.05990416	2.20861195	2.20862313
0.85	1	0.73587574	1.84052325	2.24870001	2.30150738	2.33501568
	1.1	0.71892188	1.82175475	2.21842773	2.28982006	2.31048992
	1.2	0.69728893	1.80614145	2.18322274	2.27519396	2.29534657
	1.4	0.67897490	1.77168741	2.16870824	2.23587987	2.27096577
	1.9	0.62629628	1.72273733	2.13184852	2.20356265	2.22777374
0.95	1	0.82414933	1.87127626	2.31830946	2.36707298	2.37441750
	1.1	0.73300489	1.84609224	2.28379937	2.35373760	2.35930723
	1.2	0.71834905	1.82980945	2.24083446	2.33559233	2.33776914
	1.4	0.68447266	1.80982469	2.21190242	2.28289347	2.31913452
	1.9	0.63618443	1.77131197	2.19457437	2.23111789	2.29258450

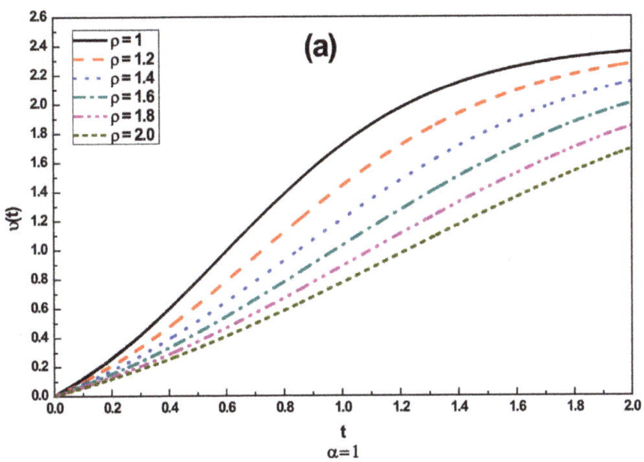

Figure 1. *Cont.*

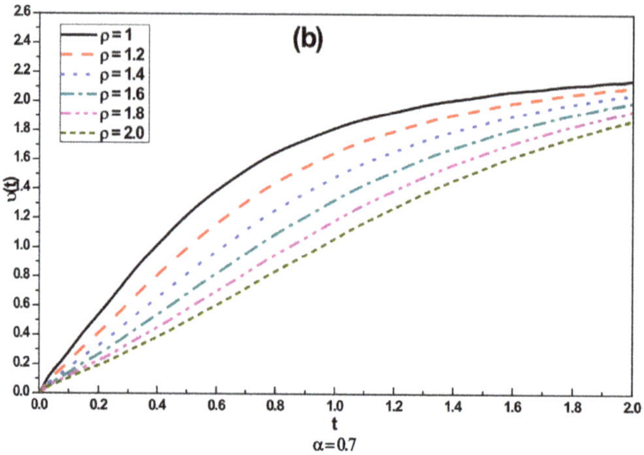

Figure 1. Numerical simulation of $\upsilon(t)$ using DSCDQM–RSK for fractional Riccati equation at different times and fraction power $(\alpha,\ \rho)$ for (**a**) $\alpha = 1$, and (**b**) $\alpha = 0.7$.

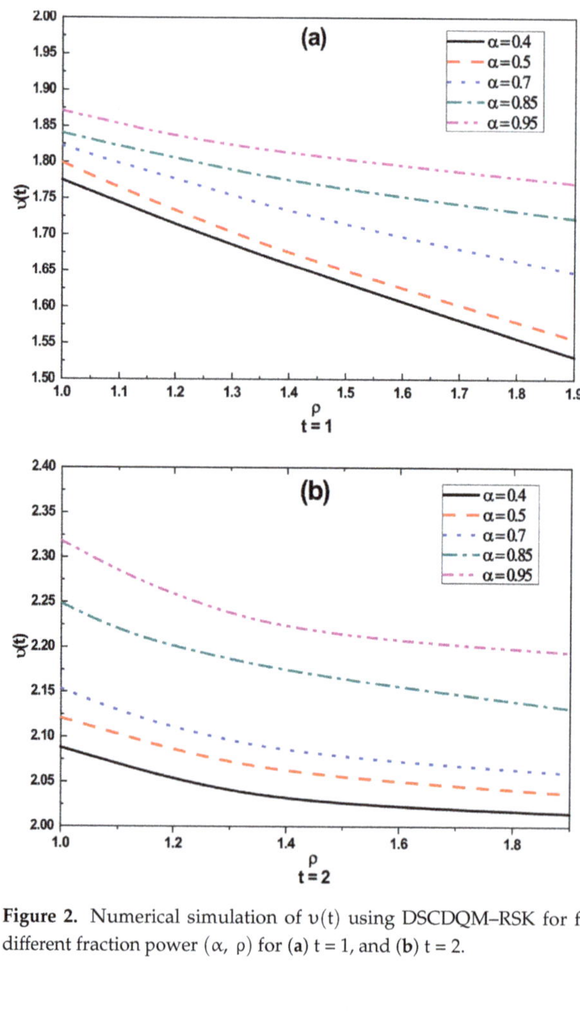

Figure 2. Numerical simulation of $\upsilon(t)$ using DSCDQM–RSK for fractional Riccati equation at different fraction power $(\alpha,\ \rho)$ for (**a**) t = 1, and (**b**) t = 2.

4.2. Problem 4.2

We deal with the fractional Lorenz system after substituting Equations (4)–(6) with Equations (19) and (20) of the proposed methods:

$$\sum_{j=1}^{L} a_{ij}^{\alpha,\rho}\, X(t_j) = \lambda\left[\sum_{j=1}^{N} \delta_{ij}\, Y(t_j) - \sum_{j=1}^{N} \delta_{ij}\, X(t_j)\right] \tag{24}$$

$$\begin{aligned} &\sum_{j=1}^{L} a_{ij}^{\alpha,\rho}\, Y(t_j) = (\phi-\lambda)\sum_{j=1}^{N} \delta_{ij}\, X(t_j) - \\ &\sum_{j=1}^{N} \delta_{ij}\, X(t_j) \sum_{j=1}^{N} \delta_{ij}\, Z(t_j) + \phi \sum_{j=1}^{N} \delta_{ij}\, Y(t_j) \end{aligned} \tag{25}$$

$$\sum_{j=1}^{L} a_{ij}^{\alpha,\rho}\, Z(t_j) = \sum_{j=1}^{N} \delta_{ij}\, X(t_j) \sum_{j=1}^{N} \delta_{ij}\, Y(t_j) - \beta \sum_{j=1}^{N} \delta_{ij}\, Z(t_j) \tag{26}$$

Dealing with the initial condition (7) is also done by substituting in the governing Equations (24)–(26). After that, we use Equation (22) to solve this system.

We will now begin to demonstrate the obtained results to explain the stability, reliability, convergence, and performance of FDQM using two types of shape functions with generalized Caputo sense, as follows:

Table 7 explains the impact of grid points (N) on the obtained results X, Y, and Z via PDQM with uniform and non-uniform grid distributions of the fractional Lorenz system with fraction $(\alpha = 1,\ \rho = 1)$. It is remarkable that non-uniform grid results are higher and more consistent with earlier solutions [62,63] and RK4 [64] at N = 11 than uniform ones at N = 13 with error $\leq 10^{-8}$, and execution time of about (0.027 s). Table 8 demonstrates the effect of control values like grid points (N), regularized Shannon factor $(\sigma = h \times \Delta)$, and bandwidth (2K + 1) on the obtained results by DSCDQM–RSK at time (T = 2), fraction $(\alpha = 1,\ \rho = 1)$. We found the best value of the regularized Shannon factor is $\sigma = 0.47 \times \Delta$, with results matching previous studies and PDQM shown in Table 7 at the fewest grid points (N = 9), bandwidth (2K + 1 = 3), and performance time of about (0.022 s). Furthermore, from Tables 7 and 8, it is noted that the maximum number of grids we use is significantly less than in previous studies (N = 1280).

Table 7. Computation of numerical solutions X, Y, Z via uniform and non-uniform PDQM for fractional Chen system (Lorenz system) with time (T = 2) and fraction $(\alpha = 1,\ \rho = 1)$ at various grid points (N). $(x_0 = 2.5, y_0 = 1, z_0 = 0.5)$ and $(\lambda = 1, \beta = 2, \phi = 1)$.

N	Uniform PDQM			CPU (s)	Non-uniform PDQM			CPU (s)
	X	Y	Z		X	Y	Z	
4	0.837919933	0.623902547	0.302407988	0.02	0.837919846	0.623902388	0.302407749	0.02
5	0.771720200	0.527485798	0.248194100	0.021	0.771720184	0.527485752	0.248193998	0.021
6	0.761378603	0.49832669	0.2415685802	0.022	0.763378566	0.522326584	0.2475685753	0.022
7	0.760223666	0.497601296	0.2409074397	0.023	0.762223591	0.515601283	0.2469074378	0.023
9	0.762203989	0.500122597	0.242400811	0.025	0.762203974	0.500122578	0.2424007951	0.024
10	0.762216222	0.500169299	0.2424081878	0.026	0.762216161	0.500169278	0.2424081821	0.025
11	0.76221575	0.500167396	0.242407838	0.027	0.76221572	0.500167392	0.242407832	0.025
12	0.76221573	0.500167394	0.2424078434	0.028	0.76221572	0.500167392	0.2424078432	0.026
13	0.76221572	0.500167392	0.2424078432	0.029	0.76221572	0.500167392	0.2424078432	0.027
	Earlier numerical solutions [62,63]							
	X		Y			Z		
1280	0.76221649		0.50016919			0.24240833		
	RK4 [64]							
	0.76221572		0.50016739			0.24240783		

Table 8. Computation of numerical solutions X, Y, Z via DSCDQM–RSK for fractional Chen system (Lorenz system) with time (T = 2) and fraction $(\alpha = 1,\ \rho = 1)$ at various grid points (N), regularized Shannon factor $(\sigma = h \times \Delta)$, and bandwidth (2K + 1). $(x_0 = 2.5, y_0 = 1, z_0 = 0.5)$ and $(\lambda = 1, \beta = 2, \phi = 1)$.

N	2K + 1	DSCDQM–RSK									CPU (s)
		σ = 0.4 × Δ			σ = 0.45 × Δ			σ = 0.47 × Δ			
		X	Y	Z	X	Y	z	X	Y	Z	
9	3	0.7738	0.5133	0.2549	0.7625	0.5008	0.2430	0.76225	0.5004	0.2425	0.01
	5	0.7735	0.5127	0.2540	0.7623	0.5006	0.2427	0.76223	0.5003	0.2424	0.012
	7	0.7732	0.5122	0.2536	0.76229	0.5005	0.2426	0.76221	0.5002	0.2424	0.014
	9	0.7732	0.5122	0.2536	0.76229	0.5005	0.2426	0.76221	0.5002	0.2424	0.016
	11	0.7732	0.5122	0.2536	0.76229	0.5005	0.2426	0.76221	0.5002	0.2424	0.018
11	3	0.7347	0.5127	0.2540	0.7623	0.5006	0.2427	0.76222	0.50023	0.2425	0.012
	5	0.734	0.5124	0.2537	0.76229	0.5005	0.2426	0.76221	0.5002	0.2424	0.014
	7	0.7732	0.5122	0.2536	0.76229	0.5005	0.2426	0.76221	0.5002	0.2424	0.016
	9	0.7732	0.5122	0.2536	0.76229	0.5005	0.2426	0.76221	0.5002	0.2424	0.018
	11	0.7732	0.5122	0.2536	0.76229	0.5005	0.2426	0.76221	0.5002	0.2424	0.020
13	3	0.7733	0.5122	0.2537	0.76231	0.5006	0.2427	0.762215	0.50026	0.24247	0.014
	5	0.7732	0.5122	0.2536	0.76229	0.5005	0.2426	0.76221	0.5002	0.2424	0.016
	7	0.7732	0.5122	0.2536	0.76229	0.5005	0.2426	0.76221	0.5002	0.2424	0.018
	9	0.7732	0.5122	0.2536	0.76229	0.5005	0.2426	0.76221	0.5002	0.2424	0.020
	11	0.7732	0.5122	0.2536	0.76229	0.5005	0.2426	0.76221	0.5002	0.2424	0.022
	Earlier numerical solutions [62,63]										
	X				Y				Z		
1280	0.76221649				0.50016919				0.24240833		
	RK4 [64]										
	0.76221572				0.50016739				0.24240783		

Figures 3 and 4 present the influence of time and fraction α on the numerical results X, Y, and Z via non-uniform PDQM and DSCDQM–RSK at $(x_0 = 2.5, y_0 = 1, z_0 = 0.5)$ and $(\lambda = 1, \beta = 2, \phi = 1)$. Thus, it is found that the dynamic behaviors of X, Y, and Z differ when the fraction α change. This means that when the value α decreases, the values of X, Y, and Z increase.

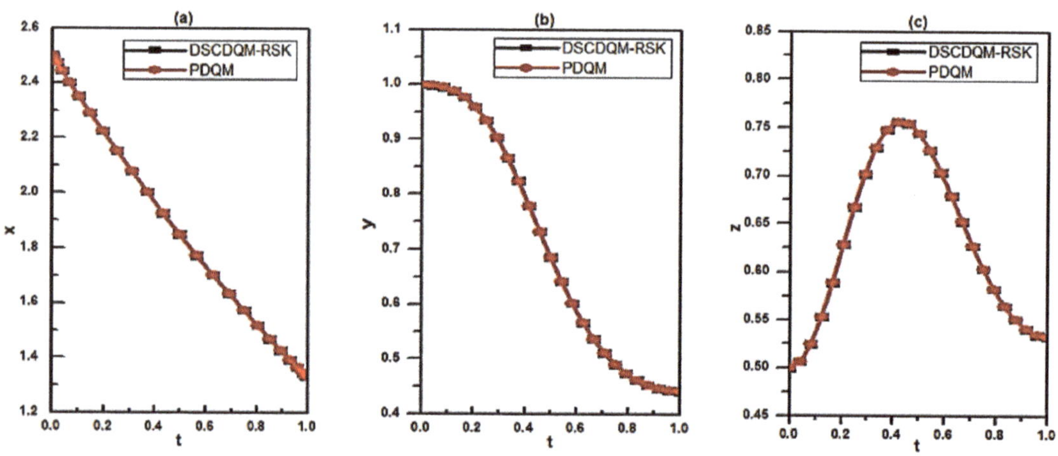

Figure 3. Variance of (**a**) X, (**b**) Y, and (**c**) Z with time (t) via non-uniform PDQM and DSCDQM–RSK for fractional Chen system with time (T = 1), fraction $(\alpha = 1,\ \rho = 1)$, $(x_0 = 2.5, y_0 = 1, z_0 = 0.5)$ and $(\lambda = 1, \beta = 2, \phi = 1)$.

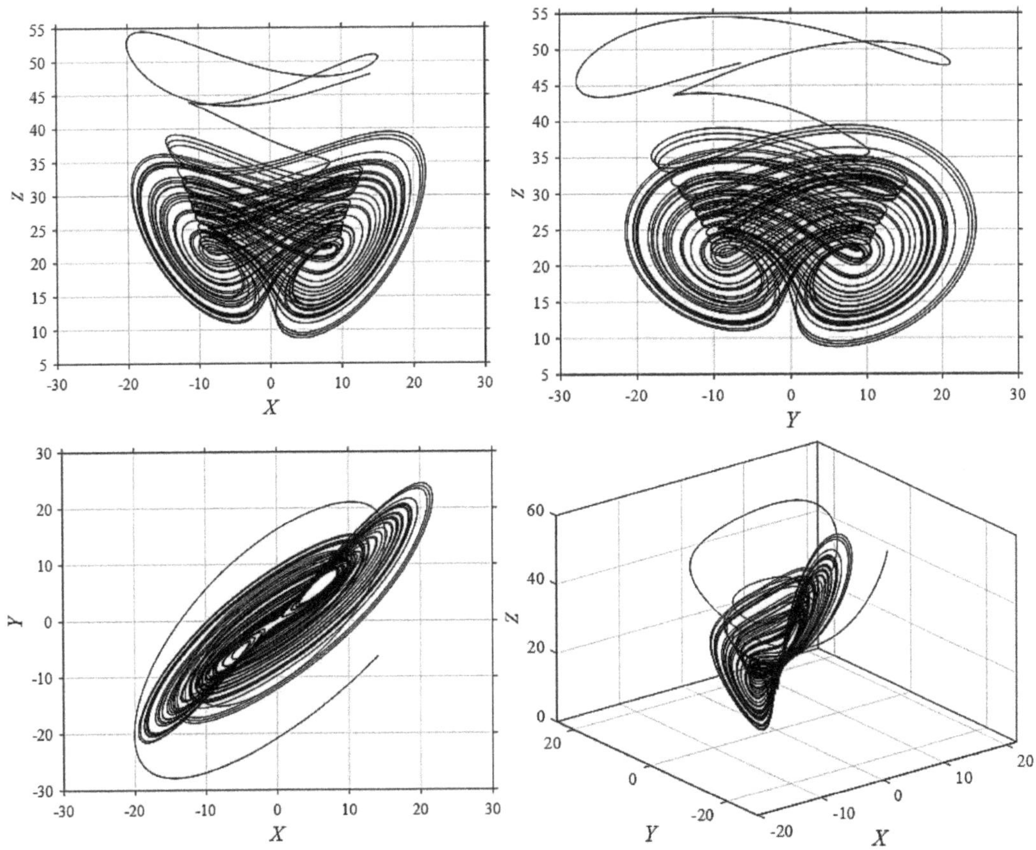

Figure 4. Chaotic attractor of fractional Lorenz system using DSCDQM–RSK with time (T = 100), fraction ($\alpha = 1,\ \rho = 1.2$), ($x_0 = 2.5, y_0 = 1, z_0 = 0.5$) and ($\lambda = 1, \beta = 2, \phi = 1$).

Also, Figures 3 and 4 show that the Lorenz system, a classic model for chaotic dynamics, can be extended to fractional-order systems. This extension introduces significant differences in the observed chaotic behavior [74,75]:

Chaotic Regimes:

- The integer-order Lorenz system exhibits a well-defined chaotic regime within a specific parameter range.
- Fractional-order Lorenz systems often exhibit chaotic behavior over a wider range of parameters and fractional orders. This can lead to more complex and diverse chaotic dynamics.

Attractor Structure:

- The integer-order Lorenz system typically has a single strange attractor.
- Fractional-order Lorenz systems can exhibit multiple strange attractors or even the coexistence of different attractors, depending on the fractional order and system parameters.

Fractal Dimension:

- The fractal dimension of the strange attractor in the integer-order Lorenz system is generally between 2 and 3.
- The fractal dimension of the strange attractors in fractional-order Lorenz systems can vary more widely, often exceeding 3. This indicates a more complex and convoluted structure.

Sensitivity to Initial Conditions:

- The integer-order Lorenz system is highly sensitive to initial conditions, leading to the butterfly effect.
- Fractional-order Lorenz systems can exhibit even greater sensitivity to initial conditions, making long-term predictions even more challenging.

Memory Effects:

- The integer-order Lorenz system does not have memory effects.
- The fractional-order Lorenz system incorporates memory effects, which can influence the system's dynamics and make it more resilient to perturbations.

So, fractional-order Lorenz systems can exhibit more complex and diverse chaotic behaviors compared to their integer-order counterparts. The increased sensitivity to initial conditions in fractional-order systems makes long-term predictions even more challenging. Fractional-order Lorenz systems can be used to model real-world phenomena with memory effects or nonlinearities that are not adequately captured by integer-order models.

Figures 4–7 show the fractional Lorenz system's dynamic behaviors as the values of fractions $(\alpha,\ \rho)$ at $(x_0 = 2.5, y_0 = 1, z_0 = 0.5)$ and $(\lambda = 1, \beta = 2, \phi = 1)$ changes. Also, in these figures, we show projections of the fractional Lorenz system attractors calculated via DSCDQM–RSK when T = 100 for some values of the fractions $(\alpha,\ \rho)$. It is observed that when the fraction ρ increases, the chaotic behavior increases more than the fraction α changes. Consequently, it is noted that the fractional Lorenz system may exhibit chaotic attractors similar to those of its integer-order counterpart when $(\alpha = 0.9,\ \rho = 0.8)$ and $(\alpha = 0.8,\ \rho = 1.2)$. Also, for smaller values of the fractions $(\alpha,\ \rho)$ the system loses its chaotic character.

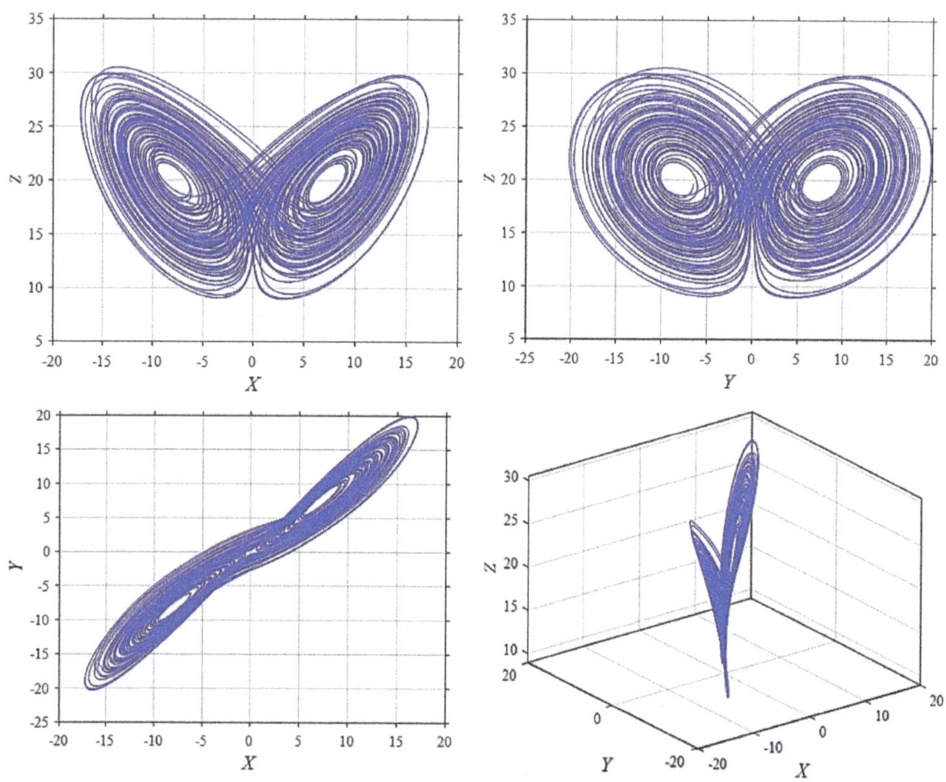

Figure 5. Chaotic attractor of fractional Lorenz system using DSCDQM–RSK with time (T = 100), fraction $(\alpha = 0.8,\ \rho = 1.2)$, $(x_0 = 2.5, y_0 = 1, z_0 = 0.5)$ and $(\lambda = 1, \beta = 2, \phi = 1)$.

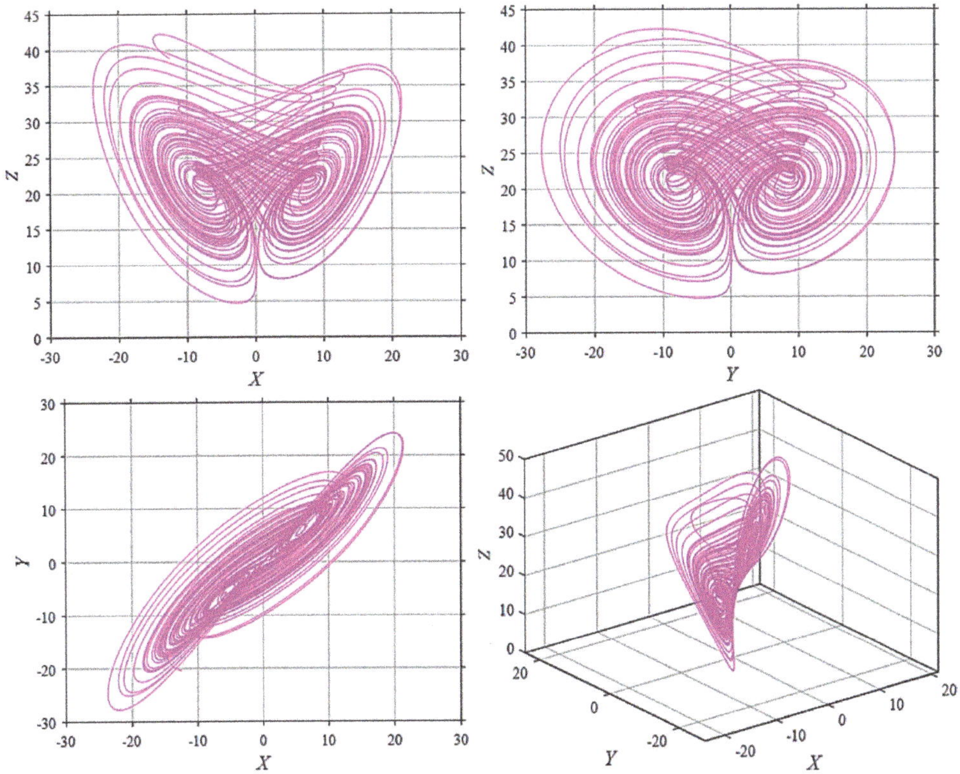

Figure 6. Chaotic attractor of fractional Lorenz system using DSCDQM–RSK with time (T = 100), fraction $(\alpha = 0.97,\ \rho = 1)$, $(x_0 = 2.5, y_0 = 1, z_0 = 0.5)$ and $(\lambda = 1, \beta = 2, \phi = 1)$.

To analyze the computational complexity of the provided code for solving the Riccati equation and the Lorenz system using the Fractional Differential Quadrature Method (FDQM), we will focus on memory space and simulation time complexities in detail. The configuration of the computer used to perform the simulation results is HP Probook 450 G8 Laptop—11th Intel Core i5-1135G7, 8 GB RAM, 512 GB PCIe NVMe SSD, 15.6″ FHD (1920 × 1080), and Intel Iris X Graphics.

1. Memory Space Complexity

Variables:

- Grid Points: The function Chebyshev grid (N) generates N Chebyshev nodes, requiring O(N) space.

The DSCDQM–RSK method demonstrated optimal performance with N = 9 grid points, a bandwidth of 2k + 1 = 7, and a regularized Shannon factor of $\sigma = 0.45 \times \Delta$ for the fractional Riccati equation. This configuration yielded a CPU time of 0.018 s. Similarly, for the fractional Lorenz system, the best results were obtained with N = 9 grid points, a bandwidth of 2k + 1 = 3, and a regularized Shannon factor of $\sigma = 0.47 \times \Delta$, achieving a CPU time of 0.02 s.

In contrast, earlier numerical methods typically required significantly more grid points, often reaching N = 640, 1280, or even 3200.

- Weighting Coefficients: The function PDQM weights (N, t) creates a matrix A of size $N \times N$. Therefore, it requires $O(N^2)$ space.
- Solution Vectors:

- The solution v, X, Y, Z vectorsfor the Riccati equation and Lorenz system are initialized as zero vectors of size N × 1, each requiring O(N) space.
- Total for all solution vectors combined: 4 × O(N) = O(N).

Total Memory Space Complexity:

- The dominant term is $O(N^2)$ from the weighting coefficients matrix. Thus, the total memory space complexity is:

$$O(N^2)$$

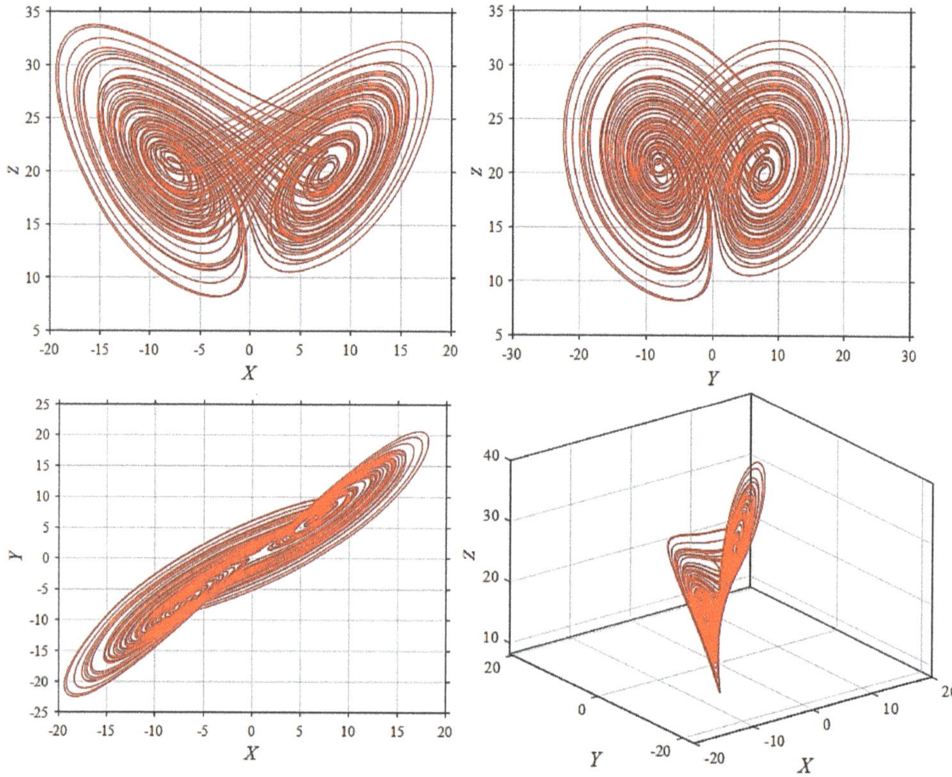

Figure 7. Chaotic attractor of fractional Lorenz system using DSCDQM–RSK with time (T = 100), fraction ($\alpha = 0.9,\ \rho = 0.8$), $(x_0 = 2.5, y_0 = 1, z_0 = 0.5)$ and $(\lambda = 1, \beta = 2, \phi = 1)$.

2. Simulation Time Complexity
For Solving the Riccati Equation:
Grid Point Generation:

- The grid points are generated in O(N) time.

Weighting Coefficients Calculation:

- The PDQM weights(N, t, 1) function computes the coefficients with a nested loop over N, resulting in $O(N^2)$ time complexity:
- Each entry in matrix A involves calculations that depend on N, leading to $O(N^2)$ complexity for the entire matrix.

Time Integration:

- The time integration loop runs for N-1 iterations, performing a constant time calculation for each iteration:

$$O(N)$$

Total Time Complexity for Riccati Equation:

- Combining these, we get:

$$O(N^2) \text{ (weighting coefficients)} + O(N) \text{ (grid points)} + O(N) \text{ (integration)} = O(N^2)$$

For Solving the Lorenz System:
Grid Point Generation:

- Again, this takes O(N) time.

Weighting Coefficients Calculation:

- The calculations for Ax, Ay, and Az each take $O(N^2)$:

$$3 \times O(N^2) = O(N^2)$$

Time Integration:

- Similar to the Riccati equation, the integration loop runs for N-1 iterations:

$$O(N)$$

Total Time Complexity for Lorenz System:

- Again combining these:

$$O(N^2) \text{ (coefficients)} + O(N) \text{ (grid points)} + O(N) \text{ (integration)} = O(N^2)$$

3. Overall Complexity Summary

- Memory Complexity: $O(N^2)$
- Time Complexity for Riccati Equation: $O(N^2)$
- Time Complexity for Lorenz System: $O(N^2)$

4. Real Numbers Example
For practical evaluation, consider the following:

- For N = 9:

Memory for weighting coefficients: 81 entries.
Memory for solution vectors: 36 entries.
Assuming each entry takes 8 bytes (for double precision), the memory usage would be:

- Weighting coefficients: $81 \times 8 = 648$ bytes (approximately 0.64 KB).
- Solution vectors: $36 \times 8 = 288$ bytes (approximately 0.28 KB).

Total memory usage for N = 9 would be approximately 1 KB.
Execution Time:

- If the operations in the loops take, say, 0.001 s per iteration:

For N = 9, the time for solving the Riccati equation and the Lorenz system would be dominated by the $O(N^2)$ term, leading to an estimated execution time of about 0.1 s (for illustration).

This detailed analysis provides insights into the computational complexity of the code, which is crucial for assessing performance in practical scenarios. The findings underscore the importance of optimizing the weighting coefficients and the iterative solvers for larger values of N.

The choice of time step in numerical methods significantly affects the accuracy of the solutions for differential equations, including those solved using the Differential Quadrature Method (DQM). Here's how:

5. Stability and Convergence:

Our numerical methods are stable because small perturbations in the initial conditions lead to small perturbations in the numerical solution.

Consider the fractional differential equation (FDE) represented in the form:

$$D_c^{\alpha} U(t) = f(t, U(t)), t \in [0, T] \tag{27}$$

where D_c^{α} is the generalized Caputo fractional derivative.

Let $U(t)$ be the exact solution and $U_n(t)$ be the numerical solution obtained through the proposed methods. Introduce a perturbation ϵ_n such that:

$$U_n(t) = U(t) + \epsilon_n \tag{28}$$

By analyzing how the perturbation evolves over time:

$$D_c^{\alpha}(U_n(t) + \epsilon_n) = f(t, U_n(t) + \epsilon_n) \tag{29}$$

This leads to the error equation:

$$D_c^{\alpha} \epsilon_n = f(t, U_n(t) + \epsilon_n) - f(t, U(t)) \tag{30}$$

Assume f satisfies a Lipschitz condition:

$$|f(t, U_1) - f(t, U_2)| \leq L|U_1 - U_2| \tag{31}$$

where L is a constant.

By applying Gronwall's inequality, show that:

$$|\epsilon_n| \leq C \cdot \Delta t^p$$

where C is a constant and p is the order of the method, ensuring that the solution remains bounded as $n \to \infty$.

Our numerical method converges because the numerical solution approaches the exact solution as the grid refinement increases.

Let:

$$\lim_{N \to \infty} \| U_n(t) - U(t) \| = 0 \tag{32}$$

By conducting an error analysis between the numerical solution and the exact

$$E_n = U_n(t) - U(t) \tag{33}$$

By using Taylor expansion around t_n to express $U(t)$:

$$U(t_n + \Delta t) = U(t_n) + \Delta t U'(t_n) + O\left(\Delta t^2\right) \tag{34}$$

Relate this to the discretized version derived from the method:

$$U_n(t_n + \Delta t) = U_n(t_n) + O(\Delta t^p) \tag{35}$$

The method is stable and the achieved convergence rates reached 10^{-8}, indicating a high level of precision in solving the nonlinear fractional initial value problems. The truncation error in our numerical methods is very small due to the Gaussian regularizer $\sigma = 0.45 \times \Delta$ which depends on a small computational domain:

6. Accuracy of the Solution:

- Each step introduces local error, which accumulates over time. Smaller time steps help minimize this accumulation, resulting in a more accurate final solution (error $\leq 10^{-8}$)
- The global error, which is the total error over the entire integration period, also tends to decrease with smaller time steps, leading to better overall accuracy.

4.3. Stability Analysis

After applying our discretization schemes to Equations (1)–(6), we obtained an equivalent set of ordinary differential equations in the time domain:

$$\frac{\mathrm{d}[U]}{\mathrm{dt}} = \mathrm{R}[U] + [\mathrm{K}] \tag{36}$$

where

1. The vector {U} represents the unknown variables at the internal grid points, where υ, X, Y, and Z are the individual components;
   - The initial conditions are stored in the vector [K];
2. R[U] is the right-hand side of Equations (1)∓(6); and
3. $a_{ij}^{(1)}$ is the weighting coefficient matrix of the first derivative:

$$a_{ij}^{(1)} = \begin{bmatrix} a_{22}^{(1)} & a_{23}^{(1)} & \cdots & a_{2(n-1)}^{(1)} \\ a_{32}^{(1)} & a_{33}^{(1)} & & a_{3(n-1)}^{(1)} \\ \vdots & & \ddots & \vdots \\ a_{(n-1)2}^{(1)} & a_{(n-1)3}^{(1)} & \cdots & a_{(n-1)(n-1)}^{(1)} \end{bmatrix}_{(N-2)\times(N-2)} \tag{37}$$

The stability of our technique was evaluated by examining system (35). We employed eigenvalue analysis of the coefficient matrices (a) to determine stability.

For the fractional differential equation represented in the form:

$$D_c^{\alpha} U(t) = f(t, U(t))$$

discretizing this using the FDQM leads to a system of equations expressed as:

$$[a][\mathrm{U}] = \mathrm{R}[U]$$

To analyze stability, we need to compute the eigenvalues λ of the matrix $[a]$. The eigenvalue problem is given by:

$$[a][\mathrm{v}] = \lambda[\mathrm{v}]$$

where v is the eigenvector associated with the eigenvalue λ.

The characteristic polynomial is obtained from:

$$\det(a - \lambda I) = 0$$

where I is the identity matrix.

The stability of the numerical method hinges on the eigenvalues of $[a]$:

1. If all eigenvalues satisfy $|\lambda| < 1$, the method is stable.
2. If any eigenvalue has $|\lambda| \geq 1$, the method may be unstable.

Figure 8 displays the stability regions for a numerical method at various fractional orders (α). Each subplot represents a different α value: 0.5, 0.7, 0.85, and 1. The plots show the eigenvalues of the coefficient matrix (a) in the complex plane (Real vs. Imaginary). At α = 0.5, the eigenvalues are all located on the real axis near −0.5. Since the magnitude of these eigenvalues is less than 1, this indicates stability for this fractional order. At α = 0.7, the eigenvalues form a V-shape, extending into both the positive and negative real axis. A portion of the eigenvalues have magnitudes greater than 1 (outside the unit circle), indicating instability in this region. The region of stability is limited to the portion of the V-shape within the unit circle. At α = 0.85, the eigenvalues form an inverted V-shape. Similar to (b), portions of the eigenvalues are outside the unit circle, indicating instability. The region of stability is again limited to the portion within the unit circle. At α = 1, the eigenvalues lie entirely on the negative real axis, forming a vertical line. All eigenvalues appear to be within the unit circle, suggesting stability for this fractional order (which corresponds to the standard integer-order case). Furthermore, Figure 9 depicts the error propagation in relation to time and fractional order.

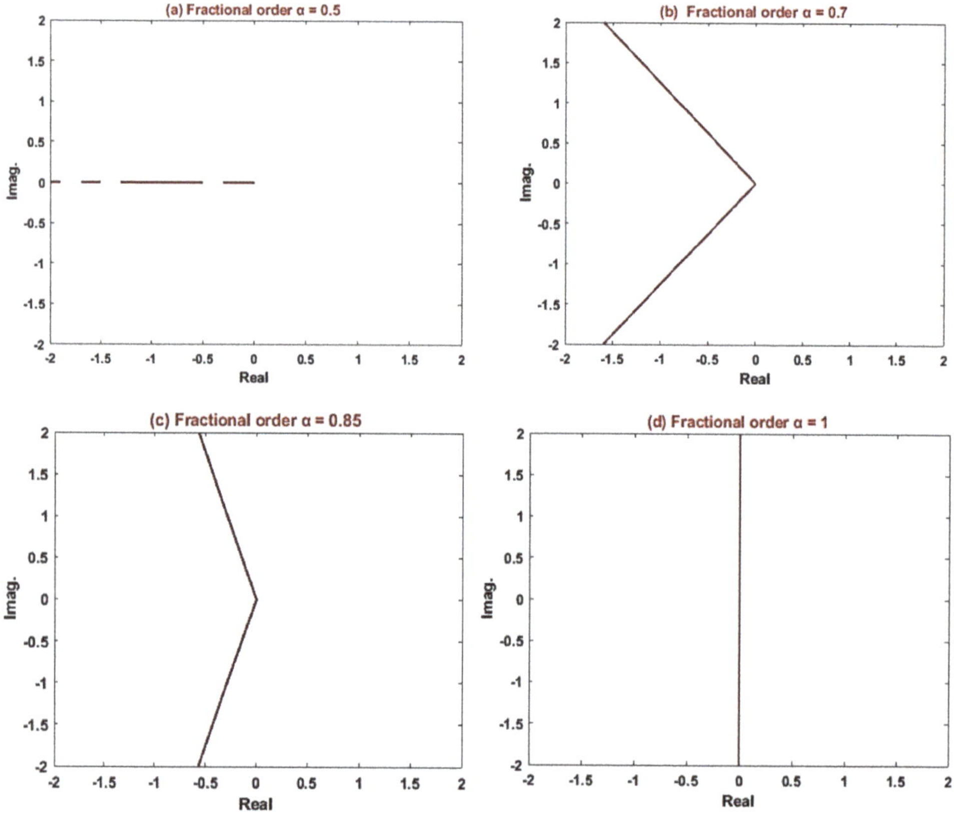

Figure 8. Regions of stability at varying fractional orders.

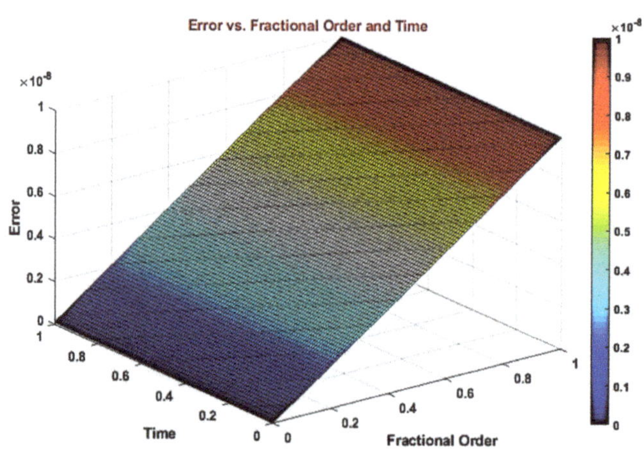

Figure 9. Propagation of errors in relation to time and fractional order.

5. Conclusions

In this present work, we have successfully investigated new numerical methods for solving the fractional Riccati equation and fractional Lorenz system. The novel numerical method is FDQM, which is based on two base functions: Lagrange interpolation polynomial and discrete singular convolution-Regularized Shannon kernel with a new generalized Caputo kind. These methods are used to transform the proposed problems into a nonlinear algebraic system. Then, the iterative method is employed to deal with the problem of nonlinearity. All numerical results were obtained using MATLAB. By comparing our results with those of existing methods, we demonstrated the superior accuracy, efficiency, and overall performance of our proposed techniques. The achieved convergence rates reached 10^{-8}, indicating a high level of precision in solving the nonlinear fractional initial value problems. Error analysis showed that non-uniform grid distributions consistently outperformed uniform distributions, with maximum errors diminishing significantly as grid points increased. Our numerical results demonstrate that the DSC-RSK method achieved significantly faster convergence rates compared to other techniques. The best results of the DSC-RSK method are achieved when grid points are N = 9, bandwidth is 2k + 1 = 7, and the regularized Shannon factor is $\sigma = 0.45 \times \Delta$ at CPU time = 0.018 s for the fractional Riccati equation. But for the fractional Lorenz system, the best results are when grid points are N = 9, bandwidth is 2k + 1 = 3, and the regularized Shannon factor is $\sigma = 0.47 \times \Delta$ at CPU time = 0.02 s. Also, the proposed techniques have been successfully employed to explain the fractional systems' dynamic behaviors. The numerical results demonstrate a strong dependence of the solution on the fractional derivative. The fractional parameters, α and ρ, offer significant advantages in studying the proposed problems with greater accuracy compared to traditional approaches. These techniques hold promise for solving more complex nonlinear equations and other differential applications involving fractional derivatives. The versatility of the FDQM was highlighted through its successful application to both the fractional Riccati equations and the fractional Lorenz system, demonstrating its potential for broader applications in fields requiring the modeling of complex dynamics. The findings suggest that further exploration of fractional orders could uncover even richer dynamics, with potential applications extending to areas such as control theory, physics, and finance.

Author Contributions: Conceptualization, M.M., O.R., M.S. and W.M.A.; methodology, M.M., O.R. and M.S.; software, M.M.; validation, M.M. and W.M.A.; formal analysis, investigation, O.R., M.S. and M.M.; resources, W.M.A.; data curation, writing—original draft preparation, O.R., M.S. and M.M.; writing—review and editing, W.M.A.; visualization, supervision, O.R. and M.S.; Funding, W.M.A. and M.M. All authors have read and agreed to the published version of the manuscript.

Funding: This research received no external funding.

Data Availability Statement: The data presented in this study are available in the article.

Conflicts of Interest: The authors declare no conflicts of interest.

References

1. Cafagna, D.; Grassi, G. Bifurcation and Chaos in the Fractional-Order Chen System via a Time-Domain Approach. *Int. J. Bifurc. Chaos* **2008**, *18*, 1845–1863. [CrossRef]
2. Petráš, I. The Fractional-Order Lorenz-Type Systems: A Review. *Fract. Calc. Appl. Anal.* **2022**, *25*, 362–377. [CrossRef]
3. Grigorenko, I.; Grigorenko, E. Chaotic Dynamics of the Fractional Lorenz System. *Phys. Rev. Lett.* **2003**, *91*, 034101. [CrossRef]
4. Deng, W.H.; Li, C.P. Chaos Synchronization of the Fractional Lü System. *Phys. A Stat. Mech. Its Appl.* **2005**, *353*, 61–72. [CrossRef]
5. Lü, J.; Chen, G. A New Chaotic Attractor Coined. *Int. J. Bifurc. Chaos* **2002**, *12*, 659–661. [CrossRef]
6. Rahman, Z.-A.S.A.; Jasim, B.H.; Al-Yasir, Y.I.A.; Hu, Y.-F.; Abd-Alhameed, R.A.; Alhasnawi, B.N. A New Fractional-Order Chaotic System with Its Analysis, Synchronization, and Circuit Realization for Secure Communication Applications. *Mathematics* **2021**, *9*, 2593. [CrossRef]
7. Aminikhah, H.; Hemmatnezhad, M. An Efficient Method for Quadratic Riccati Differential Equation. *Commun. Nonlinear Sci. Numer. Simul.* **2010**, *15*, 835–839. [CrossRef]

8. Khan, N.A.; Ara, A.; Jamil, M. An Efficient Approach for Solving the Riccati Equation with Fractional Orders. *Comput. Math. Appl.* **2011**, *61*, 2683–2689. [CrossRef]
9. Odibat, Z.; Momani, S. Modified Homotopy Perturbation Method: Application to Quadratic Riccati Differential Equation of Fractional Order. *Chaos Solitons Fractals* **2008**, *36*, 167–174. [CrossRef]
10. Cang, J.; Tan, Y.; Xu, H.; Liao, S.-J. Series Solutions of Non-Linear Riccati Differential Equations with Fractional Order. *Chaos Solitons Fractals* **2009**, *40*, 1–9. [CrossRef]
11. Tan, Y.; Abbasbandy, S. Homotopy Analysis Method for Quadratic Riccati Differential Equation. *Commun. Nonlinear Sci. Numer. Simul.* **2008**, *13*, 539–546. [CrossRef]
12. Gülsu, M.; Sezer, M. On the Solution of the Riccati Equation by the Taylor Matrix Method. *Appl. Math. Comput.* **2006**, *176*, 414–421. [CrossRef]
13. Li, Y.; Hu, L. Solving Fractional Riccati Differential Equations Using Haar Wavelet. In Proceedings of the 2010 Third International Conference on Information and Computing, Wuxi, China, 4–6 June 2010; IEEE: Piscataway, NJ, USA, 2010; Volume 1, pp. 314–317.
14. Cui, M. Combined Compact Difference Scheme for the Time Fractional Convection–Diffusion Equation with Variable Coefficients. *Appl. Math. Comput.* **2014**, *246*, 464–473. [CrossRef]
15. Gu, X.-M.; Huang, T.-Z.; Ji, C.-C.; Carpentieri, B.; Alikhanov, A.A. Fast Iterative Method with a Second-Order Implicit Difference Scheme for Time-Space Fractional Convection–Diffusion Equation. *J. Sci. Comput.* **2017**, *72*, 957–985. [CrossRef]
16. Wang, Y.-M. A Compact Finite Difference Method for a Class of Time Fractional Convection-Diffusion-Wave Equations with Variable Coefficients. *Numer. Algorithms* **2015**, *70*, 625–651. [CrossRef]
17. Salman, W.; Gavriilidis, A.; Angeli, P. A Model for Predicting Axial Mixing during Gas–Liquid Taylor Flow in Microchannels at Low Bodenstein Numbers. *Chem. Eng. J.* **2004**, *101*, 391–396. [CrossRef]
18. Xu, Q.; Hesthaven, J.S. Discontinuous Galerkin Method for Fractional Convection-Diffusion Equations. *SIAM J. Numer. Anal.* **2014**, *52*, 405–423. [CrossRef]
19. Aboelenen, T. A Direct Discontinuous Galerkin Method for Fractional Convection-Diffusion and Schrödinger-Type Equations. *Eur. Phys. J. Plus* **2018**, *133*, 316. [CrossRef]
20. Jin, B.; Lazarov, R.; Zhou, Z. A Petrov–Galerkin Finite Element Method for Fractional Convection-Diffusion Equations. *SIAM J. Numer. Anal.* **2016**, *54*, 481–503. [CrossRef]
21. Li, C.; Zeng, F. *Numerical Methods for Fractional Calculus*; CRC Press: Boca Raton, FL, USA, 2015; Volume 24, ISBN 148225381X.
22. Parvizi, M.; Eslahchi, M.R.; Dehghan, M. Numerical Solution of Fractional Advection-Diffusion Equation with a Nonlinear Source Term. *Numer. Algorithms* **2015**, *68*, 601–629. [CrossRef]
23. Saadatmandi, A.; Dehghan, M.; Azizi, M.-R. The Sinc–Legendre Collocation Method for a Class of Fractional Convection–Diffusion Equations with Variable Coefficients. *Commun. Nonlinear Sci. Numer. Simul.* **2012**, *17*, 4125–4136. [CrossRef]
24. Bhrawy, A.H.; Baleanu, D. A Spectral Legendre–Gauss–Lobatto Collocation Method for a Space-Fractional Advection Diffusion Equations with Variable Coefficients. *Rep. Math. Phys.* **2013**, *72*, 219–233. [CrossRef]
25. Tian, W.; Deng, W.; Wu, Y. Polynomial Spectral Collocation Method for Space Fractional Advection–Diffusion Equation. *Numer. Methods Partial Differ. Equ.* **2014**, *30*, 514–535. [CrossRef]
26. Badr, M.; Yazdani, A.; Jafari, H. Stability of a Finite Volume Element Method for the Time-fractional Advection-diffusion Equation. *Numer. Methods Partial Differ. Equ.* **2018**, *34*, 1459–1471. [CrossRef]
27. Gao, F.; Yuan, Y.; Du, N. An Upwind Finite Volume Element Method for Nonlinear Convection Diffusion Problem. *Am. J. Comput. Math.* **2011**, *1*, 264–270. [CrossRef]
28. Bi, Y.; Jiang, Z. The Finite Volume Element Method for the Two-Dimensional Space-Fractional Convection–Diffusion Equation. *Adv. Differ. Equ.* **2021**, *2021*, 379. [CrossRef]
29. Liu, J.; Zhang, J.; Zhang, X. Semi-Discretized Numerical Solution for Time Fractional Convection–Diffusion Equation by RBF-FD. *Appl. Math. Lett.* **2022**, *128*, 107880. [CrossRef]
30. Saadeh, R. Numerical Solutions of Fractional Convection-Diffusion Equation Using Finite-Difference and Finite-Volume Schemes. *J. Math. Comput. Sci.* **2021**, *11*, 7872–7891.
31. Tuan, N.H.; Aghdam, Y.E.; Jafari, H.; Mesgarani, H. A Novel Numerical Manner for Two-dimensional Space Fractional Diffusion Equation Arising in Transport Phenomena. *Numer. Methods Partial Differ. Equ.* **2021**, *37*, 1397–1406. [CrossRef]
32. Devshali, P.; Arora, G. Solution of Two-Dimensional Fractional Diffusion Equation by a Novel Hybrid D (TQ) Method. *Nonlinear Eng.* **2022**, *11*, 135–142. [CrossRef]
33. Khader, M.M. Numerical Treatment for Solving Fractional Riccati Differential Equation. *J. Egypt. Math. Soc.* **2013**, *21*, 32–37. [CrossRef]
34. Li, X.Y.; Wu, B.Y.; Wang, R.T. Reproducing Kernel Method for Fractional Riccati Differential Equations. *Abstr. Appl. Anal.* **2014**, *2014*, 970967. [CrossRef]
35. Sakar, M.G.; Akgül, A.; Baleanu, D. On Solutions of Fractional Riccati Differential Equations. *Adv. Differ. Equ.* **2017**, *2017*, 39. [CrossRef]
36. Agheli, B. Approximate Solution for Solving Fractional Riccati Differential Equations via Trigonometric Basic Functions. *Trans. A. Razmadze Math. Inst.* **2018**, *172*, 299–308. [CrossRef]
37. Liu, X.; Kamran; Yao, Y. Numerical Approximation of Riccati Fractional Differential Equation in the Sense of Caputo-Type Fractional Derivative. *J. Math.* **2020**, *2020*, 1274251. [CrossRef]

38. Hartley, T.T.; Lorenzo, C.F.; Qammer, H.K. Chaos in a Fractional Order Chua's System. *IEEE Trans. Circuits Syst. I Fundam. Theory Appl.* **1995**, *42*, 485–490. [CrossRef]
39. Lu, J.-G. Chaotic Dynamics of the Fractional-Order Ikeda Delay System and Its Synchronization. *Chin. Phys.* **2006**, *15*, 301–305.
40. Li, C.; Peng, G. Chaos in Chen's System with a Fractional Order. *Chaos Solitons Fractals* **2004**, *22*, 443–450. [CrossRef]
41. Diethelm, K.; Ford, N.J.; Freed, A.D. A Predictor-Corrector Approach for the Numerical Solution of Fractional Differential Equations. *Nonlinear Dyn.* **2002**, *29*, 3–22. [CrossRef]
42. Ahmadian, A.; Suleiman, M.; Salahshour, S.; Baleanu, D. A Jacobi Operational Matrix for Solving a Fuzzy Linear Fractional Differential Equation. *Adv. Differ. Equ.* **2013**, *2013*, 104. [CrossRef]
43. Yuan, L.; Yang, Q.; Zeng, C. Chaos Detection and Parameter Identification in Fractional-Order Chaotic Systems with Delay. *Nonlinear Dyn.* **2013**, *73*, 439–448. [CrossRef]
44. Luo, C.; Wang, X. Chaos in the Fractional-Order Complex Lorenz System and Its Synchronization. *Nonlinear Dyn.* **2013**, *71*, 241–257. [CrossRef]
45. Bhalekar, S.; Daftardar-Gejji, V. Fractional Ordered Liu System with Time-Delay. *Commun. Nonlinear Sci. Numer. Simul.* **2010**, *15*, 2178–2191. [CrossRef]
46. Katugampola, U.N. New Approach to a Generalized Fractional Integral. *Appl. Math. Comput.* **2011**, *218*, 860–865. [CrossRef]
47. Wang, Z.; Huang, X.; Li, N.; Song, X.-N. Image Encryption Based on a Delayed Fractional-Order Chaotic Logistic System. *Chin. Phys. B* **2012**, *21*, 050506. [CrossRef]
48. Wu, G.-C.; Baleanu, D.; Lin, Z.-X. Image Encryption Technique Based on Fractional Chaotic Time Series. *J. Vib. Control* **2016**, *22*, 2092–2099. [CrossRef]
49. Anderson, D.R.; Ulness, D.J. Properties of the Katugampola Fractional Derivative with Potential Application in Quantum Mechanics. *J. Math. Phys.* **2015**, *56*, 063502. [CrossRef]
50. Li, C.; Chen, G. Chaos in the Fractional Order Chen System and Its Control. *Chaos Solitons Fractals* **2004**, *22*, 549–554. [CrossRef]
51. Alomari, A.K. A Novel Solution for Fractional Chaotic Chen System. *J. Nonlinear Sci. Appl.* **2015**, *8*, 478–488. [CrossRef]
52. Erturk, V.S.; Kumar, P. Solution of a COVID-19 Model via New Generalized Caputo-Type Fractional Derivatives. *Chaos Solitons Fractals* **2020**, *139*, 110280. [CrossRef]
53. Xu, Y.; He, Z.; Agrawal, O.P. Numerical and Analytical Solutions of New Generalized Fractional Diffusion Equation. *Comput. Math. Appl.* **2013**, *66*, 2019–2029. [CrossRef]
54. Kumar, P.; Erturk, V.S.; Kumar, A. A New Technique to Solve Generalized Caputo Type Fractional Differential Equations with the Example of Computer Virus Model. *J. Math. Ext.* **2021**, *15*, 1–23.
55. Ragb, O.; Mohamed, M.; Matbuly, M.S. Vibration Analysis of Magneto-Electro-Thermo NanoBeam Resting on Nonlinear Elastic Foundation Using Sinc and Discrete Singular Convolution Differential Quadrature Method. *Mod. Appl. Sci.* **2019**, *13*, 49–79. [CrossRef]
56. Shu, C. *Differential Quadrature and Its Application in Engineering*; Springer Science & Business Media: London, UK, 2012; ISBN 1447104072.
57. Civalek, Ö. Free Vibration of Carbon Nanotubes Reinforced (CNTR) and Functionally Graded Shells and Plates Based on FSDT via Discrete Singular Convolution Method. *Compos. Part B Eng.* **2017**, *111*, 45–59. [CrossRef]
58. Civalek, Ö.; Kiracioglu, O. Free Vibration Analysis of Timoshenko Beams by DSC Method. *Int. J. Numer. Methods Biomed. Eng.* **2010**, *26*, 1890–1898. [CrossRef]
59. Wan, D.C.; Zhou, Y.C.; Wei, G.W. Numerical Solution of Incompressible Flows by Discrete Singular Convolution. *Int. J. Numer. Methods Fluids* **2002**, *38*, 789–810. [CrossRef]
60. Zhang, L.; Xiang, Y.; Wei, G.W. Local Adaptive Differential Quadrature for Free Vibration Analysis of Cylindrical Shells with Various Boundary Conditions. *Int. J. Mech. Sci.* **2006**, *48*, 1126–1138. [CrossRef]
61. Daftardar-Gejji, V.; Bhalekar, S.; Gade, P. Dynamics of Fractional-Ordered Chen System with Delay. *Pramana* **2012**, *79*, 61–69. [CrossRef]
62. Katugampola, U.N. Existence and Uniqueness Results for a Class of Generalized Fractional Differential Equations. *arXiv* **2014**, arXiv:1411.5229.
63. Khan, N.A.; Ara, A.; Alam Khan, N. Fractional-Order Riccati Differential Equation: Analytical Approximation and Numerical Results. *Adv. Differ. Equ.* **2013**, *2013*, 185. [CrossRef]
64. Odibat, Z.; Baleanu, D. Numerical Simulation of Initial Value Problems with Generalized Caputo-Type Fractional Derivatives. *Appl. Numer. Math.* **2020**, *156*, 94–105. [CrossRef]
65. Baleanu, D.; Wu, G.; Zeng, S. Chaos Analysis and Asymptotic Stability of Generalized Caputo Fractional Differential Equations. *Chaos Solitons Fractals* **2017**, *102*, 99–105. [CrossRef]
66. Alemu, S.; Alluvada, P.; Thelkar, A.R.; Samanvita, N.; Lemma, T.; Heyi, K. Fractional Order Sliding Mode Controller Modelling for Fractional Order SEPIC Converter. *Authorea* **2024**. [CrossRef]
67. Podlubny, I. *Fractional Differential Equations*; Academic Press: New York, NY, USA, 1999.
68. Caputo, M. Linear Models of Dissipation Whose Q Is Almost Frequency Independent—II. *Geophys. J. Int.* **1967**, *13*, 529–539. [CrossRef]
69. Ragb, O.; Wazwaz, A.; Mohamed, M.; Matbuly, M.S.; Salah, M. Fractional Differential Quadrature Techniques for Fractional Order Cauchy Reaction-diffusion Equations. *Math. Methods Appl. Sci.* **2023**, *46*, 10216–10233. [CrossRef]

70. Wei, G.W. Discrete Singular Convolution for the Solution of the Fokker–Planck Equation. *J. Chem. Phys.* **1999**, *110*, 8930–8942. [CrossRef]
71. Shao, Z.; Wei, G.W.; Zhao, S. DSC Time-Domain Solution of Maxwell's Equations. *J. Comput. Phys.* **2003**, *189*, 427–453. [CrossRef]
72. Ragb, O.; Mohamed, M.; Matbuly, M.S.; Civalek, O. An Accurate Numerical Approach for Studying Perovskite Solar Cells. *Int. J. Energy Res.* **2021**, *45*, 16456–16477. [CrossRef]
73. Ragb, O.; Mohamed, M.; Matbuly, M.S. Free Vibration of a Piezoelectric Nanobeam Resting on Nonlinear Winkler-Pasternak Foundation by Quadrature Methods. *Heliyon* **2019**, *5*, e01856. [CrossRef]
74. Gu, Y.; Li, G.; Xu, X.; Song, X.; Zhong, H. Solution of a New High-Performance Fractional-Order Lorenz System and Its Dynamics Analysis. *Nonlinear Dyn.* **2023**, *111*, 7469–7493. [CrossRef]
75. Li, H.; Shen, Y.; Han, Y.; Dong, J.; Li, J. Determining Lyapunov Exponents of Fractional-Order Systems: A General Method Based on Memory Principle. *Chaos Solitons Fractals* **2023**, *168*, 113167. [CrossRef]

fractal and fractional

MDPI

Article

Granular Fuzzy Fractional Continuous-Time Linear Systems: Roesser and Fornasini–Marchesini Models

Ghulam Muhammad [1,*], Muhammad Akram [2], Hamed Alsulami [3] and Nawab Hussain [3]

[1] Department of Mathematics, Lahore Garrison University, Lahore 54000, Pakistan
[2] Institute of Mathematics, University of the Punjab, New Campus, Lahore 54590, Pakistan; m.akram@pucit.edu.pk
[3] Department of Mathematics, King Abdulaziz University, P.O Box 80203, Jeddah 21589, Saudi Arabia; hhaalsalmi@kau.edu.sa (H.A.); nhusain@kau.edu.sa (N.H.)
* Correspondence: ghulammuhammad@lgu.edu.pk

Abstract: In this article, we introduce and investigate two classes of fuzzy fractional two-dimensional continuous-time (FFTDCT) linear systems to deal with uncertainty and fuzziness in system parameters. First, we analyze FFTDCT linear systems based on the Roesser model, incorporating fuzzy parameters into the state-space equations. The potential solution of the fuzzy fractional system is obtained using a two-dimensional granular Laplace transform approach. Second, we examine FFTDCT linear systems described by the second Fornasini–Marchesini (FM) model, where the state-space equations involve two-dimensional and one-dimensional partial fractional-order granular Caputo derivatives. We determine the fuzzy solution for this model by applying the two-dimensional granular Laplace transform. To enhance the validity of the proposed approaches, real-world applications, including signal processing systems and wireless sensor network data fusion, are solved to support the theoretical framework and demonstrate the impact of uncertainty on the system's behavior.

Keywords: granular Caputo fractional derivative; fuzzy fractional two-dimensional linear systems; granular two-dimensional Laplace transform; Roesser model; Fornasini–Marchesini second model

MSC: 34A08; 93C42; 93C55; 35R11

1. Introduction

All real-world phenomena are naturally affected by uncertainty. Developing a model, solving the problem, and analyzing the results encountered are essential tasks within the domain of fuzziness. Generally, differential equations (DEs) are commonly involved in various scientific and engineering domains [1]. These DEs typically rely on complex environments, and such complexities can be handled more precisely using fractional-order derivatives. In contrast, the model's parameters, variables, and initial or boundary conditions are assumed to be crisp for computational simplicity. Errors that arise from observations, measurements, or experiments can result in vague or incomplete descriptions of these parameters and variables. One can employ a stochastic, statistical, or fuzzy approach to deal with such uncertainty. Stochastic and statistical methods address the uncertainty due to inherent randomness in processes. Fuzzy set theory offers a framework for managing vagueness and imprecision that result from incomplete information regarding the variables and parameters of a model.

Fuzzy differential equations (FDEs) have become a valuable tool for modeling natural phenomena and are characterized by uncertainty, attracting considerable attention from researchers. The concept of FDEs was first introduced by Dubois and Prade in 1982 [2]. Many researchers have worked on FDEs by examining their existence and uniqueness (E&U), proposing novel approaches, and determining the behavior to deepen the comprehension of the models [3–5]. The solution was derived using the fuzzy Laplace transform technique [3,6,7].

The fuzzy derivatives obtained from fuzzy standard interval arithmetic (FSIA) possess some limitations. Some of them are highlighted below: (i) The solution of FDEs under fuzzy derivatives leads to CPLV [8]. Furthermore, all real-world phenomena are governed by physical laws, and these problems are often described using FDEs. However, FDEs can admit multiple fuzzy solutions, and not all of them may accurately reflect the true behavior of the physical system. Inaccurate or inappropriate solutions can lead to predictions that contradict the underlying physical principles. (ii) The fuzzy derivatives within the FSIA framework are valid only if the H-difference exists. The existence of fuzzy derivatives is restricted if the corresponding differences do not exist [9]. (iii) The n-dimensional FDEs under FSIA are transformed into a $2n$ classical system. This transformation imposes a constraint that complicates the comprehension and analysis of FDEs. (iv) FDEs under fuzzy derivatives with FSIA lead to different solutions. This phenomenon is commonly referred to as the UBM phenomenon. (v) The FDEs using FSIA frequently yield multiple or infinitely many solutions, complicating the interpretation of the results [10]. Mazandarani et al. [9] introduced the novel concept of differentiability, commonly called granular differentiability (gr-derivative), to explore the FDEs from a new perspective. This approach handles the fuzziness of FDEs by applying the fuzzy interval arithmetic based on the relative distance measure (RDM). The core innovation behind this approach is to characterize fuzzy numbers through their horizontal membership function (HMF) and to formulate the corresponding operations within this framework. This derivative is introduced to overcome the limitations of fuzzy derivatives using FSIA. FDEs based on the gr-derivative enable us to determine a unique solution to the problem. Granular differentiability (GRD) has the following main advantages when investigating FDEs: FDEs under GRD have a simple and effective solution. In FDEs involving GRD, the solution's support across the domain does not need to be intrinsically monotonic. The doubling property, multiplicity, and UBM phenomena constraints are successfully addressed and eliminated in the solutions of FDEs using GRD.

Motivation and Contribution

The modeling of complex multi-dimensional dynamical processes with memory and hereditary properties relies heavily on fractional two-dimensional continuous-time (FTDCT) linear systems. These systems are essential for studying real-world phenomena, including distributed parameter systems, thermal systems, and image processing. One effective tool for examining and managing such systems is the extension of the Roesser model to the fractional calculus. Roesser [11] introduced the most significant state-space models for two-dimensional linear systems (TDLSs). For the study of multi-dimensional systems, this model is essential. To evaluate two-dimensional linear systems (TDLSs), they offer a framework that separates the dynamics into vertical and horizontal components. Alternative state-space models for TDLSs were proposed by Fornasini and Marchesini [12] and are widely used for the study and control of multi-dimensional systems. This work extends the Roesser model and provides additional tools for understanding two-dimensional (2D) systems, particularly in the context of iterative processes and signal processing. The state-space model for TDLSs introduced by Kurek [13] is especially helpful for applications involving image processing and control systems. Kurek's approach provides a consistent framework for TDLS modeling. This model is beneficial for analyzing systems with closely related spatial dimensions, such as image filtering and thermal processes. Bose [14] examined the fundamental ideas and revelations of TDLS theory. His work mainly concentrated on signal processing applications, system realization, and stability analysis. This work laid the groundwork for understanding the structural and behavioral characteristics of TDLSs. Kaczorek [15] studied TDLSs, focusing on their mathematical formulation and solution methods. He investigated the positive systems based on the ideas previously introduced in the literature. Galkowski [16] contributed theoretically by developing the state-space realizations of TDLSs and extending them into higher-dimensional systems. Farina and Rinaldi [17] studied positive linear systems with their applications. They also extended their work in the broader context of the TDLS. Oldham and Spanier [18] presented the basic concepts, definitions, and characteristics of fractional calculus, which are essential for future studies. Miller and Ross [19] explored fractional differential equations, emphasizing their applications across various fields by establishing connections between abstract mathematics and real-world problem-solving. Podlubny [20] discussed fractional differential equations and demonstrated their importance in simulating complex systems in control theory and engineering. Kaczorek [21] introduced the concept of fractional-order discrete TDLSs, laying the groundwork for further research into fractional-order dynamics. Rogowski [22] developed a general response formula for solving the FTDCT linear system of the Roesser structure with its applications. Kaczorek and Rogowski [23] studied the descriptor case of continuous fractional-order TDLSs. Their work broadened the applicability and understanding of fractional systems in multi-dimensional contexts. Rogowski [24] studied the behavior of fractional-order TDLSs described by the Roesser type. Idczak et al. [25] examined the solution of an FTDCT linear system of the first FM type, incorporating Riemann–Liouville (RL) fractional-order partial derivatives. Their findings provided valuable insights into how such derivatives influence the dynamics and behavior of these systems. Rogowski [26] examined the FM model's positive analysis for continuous fractional-order TDLSs. Using the Roesser model, Hu et al. [27] investigated the event-triggered control methods for continuous TDLSs. Reducing communication frequency and minimizing dependency on global information are the goals of this strategy. The stability of generalized nonlinear homogeneous systems in the presence of bounded disturbances was examined by Huang et al. [28]. The conditions under which these systems maintain their stability in the face of external perturbations were carefully studied in this work. Using the concept of bounded disturbances, Ma et al. [29] investigated the estimation of the reachable set for 2D switched nonlinear positive systems, taking time-varying delays and delayed impulsive effects into account. Using the Roesser framework, Dami and Benzaouia [30] presented a new kind of 2D fractional switched system. To use state feedback controllers to stabilize the system, the study also investigated sufficient conditions (SCs). Under the Roesser framework, Huang et al. [31] examined the finite-time stability (FTS) of 2D positive systems. The study employed a co-positive Lyapunov function to construct SCs to accomplish FTS in the system. In the framework of the Roesser model, Gao et al. [32] examined the SCs for the FTS and finite-time control (FTC) of 2D systems. To mitigate the effect of stable bounded disturbance inputs on TDLSs in the Roesser framework, Ahn et al. [33] introduced a linear matrix inequality (LME) condition. The analysis used discrete Jensen inequality (DJI) and diagonally dominant matrices (DDMs). Nemati and Mamehrashi [34] developed the numerical scheme for 2D fractional optimal control systems using Legendre polynomials, the Ritz approach, and the Laplace transform technique. They also analyzed the convergence with two illustrative examples.

Zhang et al. [35] analyzed the necessary SCs for the stability of the 2D fractional first FM model. They presented these conditions with respect to polynomials and LMEs using the Kronecker product. Zhu and Lu [36] discussed the robust stability of the second 2D FM continuous fractional-order model in the presence of interval uncertainties. They determined the LMI-based stability conditions using the nominal fractional-order model, which was presented in terms of stable root clustering sets. Zhang and Wang [37] formulated the concepts of finite-region stability and boundedness of the 2D fractional-order second FM model and then analyzed the transient behavior of such systems. Benyettou et al. [38] determined the solution procedure of conformable fractional TDLSs by applying the Laplace and Sumudu transform techniques. Benyettou et al. [39] formulated the solution to the minimum energy control problem for fractional TDLSs described by the first FM model. Yan et al. [40] developed the state-space formulation for the 2D frequency transformation in the second FM model, which enables a more flexible tool for 2D zero-phase filters to prevent image distortions. Li and Hou [41] introduced the parametric controller method for TDLSs using polynomial discriminant systems and the Hurwitz theorem. The main contributions of the proposed work in this area are summarized as follows:

1. Two classes of FFTDCT linear systems are introduced and investigated to address uncertainty and fuzziness in system parameters.
2. The fuzzy solution of FFTDCT linear systems based on the Roesser model and the second FM model is obtained under one-dimensional 2D partial fractional granular Caputo derivatives.
3. The potential solution of the proposed model is determined using the 2D granular Laplace transform.
4. Real-world applications, including signal processing systems and wireless sensor network data fusion, are solved using the proposed technique.

The rest of the article is organized as follows: some fundamental concepts of the granular representation of the fuzzy number, 2D granular fractional integral (GFI), 2D granular Caputo fractional derivatives (GCFDs), and 2D granular Laplace transform are presented in Section 2. The fuzzy solution of the granular FFTDCT Roesser model using the granular 2D fuzzy Laplace transform is determined in Section 3. The fuzzy solution of the granular FFTDCT described by the second FM model is extracted in Section 4. The applications of the FFTDCT linear system described by Roesser and FM's second model are discussed in Section 5. Section 6 outlines the conclusion of the article.

2. Fuzzy Preliminaries

This section introduces the basic concepts of fuzzy analysis, including granular representations and their associated operations. Subsequently, we define the two-dimensional Riemann–Liouville (2DRL) fractional integral and the fractional derivative in Caputo sense. Moreover, we extend these concepts with the granular counterparts through the two-dimensional GFI and two-dimensional GCFD. The section further develops the theoretical framework by presenting the 2D granular Laplace transform and examining its key properties.

A fuzzy set $\mathfrak{m}$ [42] $\mathfrak{m} : [a,b] \subseteq \mathbb{R} \longrightarrow [0,1]$ is referred to as the fuzzy number (FN) if it adheres to the following properties: normal, upper semicontinuity, convex and has compact support. Let $\Xi_{\mathbb{R}}$ denote the class of all FNs on $\mathbb{R}$. The ϑ-cut of $\mathfrak{m}$ is denoted by $[\mathfrak{m}]^{\vartheta}$ and is defined by $[\mathfrak{m}]^{\vartheta} = [\mathfrak{m}^{-}_{\vartheta}, \mathfrak{m}^{+}_{\vartheta}]$, for all $0 \leq \vartheta \leq 1$.

Definition 1 ([9]). *Let $\mathfrak{m}$ be an FN; the granular representation of $\mathfrak{m}$ is defined as $\mathfrak{m}^{gr} : [0,1] \times [0,1] \longrightarrow [a,b]$, where $(\vartheta, \pi) \mapsto \mathfrak{m}^{\mathfrak{gr}}(\vartheta,\pi) = \mathfrak{m}^{-}_{\vartheta} + (\mathfrak{m}^{+}_{\vartheta} - \mathfrak{m}^{-}_{\vartheta})\pi$. Here, "gr" denotes the granular representation of $\mathfrak{m}$ over the interval $x \in [a,b]$, with $\vartheta \in [0,1]$ and $\pi \in [0,1]$. The HMF of FN $\mathfrak{m}$ is represented by $\mathbb{H}(\mathfrak{m})$ and is defined by $\mathbb{H}(\mathfrak{m}) \triangleq \mathfrak{m}^{\mathfrak{gr}}(\vartheta,\pi)$.*

We now provide Table 1, which includes various commonly used notations.

Table 1. Summary of notations.

Notation	Description	Location
$\Xi_{\mathbb{R}}$	The collection of all FNs on $\mathbb{R}$	Section 2
$\mathbb{H}(\mathfrak{m}) \triangleq \mathfrak{m}^{gr}(\vartheta, \pi)$	The HMF of the FN $\mathfrak{m} \in \Xi_{\mathbb{R}}$	Section 2
$I_{z_i}^{\alpha_i}$	The 2DRL fractional integral of order α_i regarding the variable z_i (i = 1, 2)	Definition 9
${}^{C}D_{z_i}^{\alpha_i}$	The 2D Caputo fractional derivative (CFD) of order $\alpha_i > 0$ regarding variable z_i $(i = 1, 2)$	Definition 12
$\mathcal{L}_{z_1,z_2}$	The 2D Laplace transform regarding z_1 and z_2	Definition 16
$\mathfrak{L}_{z_1,z_2}$	The 2D granular Laplace transform regarding z_1 and z_2	Definition 18
${}^{gr}\mathcal{I}_{z_i}^{\alpha_i}$	The GFI of order α_i regarding z_i (i = 1, 2)	Definition 13
${}^{gr}\mathcal{D}_{z_i}^{\alpha_i}$	The two-dimensional GCFD of order $\alpha_i > 0$ regarding z_i (i = 1, 2)	Definition 14
$I_{z_1}^{\alpha} \varkappa(z_1, z_2)$	FI of order $\alpha > 0$ of $\varkappa(z_1, z_2)$ regarding the variable z_1	Definition 8

Definition 2 ([9])**.** *The ϑ-cut of $\mathfrak{m} \in \Xi_{\mathbb{R}}$ can be represented by the following formula*

$$\mathbb{H}^{-1}(\mathfrak{m}^{gr}(\vartheta, \pi)) := [\mathfrak{m}]^{\vartheta} := \left[\inf_{\eta \geq \vartheta} \min_{\pi} \mathfrak{m}^{gr}(\eta, \pi), \sup_{\eta \geq \vartheta} \max_{\pi} \mathfrak{m}^{gr}(\eta, \pi) \right]. \tag{1}$$

Definition 3 ([9])**.** *The arithmetic operations of two FNs, $\mathfrak{m}_1$ and $\mathfrak{m}_2$, with their HMFs, $\mathbb{H}(\mathfrak{m}_1)$ and $\mathbb{H}(\mathfrak{m}_2)$, respectively, are defined by*

$$\mathbb{H}(\mathfrak{m}_1 \odot \mathfrak{m}_2) = \mathbb{H}(\mathfrak{m}_1) \bullet \mathbb{H}(\mathfrak{m}_2), \tag{2}$$

where $\odot$ and $\bullet$ denote the arithmetic operations on $\Xi_{\mathbb{R}}$ and $\mathbb{R}$, respectively, such as addition, subtraction, multiplication, or division.

Definition 4 ([9])**.** *Suppose $\varkappa : [a, b] \subseteq \mathbb{R} \to \Xi_{\mathbb{R}}$ is a fuzzy function that includes $\mathfrak{m}_1, \mathfrak{m}_2, \mathfrak{m}_3, \ldots, \mathfrak{m}_n$ FNs. The HMF of $\varkappa(z)$, represented by $\mathbb{H}(\varkappa(z)) \triangleq \varkappa^{gr}(z, \vartheta, \pi)$, is described by the given relation*

$$\varkappa^{gr} : [a, b] \times [0, 1] \times [0, 1]^n \to \mathbb{R}, \text{ where } \vartheta \in [0, 1] \text{ and } \pi \triangleq (\pi_{\mathfrak{m}_1}, \pi_{\mathfrak{m}_2}, \ldots, \pi_{\mathfrak{m}_n}). \tag{3}$$

Definition 5 ([43])**.** *Let $\mathfrak{m}_1, \mathfrak{m}_2, \mathfrak{m}_3 \in \Xi_{\mathbb{R}}$, and λ be a real number. Then, the below claims hold:*

(i). $\rho^{gr}(\mathfrak{m}_1 + \mathfrak{m}_3, \mathfrak{m}_2 + \mathfrak{m}_3) = \rho^{gr}(\mathfrak{m}_1, \mathfrak{m}_2)$.
(ii). $\rho^{gr}(\lambda \mathfrak{m}_1, \lambda \mathfrak{m}_2) = |\lambda| \rho^{gr}(\mathfrak{m}_1, \mathfrak{m}_2)$.
(iii). $\rho^{gr}(\mathfrak{m}_1 \ominus^{gr} \mathfrak{m}_2, \hat{0}) = \rho^{gr}(\mathfrak{m}_1, \mathfrak{m}_2)$.

2.1. Fuzzy Fractional Calculus

Definition 6 ([9])**.** *Let $\varkappa : (a, b) \subseteq \mathbb{R} \longrightarrow \Xi_{\mathbb{R}}$ be an FVF. The function $\varkappa$ is said to be GRD at $z \in (a, b)$ if there exists $\varkappa'_{gr}(z) \in \Xi_{\mathbb{R}}$ such that the following limit*

$$\varkappa'_{gr}(z) = \lim_{\epsilon \to 0} \frac{\varkappa(z + \epsilon) \ominus^{gr} \varkappa(z)}{\epsilon}, \tag{4}$$

exists.

Definition 7. *The fractional integral (FI) of $\varkappa \in L^1([a,b],\mathbb{R})$ of order $\alpha > 0$, denoted by $I^{\alpha}_{a^+}$, is defined by*

$$I^{\alpha}_{a^+}\varkappa(z) = \frac{1}{\Gamma(\alpha)}\int_a^z (z-\tau)^{\alpha-1}\varkappa(\tau)d\tau. \tag{5}$$

Definition 8 ([20,44]). *The FI of order $\alpha > 0$ of $\varkappa(z_1,z_2)$ regarding the variable z_1 is defined by*

$$I^{\alpha}_{z_1}\varkappa(z_1,z_2) = \frac{1}{\Gamma(\alpha)}\int_a^{z_1} (z_1-\tau)^{\alpha-1}\varkappa(\tau,z_2)d\tau. \tag{6}$$

Similarly, we can define the RL fractional integral of a 2D continuous function $\varkappa(z_1,z_2)$ regarding z_2.

Now, we define the following Definition 9 for the 2DRL fractional integral regarding the variables z_1 and z_2 based on Definition 8, as follows:

Definition 9 ([20,44]). *The two-dimensional RL fractional integral of order α_i of a continuous function $\varkappa(z_1,z_2)$ regarding variable z_i $(i=1,2)$ is given by the formula*

$$I^{\alpha_i}_{z_i}\varkappa(z_1,z_2) = \frac{1}{\Gamma(\alpha_i)}\int_a^{z_i} (z_i-\tau)^{\alpha_i-1}\varkappa(\tau)d\tau,$$

where

$$\varkappa(\tau) = \begin{cases} \varkappa(\tau,z_2) & \text{for } i=1, \\ \varkappa(z_1,\tau) & \text{for } i=2. \end{cases}$$

Definition 10. *The CFD of order $\alpha > 0$, denoted by ${}^{C}D^{\alpha}_{a^+}$, of a function $\varkappa \in C^1([a,b],\mathbb{R})$, is defined by*

$${}^{C}D^{\alpha}_{a^+}\varkappa(z) := \frac{1}{\Gamma(n-\alpha)}\int_a^z (z-\tau)^{n-\alpha-1}\varkappa^{(n)}(\tau)d\tau, \tag{7}$$

where $n \in \mathbb{N}$, such that $n-1 < \alpha < n$, and $z \in [a,b]$.

Definition 11 ([22,23]). *The CFD of order $\alpha > 0$ of a 2D continuous function $\varkappa(z_1,z_2)$ regarding variable z_1 is given by*

$${}^{C}D^{\alpha}_{a^+}\varkappa(z_1,z_2) = \frac{1}{\Gamma(n-\alpha)}\int_a^{z_1} \frac{f^{(n)}(\tau,z_2)}{(z_1-\tau)^{\alpha-n+1}}d\tau,$$

where $n-1 \leq \alpha < n$. Similarly, we can define the aforementioned CFD of a 2D continuous function $\varkappa(z_1,z_2)$ regarding z_2.

We now define the following Definition 12 for the two-dimensional Caputo fractional derivative (2DCFD) regarding the variables z_1 and z_2 based on Definition 11, as follows:

Definition 12 ([22,23]). *The 2DCFD of order $\alpha_i > 0$ of a continuous function $\varkappa(z_1,z_2)$ regarding variable z_i $(i=1,2)$ is given by*

$${}^{C}D^{\alpha_i}_{z_i}\varkappa(z_1,z_2) = \frac{1}{\Gamma(n_i-\alpha_i)}\int_a^{z_i} \frac{f^{(n_i)}(\tau)}{(z_i-\tau)^{\alpha_i-n_i+1}}d\tau,$$

where $n_i - 1 \leq \alpha_i < n_i$, *and*

$$f^{(n_i)}(\tau) = \begin{cases} \frac{\partial^{n_i}}{\partial \tau^{n_i}} \varkappa(\tau, z_2) & \text{for } i = 1, \\ \frac{\partial^{n_i}}{\partial \tau^{n_i}} \varkappa(z_1, \tau) & \text{for } i = 2. \end{cases}$$

Based on Definition 9, we present the idea of the GFI of FVFs as follows:

Definition 13. *Let* $\varkappa : [a_1, b_1] \times [a_2, b_2] \subset \mathbb{R}^2 \longrightarrow \mathbb{E}_{\mathbb{R}}$. *The GFI of order* $\alpha_i \in (0, 1]$ *of FVF is defined by*

$${}^{gr}\mathcal{I}^{\alpha_i}_{z_i} \varkappa(z_1, z_2) = \frac{1}{\Gamma(\alpha_i)} \int_a^{t_i} (t_i - \tau)^{\alpha_i - 1} \varkappa(\tau) d\tau,$$

where $\varkappa(\tau)$ *is* $\varkappa(\tau, z_2)$ *for* $i = 1$ *and* $\varkappa(z_1, \tau)$ *for* $i = 2$, *respectively.*

Remark 1. *According to Definition 13, the HMF of granular fractional integral* ${}^{gr}\mathcal{I}^{\alpha_i}_{z_i} \varkappa(z_1, z_2)$ *is defined by*

$$\begin{aligned} \mathbb{H}({}^{gr}\mathcal{I}^{\alpha_i}_{z_i} \varkappa(z_1, z_2)) &= \frac{1}{\Gamma(\alpha_i)} \int_a^{z_i} \mathbb{H}((z_i - \tau)^{\alpha_i - 1} \varkappa(\tau)) d\tau, \\ &= \frac{1}{\Gamma(\alpha_i)} \int_a^{z_i} (z_i - \tau)^{\alpha_i - 1} \mathbb{H}(\varkappa(\tau)) d\tau, \\ &= I^{\alpha_i}_{z_i} \mathbb{H}(\varkappa(\tau)). \end{aligned}$$

Thus, $\mathbb{H}({}^{gr}\mathcal{I}^{\alpha_i}_{z_i} \varkappa(z_1, z_2)) = I^{\alpha_i}_{z_i} \mathbb{H}(\varkappa(\tau))$, *where* $\varkappa(\tau)$ *is* $\varkappa(\tau, z_2)$ *for* $i = 1$ *and* $\varkappa(z_1, \tau)$ *for* $i = 2$, *respectively.*

Definition 14. *Let* $\varkappa : [a_1, b_1] \times [a_2, b_2] \subset \mathbb{R}^2 \longrightarrow \mathbb{E}_{\mathbb{R}}$. *The 2D GCFD of order* $\alpha_i \in (0, 1]$ *of the FVF* $\varkappa(z_1, z_2)$ *regarding variable* z_i $(i = 1, 2)$ *is defined by*

$${}^{gr}\mathcal{D}^{\alpha_i}_{z_i} \varkappa(z_1, z_2) = \frac{1}{\Gamma(1 - \alpha_i)} \int_a^{z_i} \frac{\varkappa'_{gr}(\tau)}{(z_i - \tau)^{\alpha_i}} d\tau,$$

where $\varkappa'_{gr}(\tau)$ *is equal to* $\frac{\partial}{\partial \tau} \varkappa_{gr}(\tau, z_2)$ *for* $i = 1$ *and* $\frac{\partial}{\partial \tau} \varkappa_{gr}(z_1, \tau)$ *for* $i = 2$, *respectively.*

Remark 2. *Similar to Remark 1, we may also infer the following:*

$$\mathbb{H}({}^{gr}\mathcal{D}^{\alpha_i}_{z_i} \varkappa(z_1, z_2)) = {}^{C}D^{\alpha_i}_{z_i} \mathbb{H}(\varkappa(z_1, z_2)). \tag{8}$$

2.2. Granular 2D Laplace Transform for FVF

First, we review some fundamental concepts and terminology related to the Laplace transform of a 2D continuous function. Next, we present the granular 2D Laplace transform of FVF and HMF.

Definition 15 ([20,23,45]). *Let* $\varkappa(p, z_2)$ *and* $\varkappa(z_1, s)$ *denote the Laplace transforms of a 2D continuous function* $\varkappa(z_1, z_2)$ *regarding* z_1 *and* z_2, *respectively. The following formulas define these transforms:*

$$\mathcal{L}_{z_1}[\varkappa(z_1, z_2)] := \int_0^{\infty} \varkappa(z_1, z_2) e^{-p z_1} dz_1, \; \mathcal{L}_{z_2}[\varkappa(z_1, z_2)] := \int_0^{\infty} \varkappa(z_1, z_2) e^{-s z_2} dz_2.$$

Definition 16 ([20,23,45]). *Suppose* $\varkappa(z_1, z_2)$ *is the real-valued continuous function from* $[0, \infty) \times [0, \infty)$ *to* $\mathbb{R}$ *such that the 2D Laplace transform of* $\varkappa(z_1, z_2)$, *denoted by* $\chi(p, s)$ *and defined by*

$$\chi(p,s) = \mathcal{L}_{z_1,z_2}\Big[\varkappa(z_1,z_2)\Big] = \mathcal{L}_{z_1}\Big\{\mathcal{L}_{z_2}\Big[\varkappa(z_1,z_2)\Big]\Big\} = \mathcal{L}_{z_2}\Big\{\mathcal{L}_{z_1}\Big[\varkappa(z_1,z_2)\Big]\Big\}$$
$$= \int_0^\infty \int_0^\infty \varkappa(z_1,z_2)e^{-pz_1-sz_2}dz_1dz_2, \tag{9}$$

for all $p, s \in \mathbb{C}$ for which the integral in Equation (9) converges.

Definition 17 ([22,23])**.** *The 2D Laplace transform of Definition 9 is given by*

$$\mathcal{L}_{z_1,z_2}[I_{z_1}^{\alpha_1}\varkappa(z_1,z_2)] = p^{-\alpha_1}\chi(p,s) \text{ and } \mathcal{L}_{z_1,z_2}[I_{z_2}^{\alpha_2}\varkappa(z_1,z_2)] = s^{-\alpha_2}\chi(p,s). \tag{10}$$

Furthermore,

$$\mathcal{L}_{z_1}\left[\frac{t_1^{\alpha_1-1}}{\Gamma(\alpha_1)}\right] = p^{-\alpha_1} \text{ and } \mathcal{L}_{z_2}\left[\frac{t_2^{\alpha_2-1}}{\Gamma(\alpha_2)}\right] = s^{-\alpha_2}, \tag{11}$$

for $\alpha_1 > 0$ and $\alpha_2 > 0$.

Theorem 1 ([22,23])**.** *The 2D Laplace transform of Definition 12 of the 2D function $\varkappa(z_1,z_2)$ regarding z_1 and z_2 is defined by*

$$\mathcal{L}_{z_1,z_2}\left[{}_{0+}^{C}D^{\alpha_1}\varkappa(z_1,z_2)\right] = p^{\alpha_1}\varkappa(p,s) - \sum_{k=1}^{n_1} p^{\alpha_1-k}F^{(k-1)}(0,s) \tag{12}$$

and

$$\mathcal{L}_{z_1,z_2}\left[{}_{0+}^{C}D^{\alpha_2}\varkappa(z_1,z_2)\right] = s^{\alpha_2}\varkappa(p,s) - \sum_{l=1}^{n_2} s^{\alpha_2-l}F^{(l-1)}(p,0), \tag{13}$$

respectively, where $F^{(k)}(0,s) = \mathcal{L}_{z_2}\left\{\frac{\partial^k}{\partial z_1^k}\varkappa(z_1,z_2)|_{z_1=0}\right\}$ and $F^{(l)}(p,0) = \mathcal{L}_{z_1}\left\{\frac{\partial^l}{\partial z_2^l}\varkappa(z_1,z_2)|_{z_2=0}\right\}$ for $k,l \in \mathbb{Z}_+$. Combining Equations (12) and (13), we get

$$\mathcal{L}_{z_1,z_2}\left[{}_{0+}^{C}D^{\alpha_1,\alpha_2}\varkappa(z_1,z_2)\right] = p^{\alpha_1}s^{\alpha_2}\varkappa(p,s) - \sum_{k=1}^{n_1}\sum_{l=1}^{n_2} p^{\alpha_1-k}s^{\alpha_2-l}F^{(k-1,l-1)}(0,0)$$
$$- p^{\alpha_1}\sum_{l=1}^{n_2} s^{\alpha_2-l}F^{(l-1)}(p,0) - s^{\alpha_2}\sum_{k=1}^{n_1} p^{\alpha_1-l}F^{(k-1)}(0,s), \tag{14}$$

where $F^{(k,l)}(0,0) = \left[\frac{\partial^k}{\partial z_1^k}\frac{\partial^l}{\partial z_2^l}\varkappa(z_1,z_2)|_{z_1=0,z_2=0}\right]$ for $k,l \in \mathbb{Z}_+$.

Definition 18. *Suppose $\varkappa(z_1,z_2)$ is the continuous FVF such that $e^{-pz_1-sz_2}\varkappa(z_1,z_2)$ is the improper fuzzy Riemann-integrable on $[0,\infty)\times[0,\infty)$, and then $\mathfrak{L}_{z_1,z_2}[\varkappa(z_1,z_2)]$ is called the granular 2D Laplace transform of $\varkappa(z_1,z_2)$ and is defined by*

$$\mathfrak{L}_{z_1,z_2}[\varkappa(z_1,z_2)] = \int_0^\infty \int_0^\infty e^{-pz_1-sz_2}\varkappa(z_1,z_2)dz_1dz_2, \tag{15}$$

where $p, s > 0$ are integers.

Remark 3. *The HMF of Definition 18 is defined by*

$$\mathbb{H}\Big(\mathfrak{L}_{z_1,z_2}[\varkappa(z_1,z_2)]\Big) = \int_0^\infty \int_0^\infty \mathbb{H}(e^{-pz_1-sz_2}\varkappa(z_1,z_2))dz_1dz_2,$$
$$= \int_0^\infty \int_0^\infty e^{-pz_1-sz_2}\mathbb{H}(\varkappa(z_1,z_2))dz_1dz_2,$$

$$= \mathcal{L}_{z_1,z_2}\left[\mathbb{H}\left(\varkappa(z_1,z_2)\right)\right]. \tag{16}$$

3. Granular FFTDCT Linear Systems in the Roesser Framework

In this section, we derive the fuzzy solution of the granular FFTDCT Roesser model using the granular 2D fuzzy Laplace transform. To achieve this, we first define the granular FFTDCT linear system governed by the following state equations:

$$\begin{bmatrix} {}^{gr}_{0^+}\mathcal{D}^{\alpha_1}\varkappa_1(z_1,z_2) \\ {}^{gr}_{0^+}\mathcal{D}^{\alpha_2}\varkappa_2(z_1,z_2) \end{bmatrix} = A\begin{bmatrix} \varkappa_1(z_1,z_2) \\ \varkappa_2(z_1,z_2) \end{bmatrix} + Bu(z_1,z_2), \tag{17}$$

$$y(z_1,z_2) = C\begin{bmatrix} \varkappa_1(z_1,z_2) \\ \varkappa_2(z_1,z_2) \end{bmatrix} + Du(z_1,z_2), \tag{18}$$

where $A = [a_{ij}]$, $B = [b_i]$ for $i,j = 1,2$, $\varkappa_1(z_1,z_2) \in \Xi_{\mathbb{R}}^{n_1}$, and $\varkappa_2(z_1,z_2) \in \Xi_{\mathbb{R}}^{n_2}$ $(n = n_1 + n_2)$ are the fuzzy horizontal and fuzzy vertical state vectors, respectively. Moreover, $u(z_1,z_2) \in \Xi_{\mathbb{R}}^{m}$ and $y(z_1,z_2) \in \Xi_{\mathbb{R}}^{p}$ are the fuzzy inputs and output vectors of the system. Furthermore, $A \in \Xi_{\mathbb{R}}^{n_i\times j}$, $B \in \Xi_{\mathbb{R}}^{n_i\times m}$, $C \in \Xi_{\mathbb{R}}^{p\times n}$, and $D \in \Xi_{\mathbb{R}}^{p\times m}$ are the fuzzy matrices. For simplicity, we consider the system (17) with fractional orders $\alpha_1,\alpha_2 \in (0,1)$.

Note 1. *Let $\Xi_{\mathbb{R}}^{n\times n}$ be the class of all fuzzy matrices of size n and $\Xi_{\mathbb{R}}^{n} = \Xi_{\mathbb{R}}^{n\times 1}$. Moreover, I_n is the identity matrix of size n.*

Theorem 2. *The HMF of the fuzzy solution of system (17) with fractional orders $0 < \alpha_1 < 1$, $0 < \alpha_2 < 1$ for arbitrary fuzzy input $u(z_1,z_2)$ is given by the following*

$$\begin{aligned}
\begin{bmatrix} \mathbb{H}(\varkappa_1(z_1,z_2)) \\ \mathbb{H}(\varkappa_2(z_1,z_2)) \end{bmatrix} &= \sum_{i=0}^{\infty}\sum_{j=1}^{\infty}\mathbb{H}(T_{ij})\left(\begin{bmatrix} \frac{z_1^{i\alpha_1}}{\Gamma(1+i\alpha_1)}\frac{1}{\Gamma((j\alpha_2))}\int_0^{z_2}(z_2-\tau_2)^{j\alpha_2-1}\mathbb{H}(\varkappa_1(0,\tau_2))d\tau_2 \\ 0 \end{bmatrix}\right. \\
&+\left.\begin{bmatrix} \frac{\mathbb{H}(b_1)}{\Gamma((i+1)\alpha_1)\Gamma(j\alpha_2)}\int_0^{z_1}\int_0^{z_2}(z_1-\tau_1)^{(i+1)\alpha_1-1}(z_2-\tau_2)^{j\alpha_2-1}\mathbb{H}(u(\tau_1,\tau_2))d\tau_2 d\tau_1 \\ 0 \end{bmatrix}\right) \\
&+\sum_{i=0}^{\infty}\mathbb{H}(T_{i0})\left(\begin{bmatrix} \frac{z_1^{i\alpha_1}}{\Gamma(1+i\alpha_1)}\mathbb{H}(\varkappa_1(0,z_2)) \\ 0 \end{bmatrix} + \begin{bmatrix} \frac{\mathbb{H}(b_1)}{\Gamma((i+1)\alpha_1)}\int_0^{z_1}(z_1-\tau_1)^{(i+1)\alpha_1-1}\mathbb{H}(u(\tau_1,z_2))d\tau_1 \\ 0 \end{bmatrix}\right) \\
&+\sum_{i=1}^{\infty}\sum_{j=0}^{\infty}\mathbb{H}(T_{ij})\left(\begin{bmatrix} 0 \\ \frac{z_2^{j\alpha_2}}{\Gamma(1+j\alpha_2)}\frac{1}{\Gamma((i\alpha_1))}\int_0^{z_1}(z_1-\tau_1)^{i\alpha_1-1}\mathbb{H}(\varkappa_2(\tau_1,0))d\tau_1 \end{bmatrix}\right. \\
&+\left.\begin{bmatrix} 0 \\ \frac{\mathbb{H}(b_2)}{\Gamma(i\alpha_1)\Gamma((j+1)\alpha_2)}\int_0^{z_1}\int_0^{z_2}(z_1-\tau_1)^{i\alpha_1-1}(z_2-\tau_2)^{(j+1)\alpha_2-1}\mathbb{H}(u(\tau_1,\tau_2))d\tau_2 d\tau_1 \end{bmatrix}\right) \\
&+\sum_{i=0}^{\infty}\mathbb{H}(T_{0j})\left(\begin{bmatrix} 0 \\ \frac{z_1^{j\alpha_2}}{\Gamma(1+j\alpha_2)}\mathbb{H}(\varkappa_2(z_1,0)) \end{bmatrix} + \begin{bmatrix} 0 \\ \frac{\mathbb{H}(b_2)}{\Gamma((j+1)\alpha_2)}\int_0^{z_2}(z_2-\tau_2)^{(j+1)\alpha_2-1}\mathbb{H}(u(z_1,\tau_2))d\tau_2 \end{bmatrix}\right).
\end{aligned} \tag{19}$$

with the fuzzy transition matrices given in Equation (29).

Proof. For each $z_1, z_2 \in [0, T]$, applying the 2D FLT on both sides to the system (17) and using the Linearity property, we get

$$\begin{bmatrix} \mathfrak{L}_{z_1,z_2}\left[{}^{gr}_{0+}\mathcal{D}^{\alpha_1}\varkappa_1(z_1,z_2)\right] \\ \mathfrak{L}_{z_1,z_2}\left[{}^{gr}_{0+}\mathcal{D}^{\alpha_2}\varkappa_2(z_1,z_2)\right] \end{bmatrix} = \begin{bmatrix} a_{11} & a_{12} \\ a_{21} & a_{22} \end{bmatrix} \begin{bmatrix} \mathfrak{L}_{z_1,z_2}[\varkappa_1(z_1,z_2)] \\ \mathfrak{L}_{z_1,z_2}[\varkappa_2(z_1,z_2)] \end{bmatrix} + \begin{bmatrix} b_1 \\ b_2 \end{bmatrix} \mathfrak{L}_{z_1,z_2}[u(z_1,z_2)]. \quad (20)$$

Applying the HMF to Equation (20) and utilizing Remark 3, we get

$$\begin{bmatrix} \mathcal{L}_{z_1,z_2}\left[\mathbb{H}\left({}^{gr}_{0+}\mathcal{D}^{\alpha_1}\varkappa_1\right)(z_1,z_2)\right] \\ \mathcal{L}_{z_1,z_2}\left[\mathbb{H}\left({}^{gr}_{0+}\mathcal{D}^{\alpha_2}\varkappa_2\right)(z_1,z_2)\right] \end{bmatrix} = \begin{bmatrix} \mathbb{H}(a_{11}) & \mathbb{H}(a_{12}) \\ \mathbb{H}(a_{21}) & \mathbb{H}(a_{22}) \end{bmatrix} \begin{bmatrix} \mathcal{L}_{z_1,z_2}[\mathbb{H}(\varkappa_1(z_1,z_2))] \\ \mathcal{L}_{z_1,z_2}[\mathbb{H}(\varkappa_2(z_1,z_2))] \end{bmatrix} + \begin{bmatrix} \mathbb{H}(b_1) \\ \mathbb{H}(b_2) \end{bmatrix} \mathcal{L}_{z_1,z_2}[\mathbb{H}(u(z_1,z_2))]. \quad (21)$$

Using Remark 2, the above Equation (21) transforms into the following equation

$$\begin{bmatrix} \mathcal{L}_{z_1,z_2}\left[{}^{C}_{0+}D^{\alpha_1}\mathbb{H}(\varkappa_1(z_1,z_2))\right] \\ \mathcal{L}_{z_1,z_2}\left[{}^{C}_{0+}D^{\alpha_2}\mathbb{H}(\varkappa_2(z_1,z_2))\right] \end{bmatrix} = \begin{bmatrix} \mathbb{H}(a_{11}) & \mathbb{H}(a_{12}) \\ \mathbb{H}(a_{21}) & \mathbb{H}(a_{22}) \end{bmatrix} \begin{bmatrix} \mathcal{L}_{z_1,z_2}[\mathbb{H}(\varkappa_1(z_1,z_2))] \\ \mathcal{L}_{z_1,z_2}[\mathbb{H}(\varkappa_2(z_1,z_2))] \end{bmatrix} + \begin{bmatrix} \mathbb{H}(b_1) \\ \mathbb{H}(b_2) \end{bmatrix} \mathcal{L}_{z_1,z_2}[\mathbb{H}(u(z_1,z_2))]. \quad (22)$$

Applying Theorem 1, Equation (22) can be written in the following form

$$\begin{bmatrix} p^{\alpha_1}\mathbb{H}(\chi_1(p,s)) - p^{\alpha_1-1}\mathbb{H}(\chi_1(0,s)) \\ s^{\alpha_2}\mathbb{H}(\chi_2(p,s)) - s^{\alpha_2-1}\mathbb{H}(\chi_2(p,0)) \end{bmatrix} = \begin{bmatrix} \mathbb{H}(a_{11}) & \mathbb{H}(a_{12}) \\ \mathbb{H}(a_{21}) & \mathbb{H}(a_{22}) \end{bmatrix} \begin{bmatrix} \mathbb{H}(\chi_1(p,s)) \\ \mathbb{H}(\chi_2(p,s)) \end{bmatrix} + \begin{bmatrix} \mathbb{H}(b_1) \\ \mathbb{H}(b_2) \end{bmatrix} \mathbb{H}(\mathcal{U}(p,s)), \quad (23)$$

where $\mathbb{H}(\chi_1(p,s)) = \mathcal{L}_{z_1,z_2}\{\mathbb{H}(\varkappa_1(z_1,z_2))\}$, $\mathbb{H}(\chi_2(p,s)) = \mathcal{L}_{z_1,z_2}\{\mathbb{H}(\varkappa_2(z_1,z_2))\}$, $\mathbb{H}(\chi_2(p,0)) = \mathcal{L}_{z_1}\{\mathbb{H}(\varkappa_2(z_1,0))\}$, and $\mathbb{H}(\chi_1(0,s)) = \mathcal{L}_{z_2}\{\mathbb{H}(\varkappa_1(0,z_2))\}$. Pre-multiply Equation (23) by the matrix $\begin{bmatrix} p^{-\alpha_1}I_{n_1} & 0 \\ 0 & p^{-\alpha_2}I_{n_2} \end{bmatrix}$. Here, I_{n_1} and I_{n_2} are the identity matrices of orders $n_1 \times n_1$ and $n_2 \times n_2$, respectively. We obtain

$$\begin{bmatrix} \mathbb{H}(\chi_1(p,s)) \\ \mathbb{H}(\chi_2(p,s)) \end{bmatrix} = \begin{bmatrix} I_{n_1} - p^{-\alpha_1}a_{11} & -p^{-\alpha_1}A_{12} \\ -s^{-\alpha_2}A_{21} & I_{n_2} - s^{-\alpha_2}a_{22} \end{bmatrix}^{-1} \times \left(\begin{bmatrix} -p^{-1}\mathbb{H}(\chi_1(0,s)) \\ -s^{-1}\mathbb{H}(\chi_2(p,0)) \end{bmatrix} + \begin{bmatrix} p^{-\alpha_1}\mathbb{H}(b_1) \\ s^{-\alpha_2}\mathbb{H}(b_2) \end{bmatrix} \mathbb{H}(\mathcal{U}(p,s)) \right). \quad (24)$$

Suppose

$$Q(p,s) = \begin{bmatrix} I_{n_1} - p^{-\alpha_1}a_{11} & -p^{-\alpha_1}A_{12} \\ -s^{-\alpha_2}A_{21} & I_{n_2} - s^{-\alpha_2}a_{22} \end{bmatrix}. \quad (25)$$

Equation (24) can be written in the following form

$$\begin{bmatrix} \mathbb{H}(\chi_1(p,s)) \\ \mathbb{H}(\chi_2(p,s)) \end{bmatrix} = Q^{-1}(p,s) \times \left(\begin{bmatrix} -p^{-1}\mathbb{H}(\chi_1(0,s)) \\ -s^{-1}\mathbb{H}(\chi_2(p,0)) \end{bmatrix} + \begin{bmatrix} p^{-\alpha_1}\mathbb{H}(b_1) \\ s^{-\alpha_2}\mathbb{H}(b_2) \end{bmatrix} \mathbb{H}(\mathcal{U}(p,s)) \right). \quad (26)$$

Let

$$Q^{-1}(p,s) = \sum_{i=0}^{\infty}\sum_{j=0}^{\infty} \mathbb{H}(T_{ij})p^{-i\alpha_1}s^{-j\alpha_2}, \tag{27}$$

where $\mathbb{H}(T_{ij})$ is zero fuzzy matrix when $i,j < 0$ and $\mathbb{H}(T_{ij}) \in \Xi_{\mathbb{R}}^{n\times n}$ for other cases. We know that the product of Equations (25) and (27) is the identity matrix. So, from these two equations, we have

$$\sum_{i=0}^{\infty}\sum_{j=0}^{\infty}\Big(\mathbb{H}(T_{ij}) - \mathbb{H}(T_{01})\mathbb{H}(T_{i,j-1}) - \mathbb{H}(T_{10})\mathbb{H}(T_{i-1,j})\Big)p^{-i\alpha_1}s^{-j\alpha_2} = I_n. \tag{28}$$

Comparing the coefficients p and s in Equation (28), we get

$$\mathbb{H}(T_{ij}) = \begin{cases} I_n, & i,j=0, \\ 0, & i<0 \text{ and/or } j<0, \\ \mathbb{H}(T_{01})\mathbb{H}(T_{i,j-1}) + \mathbb{H}(T_{10})\mathbb{H}(T_{i-1,j}), & i,j>0, \end{cases} \tag{29}$$

and

$$\mathbb{H}(T_{01}) = \begin{bmatrix} 0 & 0 \\ \mathbb{H}(a_{21}) & \mathbb{H}(a_{22}) \end{bmatrix}, \ \mathbb{H}(T_{10}) = \begin{bmatrix} \mathbb{H}(a_{11}) & \mathbb{H}(a_{12}) \\ 0 & 0 \end{bmatrix}. \tag{30}$$

Substituting Equation (27) into Equation (26), and taking into account Equation (29), we get

$$\begin{aligned} \begin{bmatrix} \mathbb{H}(\chi_1(p,s)) \\ \mathbb{H}(\chi_2(p,s)) \end{bmatrix} = \sum_{i=0}^{\infty}\sum_{j=0}^{\infty} \mathbb{H}(T_{ij})\Bigg(&\begin{bmatrix} p^{-i\alpha_1-1}s^{-j\alpha_2}\mathbb{H}(\chi_1(0,s)) \\ p^{-i\alpha_1}s^{-j\alpha_2-1}\mathbb{H}(\chi_2(p,0)) \end{bmatrix} \\ &+ \begin{bmatrix} p^{-(i+1)\alpha_1}s^{-j\alpha_2}\mathbb{H}(b_1) \\ p^{-i\alpha_1}s^{-(j+1)\alpha_2}\mathbb{H}(b_2) \end{bmatrix}\mathbb{H}(\mathcal{U}(p,s))\Bigg). \end{aligned} \tag{31}$$

Applying the two-dimensional inverse Laplace transform to Equation (31) and using Definition 17, we get

$$\begin{aligned} \begin{bmatrix} \mathbb{H}(\varkappa_1(z_1,z_2)) \\ \mathbb{H}(\varkappa_2(z_1,z_2)) \end{bmatrix} &= \sum_{i=0}^{\infty}\sum_{j=1}^{\infty} \mathbb{H}(T_{ij})\Bigg(\begin{bmatrix} \frac{z_1^{i\alpha_1}}{\Gamma(1+i\alpha_1)}\frac{1}{\Gamma((j\alpha_2))}\int_0^{z_2}(z_2-\tau_2)^{j\alpha_2-1}\mathbb{H}(\varkappa_1(0,\tau_2))d\tau_2 \\ 0 \end{bmatrix} \\ &+ \begin{bmatrix} \frac{\mathbb{H}(b_1)}{\Gamma((i+1)\alpha_1)\Gamma(j\alpha_2)}\int_0^{z_1}\int_0^{z_2}(z_1-\tau_1)^{(i+1)\alpha_1-1}(z_2-\tau_2)^{j\alpha_2-1}\mathbb{H}(u(\tau_1,\tau_2))d\tau_2 d\tau_1 \\ 0 \end{bmatrix}\Bigg) \\ &+ \sum_{i=0}^{\infty}\mathbb{H}(T_{i0})\Bigg(\begin{bmatrix} \frac{z_1^{i\alpha_1}}{\Gamma(1+i\alpha_1)}\mathbb{H}(\varkappa_1(0,z_2)) \\ 0 \end{bmatrix} + \begin{bmatrix} \frac{\mathbb{H}(b_1)}{\Gamma((i+1)\alpha_1)}\int_0^{z_1}(z_1-\tau_1)^{(i+1)\alpha_1-1}\mathbb{H}(u(\tau_1,z_2))d\tau_1 \\ 0 \end{bmatrix}\Bigg) \\ &+ \sum_{i=1}^{\infty}\sum_{j=0}^{\infty}\mathbb{H}(T_{ij})\Bigg(\begin{bmatrix} 0 \\ \frac{z_2^{j\alpha_2}}{\Gamma(1+j\alpha_2)}\frac{1}{\Gamma((i\alpha_1))}\int_0^{z_1}(z_1-\tau_1)^{i\alpha_1-1}\mathbb{H}(\varkappa_2(\tau_1,0))d\tau_1 \end{bmatrix} \\ &+ \begin{bmatrix} 0 \\ \frac{\mathbb{H}(b_2)}{\Gamma(i\alpha_1)\Gamma((j+1)\alpha_2)}\int_0^{z_1}\int_0^{z_2}(z_1-\tau_1)^{i\alpha_1-1}(z_2-\tau_2)^{(j+1)\alpha_2-1}\mathbb{H}(u(\tau_1,\tau_2))d\tau_2 d\tau_1 \end{bmatrix}\Bigg) \end{aligned}$$

$$
+\sum_{i=0}^{\infty}\mathbb{H}(T_{0j})\left(\begin{bmatrix} 0 \\ \frac{z_1^{j\alpha_2}}{\Gamma(1+j\alpha_2)}\mathbb{H}(\varkappa_2(z_1,0)) \end{bmatrix}+\begin{bmatrix} 0 \\ \frac{\mathbb{H}(b_2)}{\Gamma((j+1)\alpha_2)}\int_0^{z_2}(z_2-\tau_2)^{(j+1)\alpha_2-1}\mathbb{H}(u(z_1,\tau_2))d\tau_2 \end{bmatrix}\right). \tag{32}
$$

This completes the proof. □

4. Granular Fuzzy Fractional 2D Continuous Linear Systems: A Fornasini–Marchesini Second Model Approach

Consider the state-space equation for the granular FFTDCT linear system

$$
\begin{aligned}
{}_{0^+}^{gr}\mathcal{D}^{\alpha_1,\alpha_2}\varkappa(z_1,z_2) &= A_1{}_{0^+}^{gr}\mathcal{D}^{\alpha_1}\varkappa(z_1,z_2)+A_2{}_{0^+}^{gr}\mathcal{D}^{\alpha_2}\varkappa(z_1,z_2)+B_1{}_{0^+}^{gr}\mathcal{D}^{\alpha_1}u(z_1,z_2)\\
&\quad + B_2{}_{0^+}^{gr}\mathcal{D}^{\alpha_2}u(z_1,z_2),
\end{aligned} \tag{33}
$$

where ${}_{0^+}^{gr}\mathcal{D}^{\alpha_1,\alpha_2}$ represents the granular Caputo fractional partial derivative of order α_i for $i=1,2$. $\mathcal{D}^{\alpha_1}$ and $\mathcal{D}^{\alpha_2}$ are the GCFDs of order α_1 and α_2, respectively. $\varkappa(z_1,z_2)\in\Xi_{\mathbb{R}}^n$ is a fuzzy state vector, and $u(z_1,z_2)\in\Xi_{\mathbb{R}}^m$ is a fuzzy input vector of the system. Regarding fuzzy matrices $A_1,A_2\in\Xi_{\mathbb{R}}^{n\times n}$ and $B_1,B_2\in\Xi_{\mathbb{R}}^{n\times m}$, the system (33) with fractional orders $\alpha_1,\alpha_2\in(0,1)$ is taken into consideration for simplicity.

Theorem 3. *The solution of the fuzzy system (33) with fractional orders $0<\alpha_1<1, 0<\alpha_2<1$ for arbitrary fuzzy input $u(z_1,z_2)$ with the uncertain initial condition $\varkappa(0,0)$ and the boundary conditions $\varkappa(z_1,0)$, $\varkappa(0,z_2)$ is given by the following*

$$
\begin{aligned}
\mathbb{H}(\varkappa(z_1,z_2)) :=& \sum_{i=0}^{\infty}\sum_{j=0}^{\infty}\Bigg(-\mathbb{H}(T_{ij})\frac{t_1^{i\alpha_1}}{\Gamma(i\alpha_1+1)}\frac{t_2^{j\alpha_2}}{\Gamma(i\alpha_2+1)}\varkappa(0,0)-\mathbb{H}(T_{ij})\mathbb{H}(B_1)\frac{t_1^{i\alpha_1}}{\Gamma(i\alpha_1+1)}\frac{1}{\Gamma((j+1)\alpha_2)}\int_0^{z_2}(z_2-\tau_2)^{(j+1)\alpha_2-1}\mathbb{H}(u(0,\tau_2))d\tau_2\\
&-\mathbb{H}(T_{ij})\mathbb{H}(B_2)\frac{t_2^{j\alpha_2}}{\Gamma(j\alpha_2+1)}\frac{1}{\Gamma((i+1)\alpha_1)}\int_0^{z_1}(z_1-\tau_1)^{(i+1)\alpha_1-1}\mathbb{H}(u(\tau_1,0))d\tau_1\\
&+\mathbb{H}(T_{i,j-1})\mathbb{H}(A_1)\frac{t_2^{j\alpha_2}}{\Gamma(j\alpha_2+1)}\frac{1}{\Gamma((i\alpha_1))}\int_0^{z_1}(z_1-\tau_1)^{i\alpha_1-1}\mathbb{H}(\varkappa(\tau_1,0))d\tau_1\\
&+\mathbb{H}(T_{i-1,j})\mathbb{H}(A_2)\frac{t_1^{i\alpha_1}}{\Gamma(i\alpha_1+1)}\frac{1}{\Gamma((j\alpha_2))}\int_0^{z_2}(z_2-\tau_2)^{j\alpha_2-1}\mathbb{H}(\varkappa(0,\tau_2))d\tau_2\\
&+[\mathbb{H}(T_{i,j-1})\mathbb{H}(B_1)+\mathbb{H}(T_{i-1,j})\mathbb{H}(B_2)]\frac{1}{\Gamma(i\alpha_1)\Gamma(j\alpha_2)}\int_0^{z_1}\int_0^{z_2}(z_1-\tau_1)^{i\alpha_1-1}(z_2-\tau_2)^{j\alpha_2-1}\mathbb{H}(u(\tau_1,\tau_2))d\tau_1 d\tau_2.
\end{aligned} \tag{34}
$$

with the transition matrices given in Equation (43).

Proof. For each $z_1,z_2\in[0,T]$, applying the 2D FLT on both sides to the system (33) and using the Linearity property, we get

$$
\begin{aligned}
\mathfrak{L}_{z_1,z_2}\left[{}_{0^+}^{gr}\mathcal{D}^{\alpha_1,\alpha_2}\varkappa(z_1,z_2)\right] &= A_1\mathfrak{L}_{z_1,z_2}\left[{}_{0^+}^{gr}\mathcal{D}^{\alpha_1}\varkappa(z_1,z_2)\right]+A_2\mathfrak{L}_{z_1,z_2}\left[{}_{0^+}^{gr}\mathcal{D}^{\alpha_2}\varkappa(z_1,z_2)\right]\\
&\quad + B_1\mathfrak{L}_{z_1,z_2}\left[{}_{0^+}^{gr}\mathcal{D}^{\alpha_1}u(z_1,z_2)\right]+B_2\mathfrak{L}_{z_1,z_2}\left[{}_{0^+}^{gr}\mathcal{D}^{\alpha_2}u(z_1,z_2)\right].
\end{aligned} \tag{35}
$$

Applying the HMF to Equation (35), and utilizing Remark 3, we get

$$
\begin{aligned}
\mathcal{L}_{z_1,z_2}\left[\mathbb{H}\left({}_{0^+}^{gr}\mathcal{D}^{\alpha_1,\alpha_2}\varkappa(z_1,z_2)\right)\right] =& \mathbb{H}(A_1)\mathcal{L}_{z_1,z_2}\left[\mathbb{H}\left({}_{0^+}^{gr}\mathcal{D}^{\alpha_1}\varkappa(z_1,z_2)\right)\right]+\mathbb{H}(A_2)\mathcal{L}_{z_1,z_2}\left[\mathbb{H}\left({}_{0^+}^{gr}\mathcal{D}^{\alpha_2}\varkappa(z_1,z_2)\right)\right]\\
&+\mathbb{H}(B_1)\mathcal{L}_{z_1,z_2}\left[\mathbb{H}\left({}_{0^+}^{gr}\mathcal{D}^{\alpha_1}u(z_1,z_2)\right)\right]+\mathbb{H}(B_2)\mathcal{L}_{z_1,z_2}\left[\mathbb{H}\left({}_{0^+}^{gr}\mathcal{D}^{\alpha_2}u(z_1,z_2)\right)\right].
\end{aligned} \tag{36}
$$

Using Remark 2, the above Equation (36) transforms into the following equation

$$
\begin{aligned}
\mathcal{L}_{z_1,z_2}\left[{}_{0^+}^{C}\mathcal{D}^{\alpha_1,\alpha_2}\mathbb{H}(\varkappa(z_1,z_2))\right] =& \mathbb{H}(A_1)\mathcal{L}_{z_1,z_2}\left[{}_{0^+}^{C}\mathcal{D}^{\alpha_1}\mathbb{H}(\varkappa(z_1,z_2))\right]+\mathbb{H}(A_2)\mathcal{L}_{z_1,z_2}\left[{}_{0^+}^{C}\mathcal{D}^{\alpha_2}\mathbb{H}(\varkappa(z_1,z_2))\right]\\
&+\mathbb{H}(B_1)\mathcal{L}_{z_1,z_2}\left[{}_{0^+}^{C}\mathcal{D}^{\alpha_1}\mathbb{H}(u(z_1,z_2))\right]+\mathbb{H}(B_2)\mathcal{L}_{z_1,z_2}\left[{}_{0^+}^{C}\mathcal{D}^{\alpha_2}\mathbb{H}(u(z_1,z_2))\right].
\end{aligned} \tag{37}
$$

Applying Theorem 1, Equation (37) can be expressed as

$$\begin{aligned}[][p^{\alpha_1}s^{\alpha_2}I_n - p^{\alpha_1}\mathbb{H}(A_1) - s^{\alpha_2}\mathbb{H}(A_2)]\mathbb{H}(\chi(p,s)) &= s^{\alpha_2-1}[p^{\alpha_1}I_n - \mathbb{H}(A_2)]\mathbb{H}(\chi(p,0)) + p^{\alpha_1-1}[s^{\alpha_2}I_n - \mathbb{H}(A_1)]\mathbb{H}(\chi(0,s)) \\ &- p^{\alpha_1-1}s^{\alpha_2-1}\mathbb{H}(\varkappa(0,0)) + \mathbb{H}(B_1)[p^{\alpha_1}\mathbb{H}(\mathcal{U}(p,s)) - p^{\alpha_1-1}\mathbb{H}(\mathcal{U}(0,s))] + \mathbb{H}(B_2)[s^{\alpha_2}\mathbb{H}(\mathcal{U}(p,s)) - s^{\alpha_2-1}\mathbb{H}(\mathcal{U}(p,0))],\end{aligned} \tag{38}$$

where $\mathbb{H}(\chi(p,s)) = \mathcal{L}_{z_1,z_2}\{\mathbb{H}(\varkappa(z_1,z_2))\}$, $\mathbb{H}(\chi(p,0)) = \mathcal{L}_{z_1}\{\mathbb{H}(\varkappa(z_1,0))\}$, and $\mathbb{H}(\chi(0,s)) = \mathcal{L}_{z_2}\{\mathbb{H}(\varkappa(0,z_2))\}$.

Let us suppose the polynomial matrix

$$Q(p,s) = [p^{\alpha_1}s^{\alpha_2}I_n - p^{\alpha_1}\mathbb{H}(A_1) - s^{\alpha_2}\mathbb{H}(A_2)]. \tag{39}$$

The inverse of the matrix given in Equation (39) can be expressed as

$$Q^{-1}(p,s) = \sum_{i=0}^{\infty}\sum_{j=0}^{\infty}\mathbb{H}(T_{ij})p^{-(i+1)\alpha_1}s^{-(j+1)\alpha_2}, \tag{40}$$

where $\mathbb{H}(T_{ij})$ is zero fuzzy matrix when $i,j<0$ and $\mathbb{H}(T_{ij}) \in \Xi_{\mathbb{R}}^{n\times n}$ for other cases.

We know that the product of Equations (39) and (40) is the identity matrix. So, from these two equations, we have

$$\left[\sum_{i=0}^{\infty}\sum_{j=0}^{\infty}\mathbb{H}(T_{ij})p^{-(i+1)\alpha_1}s^{-(j+1)\alpha_2}\right]\left[p^{\alpha_1}s^{\alpha_2}I_n - p^{\alpha_1}\mathbb{H}(A_1) - s^{\alpha_2}\mathbb{H}(A_2)\right] = I_n, \tag{41}$$

or Equation (41) is written more precisely as

$$\sum_{i=0}^{\infty}\sum_{j=0}^{\infty}\Big(\mathbb{H}(T_{ij}) - \mathbb{H}(T_{i,j-1})\mathbb{H}(A_1) - \mathbb{H}(T_{i-1,j})\mathbb{H}(A_2)\Big)p^{-i\alpha_1}s^{-j\alpha_2} = I_n. \tag{42}$$

Comparing the coefficients p and s in Equation (42), we get

$$\mathbb{H}(T_{ij}) = \begin{cases} I_n, & i,j=0, \\ 0, & i<0 \text{ and/or } j<0, \\ \mathbb{H}(A_1)\mathbb{H}(T_{i,j-1}) + \mathbb{H}(A_2)\mathbb{H}(T_{i-1,j}), & i,j>0. \end{cases} \tag{43}$$

Multiplying Equation (38) by Equation (40), and taking into account Equation (43), we get

$$\begin{aligned}\mathbb{H}(\chi(p,s)) = \sum_{i=0}^{\infty}\sum_{j=0}^{\infty}\Big(&-\mathbb{H}(T_{ij})p^{-(i\alpha_1+1)}s^{-(j\alpha_2+1)}\varkappa(0,0) - \mathbb{H}(T_{ij})p^{-(i\alpha_1+1)}s^{-(j+1)\alpha_2}\mathbb{H}(B_1)\mathbb{H}(\mathcal{U}(0,s)) \\ &- \mathbb{H}(T_{ij})p^{-(i+1)\alpha_1}s^{-(j\alpha_2+1)}\mathbb{H}(B_2)\mathbb{H}(\mathcal{U}(p,0)) + \mathbb{H}(T_{i,j-1})p^{-i\alpha_1}s^{-(j\alpha_2+1)}\mathbb{H}(A_1)\mathbb{H}(\chi(p,0)) \\ &+ \mathbb{H}(T_{i-1,j})p^{-(i\alpha_1+1)}s^{-j\alpha_2}\mathbb{H}(A_2)\mathbb{H}(\chi(0,s)) + [\mathbb{H}(T_{i,j-1})\mathbb{H}(B_1) + \mathbb{H}(T_{i-1,j})\mathbb{H}(B_2)]p^{-i\alpha_1}s^{-j\alpha_2}\mathbb{H}(\mathcal{U}(p,s))\Big).\end{aligned} \tag{44}$$

Applying the two-dimensional inverse Laplace transform to Equation (44) and using Definition 17, we get

$$\begin{aligned}\mathbb{H}(\varkappa(z_1,z_2)) = \sum_{i=0}^{\infty}\sum_{j=0}^{\infty}\Big(&-\mathbb{H}(T_{ij})\frac{t_1^{i\alpha_1}}{\Gamma(i\alpha_1+1)}\frac{t_2^{j\alpha_2}}{\Gamma(i\alpha_2+1)}\varkappa(0,0) - \mathbb{H}(T_{ij})\mathbb{H}(B_1)\frac{t_1^{i\alpha_1}}{\Gamma(i\alpha_1+1)}\frac{1}{\Gamma((j+1)\alpha_2)}\int_0^{z_2}(z_2-\tau_2)^{(j+1)\alpha_2-1}\mathbb{H}(u(0,\tau_2))d\tau_2 \\ &- \mathbb{H}(T_{ij})\mathbb{H}(B_2)\frac{t_2^{j\alpha_2}}{\Gamma(j\alpha_2+1)}\frac{1}{\Gamma((i+1)\alpha_1)}\int_0^{z_1}(z_1-\tau_1)^{(i+1)\alpha_1-1}\mathbb{H}(u(\tau_1,0))d\tau_1\end{aligned}$$

$$+\mathbb{H}(T_{i,j-1})\mathbb{H}(A_1)\frac{t_2^{j\alpha_2}}{\Gamma(j\alpha_2+1)}\frac{1}{\Gamma((i\alpha_1))}\int_0^{z_1}(z_1-\tau_1)^{i\alpha_1-1}\mathbb{H}(\varkappa(\tau_1,0))d\tau_1$$

$$+\mathbb{H}(T_{i-1,j})\mathbb{H}(A_2)\frac{t_1^{i\alpha_1}}{\Gamma(i\alpha_1+1)}\frac{1}{\Gamma((j\alpha_2))}\int_0^{z_2}(z_2-\tau_2)^{j\alpha_2-1}\mathbb{H}(\varkappa(0,\tau_2))d\tau_2$$

$$+[\mathbb{H}(T_{i,j-1})\mathbb{H}(B_1)+\mathbb{H}(T_{i-1,j})\mathbb{H}(B_2)]\frac{1}{\Gamma(i\alpha_1)\Gamma(j\alpha_2)}\int_0^{z_1}\int_0^{z_2}(z_1-\tau_1)^{i\alpha_1-1}(z_2-\tau_2)^{j\alpha_2-1}\mathbb{H}(u(\tau_1,\tau_2))d\tau_1 d\tau_2. \quad (45)$$

This completes the proof. □

Now, we consider the following example to illustrate the general result. The purpose of this example is to illustrate the aforementioned Theorem 3.

Example 1. *Consider the granular fuzzy fractional 2D linear system (33) with $\alpha_1 = 0.9$, $\alpha_2 = 0.8$, and the fuzzy matrices*

$$A_1 = \begin{bmatrix} \tilde{1} & \hat{0} \\ \hat{0} & \tilde{1} \end{bmatrix},\ A_2 = \begin{bmatrix} \tilde{1} & \tilde{1} \\ \tilde{1} & \hat{0} \end{bmatrix},\ B_1 = \begin{bmatrix} \tilde{1} \\ \hat{0} \end{bmatrix},\ B_2 = \begin{bmatrix} \hat{0} \\ \tilde{1} \end{bmatrix}, \quad (46)$$

where $\tilde{1} = (0.5, 1, 1.5)$ and $\hat{0} = (0,0,0)$. The HMFs of the fuzzy matrices given in Equation (46) are

$$\mathbb{H}(A_1) = \begin{bmatrix} \frac{1}{2}+\frac{\vartheta}{2}+(1-\vartheta)\pi & 0 \\ 0 & \frac{1}{2}+\frac{\vartheta}{2}+(1-\vartheta)\pi \end{bmatrix},$$

$$\mathbb{H}(A_2) = \begin{bmatrix} \frac{1}{2}+\frac{\vartheta}{2}+(1-\vartheta)\pi & \frac{1}{2}+\frac{\vartheta}{2}+(1-\vartheta)\pi \\ \frac{1}{2}+\frac{\vartheta}{2}+(1-\vartheta)\pi & 0 \end{bmatrix},$$

$$\mathbb{H}(B_1) = \begin{bmatrix} \frac{1}{2}+\frac{\vartheta}{2}+(1-\vartheta)\pi \\ 0 \end{bmatrix},\ \mathbb{H}(B_2) = \begin{bmatrix} 0 \\ \frac{1}{2}+\frac{\vartheta}{2}+(1-\vartheta)\pi \end{bmatrix}, \quad (47)$$

We consider the initial condition $\varkappa(0,0) = \hat{0}$, boundary conditions $\varkappa(z_1,0) = \varkappa(0,z_2) = \hat{0}$, and the fuzzy input is

$$u(z_1,z_2) := \begin{cases} \hat{0}, & z_1, z_2 < 0, \\ \hat{1}, & z_1, z_2 \geq 0. \end{cases} \quad (48)$$

The HMF of the fuzzy input function is

$$\mathbb{H}(u(z_1,z_2)) = \begin{cases} 0, & z_1 < 0 \text{ and/or } z_2 < 0, \\ 1, & z_1, z_2 \geq 0. \end{cases} \quad (49)$$

According to Theorem 3, the fuzzy solution is given in the following

$$\mathbb{H}(\varkappa(z_1,z_2)) = \sum_{i=0}^{\infty}\sum_{j=0}^{\infty}\Bigg(-\mathbb{H}(T_{ij})\mathbb{H}(B_1)\frac{t_1^{i\alpha_1}}{\Gamma(i\alpha_1+1)}\frac{1}{\Gamma((j+1)\alpha_2)}\int_0^{z_2}(z_2-\tau_2)^{(j+1)\alpha_2-1}d\tau_2$$

$$-\mathbb{H}(T_{ij})\mathbb{H}(B_2)\frac{t_2^{j\alpha_2}}{\Gamma(j\alpha_2+1)}\frac{1}{\Gamma((i+1)\alpha_1)}\int_0^{z_1}(z_1-\tau_1)^{(i+1)\alpha_1-1}d\tau_1$$

$$+[\mathbb{H}(T_{i,j-1})\mathbb{H}(B_1)+\mathbb{H}(T_{i-1,j})\mathbb{H}(B_2)]\frac{1}{\Gamma(i\alpha_1)\Gamma(j\alpha_2)}\int_0^{z_1}\int_0^{z_2}(z_1-\tau_1)^{i\alpha_1-1}(z_2-\tau_2)^{j\alpha_2-1}d\tau_1 d\tau_2\Bigg)$$

$$=\sum_{i=0}^{\infty}\sum_{j=0}^{\infty}\Bigg(-\mathbb{H}(T_{ij})\mathbb{H}(B_1)\frac{t_1^{i\alpha_1}t_2^{(j+1)\alpha_2}}{\Gamma(i\alpha_1+1)\Gamma((j+1)\alpha_2)}\mathbb{H}(T_{ij})\mathbb{H}(B_2)\frac{t_1^{(i+1)\alpha_1}t_2^{j\alpha_2}}{\Gamma(j\alpha_2+1)\Gamma((i+1)\alpha_1)}$$

$$+[\mathbb{H}(T_{i,j-1})\mathbb{H}(B_1)+\mathbb{H}(T_{i-1,j})\mathbb{H}(B_2)]\frac{t_1^{i\alpha_1}t_2^{j\alpha_2}}{\Gamma(i\alpha_1+1)\Gamma(j\alpha_2+1)}\Bigg). \tag{50}$$

The graphical representation of the fuzzy solution for Example 1 is presented in Figures 1–3. Each figure highlights the various aspects of the fuzzy solutions and their associated fuzziness. The graphical representation of the HMF of fuzzy solution $\varkappa_1$ is presented in Figure 1. The time variables z_1 and z_2 are fixed at 1 on the left side, which allows us to observe the fuzziness in $\varkappa_1$ at a specific time instance. The HMF illustrates how this fuzzy solution varies regarding the ϑ-cut and π, with the spread of the function indicating the degree of uncertainty. Higher uncertainty is associated with a greater spread, whereas a narrower spread suggests a more precise solution. When ϑ and π are fixed to 1, the variation of z_1 and z_2 is displayed on the right side of Figure 1. This plot shows how $\varkappa_1$ changes dynamically over time, highlighting how the uncertainty changes as the system behavior changes. Fuzziness and time interact, demonstrating that the system's uncertainty is dynamic and changes over time. Likewise, Figure 2 displays the graphical representations of fuzzy solutions under the HMF and its temporal variation, $\varkappa_2$. The variables z_1 and z_2 are fixed to 1 on the left side to provide the graphical depiction of the HMF of $\varkappa_2$, whereas $\varkappa_1$ shows that the fuzziness is not evenly distributed across the system; the spread of the membership function for $\varkappa_2$ shows the degree of uncertainty. Holding the horizontal membership parameters constant allows the variation in $\varkappa_2$ regarding z_1 and z_2, displayed on the right side of Figure 2. This figure shows the evolution of $\varkappa_2$ and its fuzziness. The temporal variables $\varkappa_1$ and $\varkappa_2$ behave differently, suggesting that the properties of each solution significantly influence the fuzziness of the systems. Figure 3 shows fuzzy solutions $\varkappa_1$ and $\varkappa_2$ in three dimensions. The uncertainty in $\varkappa_1$ is affected by time and the degree of membership, as seen in $\varkappa_1$. Additionally, it illustrates the ambiguity between time and fuzziness. By revealing complex patterns in the system's behavior, the graph emphasizes the need to consider several dimensions while assessing fuzzy systems. On the right side of Figure 3, plotting $\varkappa_2$ under the same conditions provides an alternative perspective regarding the system's response. This figure highlights the intricate connection between time, fuzziness, and the system's dynamics. It also provides a more in-depth understanding of the model's uncertainty. The results demonstrate the importance of considering fuzziness in analyzing continuous fuzzy systems. It is clear from the graphical representations how uncertainty spreads and evolves and the behavior of both time-dependent features and the degree of membership influence the system's behavior.

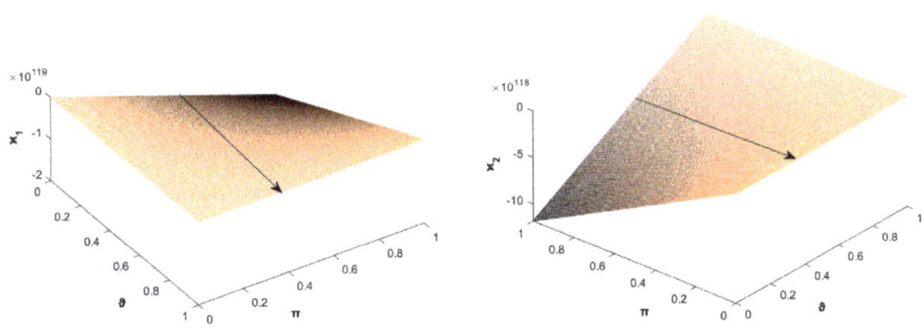

Figure 1. The **left** figure shows HMFs of $\varkappa_1(z_1, z_2)$, and the **right** figure shows the HMFs of $\varkappa_2(z_1, z_2)$ for different values of ϑ and π by fixing $z_1 = z_2 = 1$.

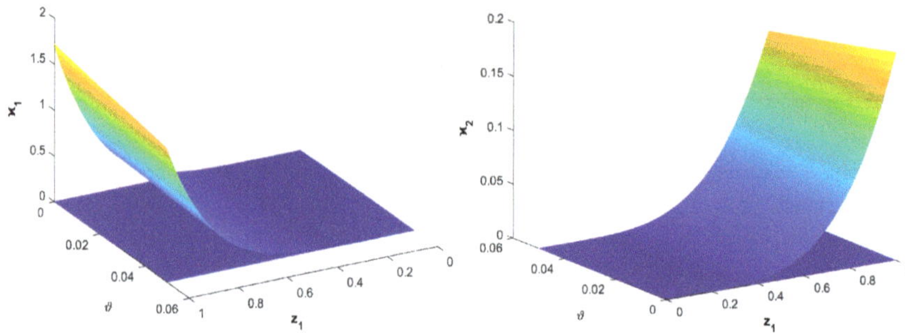

Figure 2. Graphical representations of fuzzy solutions $\varkappa_1(z_1, 1, \vartheta)$ and $\varkappa_2(z_1, 1, \vartheta)$, respectively.

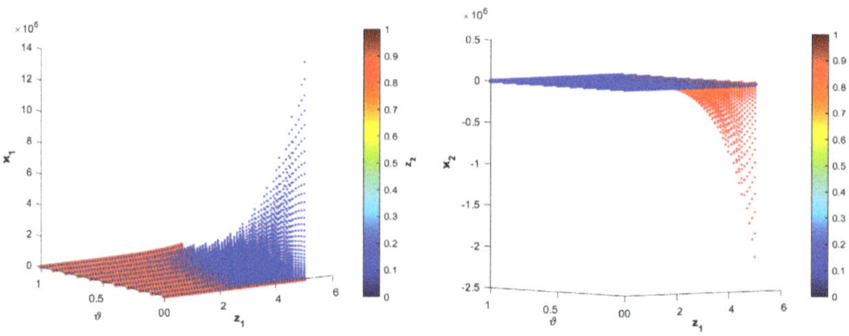

Figure 3. The **left** and **right** figures show the four-dimensional scatter plots of fuzzy solutions $\varkappa_1(z_1, z_2, \vartheta)$ and $\varkappa_2(z_1, z_2, \vartheta)$, respectively. The red points represent the left bound, and the blue points represent the right bound of the ϑ-cut of the FVF.

5. Applications of FFTDCT Linear System

This section discusses the real-world applications of the proposed granular FFTDCT linear system. The Roesser model is used in signal processing systems because the fuzzy fractional framework efficiently represents the inherent uncertainty of signal components. The second FM model, on the other hand, addresses the challenges of sensor data fusion (SDF) in wireless sensor networks (WSNs) as the reconstruction of the fused sensor state is highly dependent on temporal and spatial uncertainties.

5.1. Application of FFTDCT Linear System Described by the Roesser Model in Signal Processing System

Echo suppression and signal filtering play a crucial role in digital communication and image processing, particularly when uncertainty, fuzziness, memory effects, and spatial distributions influence signal propagation. To model this situation, we consider the Roesser-type granular FFTDCT linear system (17), where the components $\varkappa_1(z_1, z_2)$ and $\varkappa_2(z_1, z_2)$ represent the horizontal and vertical signal flow, respectively. Moreover, $u(z_1, z_2)$ represents the incoming echo/background noise. The matrices A and B are modeled as fuzzy matrices, and the memory effect of the system is described by the fractional orders $\alpha_1 = 0.9$ and $\alpha_2 = 0.8$. This is an important feature in media, where the behavior of the past signals influences the present state. The fuzzy matrices are defined as

$$A_1 = \begin{bmatrix} \tilde{1} & \tilde{2} \\ \hat{0} & \tilde{1} \end{bmatrix}, \text{ and } B_1 = \begin{bmatrix} \tilde{1} \\ \tilde{2} \end{bmatrix}, \tag{51}$$

where $\tilde{1} = (0.5, 1, 1.5)$, $\tilde{2} = (1.5, 2, 2.5)$, and $\hat{0} = (0, 0, 0)$. The matrix A_1 characterizes the impact of the current state and neighboring signal states on the system at every point (z_1, z_2), analogous to echo weights in 2D spatial domains. The matrix B_1 captures how the external inputs, including environmental disturbances, influence the system state. The HMFs of the fuzzy matrices given in Equation (51) are

$$\mathbb{H}(A_1) = \begin{bmatrix} \frac{1}{2} + \frac{\vartheta}{2} + (1-\vartheta)\pi & \frac{3}{2} + \frac{\vartheta}{2} + (1-\vartheta)\pi \\ 0 & \frac{1}{2} + \frac{\vartheta}{2} + (1-\vartheta)\pi \end{bmatrix}, \quad \mathbb{H}(B_1) = \begin{bmatrix} \frac{1}{2} + \frac{\vartheta}{2} + (1-\vartheta)\pi \\ \frac{3}{2} + \frac{\vartheta}{2} + (1-\vartheta)\pi \end{bmatrix}. \tag{52}$$

The uncertain initial condition $\varkappa(0,0) = \tilde{1}$ represents the signal uncertainty due to measurement errors or external disturbance. The boundary conditions $\varkappa(z_1, 0) = (z_1, 2z_1, 3z_1)$ and $\varkappa(0, z_2) = (e^{z_2}, 2e^{z_2}, 3e^{z_2})$ define the signal profiles at the boundaries, capturing how the horizontal and vertical input influence propagation. The fuzzy input function simulates an environment with sporadic background signals, including noise bursts or intermittent interference:

$$u(z_1, z_2) = \begin{cases} \hat{0}, & z_1, z_2 < 0, \\ \hat{1}, & z_1, z_2 \geq 0. \end{cases} \tag{53}$$

The HMF of the fuzzy input function is

$$\mathbb{H}(u(z_1, z_2)) = \begin{cases} 0, & z_1, z_2 < 0, \\ 1, & z_1, z_2 \geq 0. \end{cases} \tag{54}$$

The following is the fuzzy solution based on Theorem 3

$$\begin{aligned} \begin{bmatrix} \mathbb{H}(\varkappa_1(z_1, z_2)) \\ \mathbb{H}(\varkappa_2(z_1, z_2)) \end{bmatrix} &= \sum_{i=0}^{\infty}\sum_{j=1}^{\infty} \mathbb{H}(T_{ij}) \left(\begin{bmatrix} \frac{z_1^{i\alpha_1}}{\Gamma(1+i\alpha_1)}(1+\vartheta+2(1-\vartheta)\pi)e^{z_2} \\ 0 \end{bmatrix} + \begin{bmatrix} \frac{\mathbb{H}(b_1)}{\Gamma((i+1)\alpha_1+1)\Gamma(j\alpha_2+1)} z_1^{(i+1)\alpha_1} z_2^{j\alpha_2} \\ 0 \end{bmatrix} \right) \\ &+ \sum_{i=0}^{\infty} \mathbb{H}(T_{i0}) \left(\begin{bmatrix} \frac{z_1^{i\alpha_1}}{\Gamma(1+i\alpha_1)}(1+\vartheta+2(1-\vartheta)\pi)e^{z_2} \\ 0 \end{bmatrix} + \begin{bmatrix} \frac{\mathbb{H}(b_1)}{\Gamma((i+1)\alpha_1+1)} z_1^{(i+1)\alpha_1} \\ 0 \end{bmatrix} \right) \\ &+ \sum_{i=1}^{\infty}\sum_{j=0}^{\infty} \mathbb{H}(T_{ij}) \left(\begin{bmatrix} 0 \\ \frac{z_2^{j\alpha_2}}{\Gamma(1+j\alpha_2)} \frac{(1+\vartheta+2(1-\vartheta)\pi)z_1^{1+i\alpha_1}}{\Gamma(2+i\alpha_1)} \end{bmatrix} + \begin{bmatrix} 0 \\ \frac{\mathbb{H}(b_2)}{\Gamma(i\alpha_1+1)\Gamma((j+1)\alpha_2+1)} z_1^{i\alpha_1} z_2^{(j+1)\alpha_2} \end{bmatrix} \right) \\ &+ \sum_{i=0}^{\infty} \mathbb{H}(T_{0j}) \left(\begin{bmatrix} 0 \\ \frac{z_1^{j\alpha_2}}{\Gamma(1+j\alpha_2)}(1+\vartheta+2(1-\vartheta)\pi)z_1 \end{bmatrix} + \begin{bmatrix} 0 \\ \frac{\mathbb{H}(b_2)}{\Gamma((j+1)\alpha_2+1)} z_2^{(j+1)\alpha_2} \end{bmatrix} \right). \end{aligned} \tag{55}$$

The plots of the aforementioned fuzzy solution are provided in Figures 4–6 with values of $i = 25$ and $j = 25$.

To validate the accuracy of the proposed approach, we compare the analytical fuzzy solution derived in Equation (55) with the approximate solution obtained using the fuzzy fractional forward Euler method. The values of the fractional orders, fuzzy parameters, and uncertain initial and boundary conditions used in this comparison are specified in Section 5.1. Table 2 presents the numerical results for both the analytical and approximate solutions of $\varkappa_1(z_1, z_2, \vartheta, \pi)$ (hereafter referred to as $\varkappa_1$) and $\varkappa_2(z_1, z_2, \vartheta, \pi)$ (hereafter referred to as $\varkappa_2$). In the table, $\varkappa_{1-\text{Analytic}}$ and $\varkappa_{2-\text{Analytic}}$ denote the analytical solutions of

$\varkappa_1$ and $\varkappa_2$, respectively, while $\varkappa_{1-mathrmApprox.}$ and $\varkappa_{2-\mathrm{Approx.}}$ represent the corresponding approximate solutions obtained via the numerical method.

Table 2. The numerical values of the analytical and approximate solutions of $\varkappa_1$ and $\varkappa_2$.

z_1	z_2	ϑ	π	$\varkappa_{1-}$**Analytic**	$\varkappa_{2-}$**Analytic**	$\varkappa_{1-}$**Approx.**	$\varkappa_{2-}$**Approx.**
0.0	0.0	0.0	0.0	0.5123	0.5101	0.5112	0.5100
0.1	0.1	0.1	0.1	0.2439	0.3501	0.2422	0.3452
0.2	0.2	0.2	0.2	0.7201	0.8112	0.7199	0.8108
0.3	0.3	0.3	0.3	1.5607	1.4140	1.5602	1.4112
0.4	0.4	0.4	0.4	2.8969	2.1715	2.8950	2.1612
0.5	0.5	0.5	0.5	4.8501	3.1839	4.8499	3.1822
0.6	0.6	0.6	0.6	7.5899	4.1930	7.5812	4.1901
0.7	0.7	0.7	0.7	11.1483	5.3929	11.1460	5.3924
0.8	0.8	0.8	0.8	15.5037	6.6530	15.5001	6.6501
0.9	0.9	0.9	0.9	20.9987	7.8535	20.9940	7.8427
1.0	1.0	1.0	1.0	24.9339	8.8185	24.8312	8.8130

Now, we calculate the pointwise absolute and relative errors between the analytical and approximate solutions. Table 3 presents the error analysis results for both $\varkappa_1$ and $\varkappa_2$. The pointwise absolute error (AE) is computed using the formula

$$\mathrm{AE} = \left|\varkappa_{\mathrm{Analytic}} - \varkappa_{\mathrm{Approx.}}\right|,$$

while the pointwise relative error (RE) is given by

$$\mathrm{RE} = \frac{\left|\varkappa_{\mathrm{Analytic}} - \varkappa_{\mathrm{Approx.}}\right|}{\left|\varkappa_{\mathrm{Analytic}}\right|}.$$

These metrics enable a quantitative comparison of the numerical approximation with the exact fuzzy analytical solution.

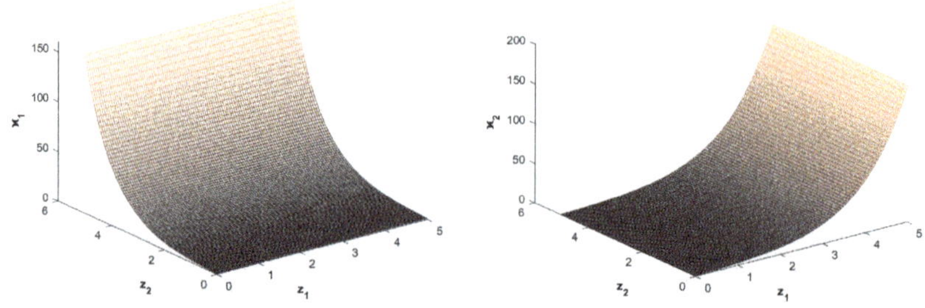

Figure 4. The **left** and **right** figures show the graphical representations of $\varkappa_1(z_1, z_2)$ and $\varkappa_2(z_1, z_2)$ for different values of z_1 and z_2 by fixing ϑ and π.

Figure 4 shows the graphical visualization of the components $\varkappa_1(z_1, z_2)$ and $\varkappa_2(z_1, z_2)$ by taking $\vartheta = 1$ and $\pi = 1$. These figures illustrate the evolution of the fuzzy fractional signal under uncertain environments. Here, $\pi = 1$ ensures that the horizontal membership distribution spans its entire range, indicating the system's maximum predicted response. In this scenario, $\vartheta = 1$ captures the crisp core of the fuzzy solution. Both $\varkappa_1(z_1, z_2)$ and $\varkappa_2(z_1, z_2)$ represent distinct components of a processed signal, each influenced by internal system feedback and external disturbances, with their behavior modeled using fuzzy and fractional parameters. The smooth and increasing trend of both surfaces shows a stable signal evolution, where the system efficiently captures both attenuation and amplification in response to changes in z_1 and z_2. This behavior represents the signal processing scenario in an uncertain environment, including echo suppression, where the memory effect and fuzziness are inherent. The graphical representation indicates that the system remains bounded and predictable, which is essential for practical signal reconstruction and enhancement. Figure 5 represents the graphical behavior of the fuzzy solutions of the components $\varkappa_1(z_1, 1, \vartheta)$ and $\varkappa_2(1, z_2, \vartheta)$, indicating the smooth and continuous surfaces. This confirms the stable behavior of the system with fractional orders $\alpha_1 = 0.9$ and $\alpha_2 = 0.8$. The proposed solution captures the expected uncertainty propagation in a fuzzy environment. These graphical representations demonstrate that the fractional orders and fuzzy parameters jointly influence the flexibility of the system and memory effect. Figure 6 provides graphical representations of fuzzy solutions $\varkappa_1(z_1, z_2, \vartheta)$ and $\varkappa_2(z_1, z_2, \vartheta)$. The left and right figures show the four-dimensional scatter plots of fuzzy solutions $\varkappa_1(z_1, z_2, \vartheta)$ and $\varkappa_2(z_1, z_2, \vartheta)$, respectively. In Figure 6, the red points represent the left bound, and the blue points represent the right bound of the ϑ-cut of the FVF. This graphical representation illustrates how the uncertainty varies between input parameters for fixed fractional orders $\alpha_1 = 0.9$ and $\alpha_2 = 0.8$, offering insight into its spread and behavior.

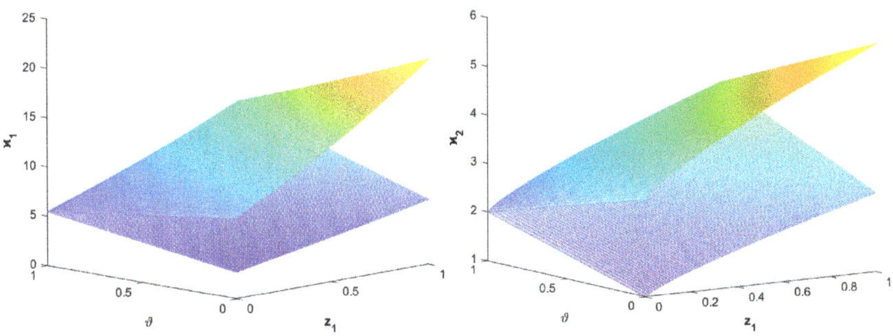

Figure 5. The **left** and **right** figures show the graphical representations of fuzzy solutions $\varkappa_1(z_1 1, \vartheta)$ and $\varkappa_2(1, z_2, \vartheta)$, respectively.

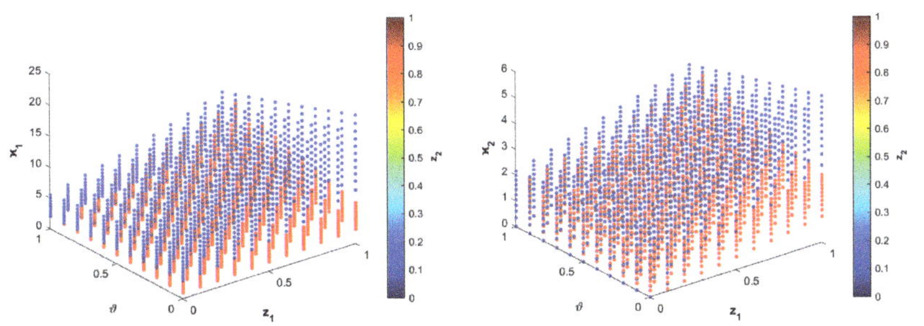

Figure 6. The **left** and **right** figures show the four-dimensional scatter plots of fuzzy solutions $\varkappa_1(z_1, z_2, \vartheta)$ and $\varkappa_2(z_1, z_2, \vartheta)$, respectively. The red points represent the left bound, and the blue points represent the right bound of the ϑ-cut of the FVF.

Table 3. Absolute and relative errors between analytical and approximate solutions of $\varkappa_1$ and $\varkappa_2$.

$\varkappa_1$-Analytic	$\varkappa_1$-Approx.	AE $\varkappa_1$	RE $\varkappa_1$	$\varkappa_2$-Analytic	$\varkappa_2$-Approx.	AE $\varkappa_2$	RE $\varkappa_2$
0.5123	0.5112	0.0011	0.002147	0.5101	0.5100	0.0001	0.000196
0.2439	0.2422	0.0017	0.006970	0.3501	0.3452	0.0049	0.014000
0.7201	0.7199	0.0002	0.000278	0.8112	0.8108	0.0004	0.000493
1.5607	1.5602	0.0005	0.000320	1.4140	1.4112	0.0028	0.001982
2.8969	2.8950	0.0019	0.000656	2.1715	2.1612	0.0103	0.004740
4.8501	4.8499	0.0002	0.000041	3.1839	3.1822	0.0017	0.000533
7.5899	7.5812	0.0087	0.001146	4.1930	4.1901	0.0029	0.000693
11.1483	11.1460	0.0023	0.000206	5.3929	5.3924	0.0005	0.000093
15.5037	15.5001	0.0036	0.000232	6.6530	6.6501	0.0029	0.000437
20.9987	20.9940	0.0047	0.000224	7.8535	7.8427	0.0108	0.001375
24.9339	24.8312	0.1027	0.004119	8.8185	8.8130	0.0055	0.000623

5.2. Application of FFTDCT Linear System in Wireless Sensor Network Data Fusion

Now, we apply the proposed model (33) to describe the problem of SDF in WSNs in a fuzzy environment. In real-world applications, spatially distributed sensors in a geographic region monitor conditions, including temperature, air quality, or humidity in a 2D space. Sensor readings usually exhibit uncertainty due to hardware constraints, latency in data transmission, and external interference. These properties are naturally described using fuzzy numbers, while fractional-order derivatives well model the memory-dependent characteristic of physical processes. The uncertain dynamics of the SDF of the WSN can be well captured by the proposed system (33), where $\varkappa(z_1, z_2)$ represents the fused sensor state within the spatial coordinates z_1 and z_2. $u(z_1, z_2)$ describes an external control or input source, including the sensor reading's emission signal or distributed activations. In our simulation, we assume the fractional orders $\alpha_1 = 0.9$ and $\alpha_2 = 0.8$ to capture the inherent long-memory dynamics and the delayed spatial interaction observed in transmission of WSN data. The fuzzy system matrices and its HMF are defined in Equations (46) and (47), where $\tilde{1} = (0.5, 1, 1.5)$ in Equation (46) represents fuzzy measurements and $\hat{0} = (0, 0, 0)$ indicates perfect certainty at zero. We consider the fuzzy initial condition $\varkappa(0, 0) = \tilde{1}$ and the fuzzy boundary conditions $\varkappa(z_1, 0) = (z_1, 2z_1, 3z_1)$ and $\varkappa(0, z_2) = (e^{z_2}, 2e^{z_2}, 3e^{z_2})$ for the SDF problem in WSNs to describe the initial uncertainty and horizontal and vertical boundary profile, respectively. The fuzzy input formulation in Equation (54) describes the activation state of the sensors when $z_1, z_2 \geq 0$ and their inactivity in unobservable regions. The HMF of the fuzzy input function is given in Equation (54). According to Theorem 3, the fuzzy solution is given in the following:

$$
\begin{aligned}
\mathbb{H}(\varkappa(z_1, z_2)) = \sum_{i=0}^{\infty}\sum_{j=0}^{\infty}\Bigg(& -\mathbb{H}(T_{ij})\frac{(\frac{1}{2}+\frac{\vartheta}{2}(1-\vartheta)\pi)t_1^{i\alpha_1}t_2^{j\alpha_2}}{\Gamma(i\alpha_1+1)\Gamma(i\alpha_2+1)} - \mathbb{H}(T_{ij})\mathbb{H}(B_1)\frac{t_1^{i\alpha_1}}{\Gamma(i\alpha_1+1)}\frac{1}{\Gamma((j+1)\alpha_2)}\int_0^{z_2}(z_2-\tau_2)^{(j+1)\alpha_2-1}d\tau_2 \\
& -\mathbb{H}(T_{ij})\mathbb{H}(B_2)\frac{t_2^{j\alpha_2}}{\Gamma(j\alpha_2+1)}\frac{1}{\Gamma((i+1)\alpha_1)}\int_0^{z_1}(z_1-\tau_1)^{(i+1)\alpha_1-1}d\tau_1 \\
& +\mathbb{H}(T_{i,j-1})\mathbb{H}(A_1)\frac{t_2^{j\alpha_2}}{\Gamma(j\alpha_2+1)}\frac{1}{\Gamma((i\alpha_1))}\int_0^{z_1}(z_1-\tau_1)^{i\alpha_1-1}(1+\vartheta+2(1-\vartheta)\pi)\tau_1 d\tau_1 \\
& +\mathbb{H}(T_{i-1,j})\mathbb{H}(A_2)\frac{t_1^{i\alpha_1}}{\Gamma(i\alpha_1+1)}\frac{1}{\Gamma((j\alpha_2))}\int_0^{z_2}(z_2-\tau_2)^{j\alpha_2-1}(1+\vartheta+2(1-\vartheta)\pi)e^{\tau_2}d\tau_2 \\
& +[\mathbb{H}(T_{i,j-1})\mathbb{H}(B_1)+\mathbb{H}(T_{i-1,j})\mathbb{H}(B_2)]\frac{1}{\Gamma(i\alpha_1)\Gamma(j\alpha_2)}\int_0^{z_1}\int_0^{z_2}(z_1-\tau_1)^{i\alpha_1-1}(z_2-\tau_2)^{j\alpha_2-1}d\tau_1 d\tau_2\Bigg).
\end{aligned}
\tag{56}
$$

After performing the integral in Equation (56) and simplifying the resulting expression, we obtain the following:

$$\begin{aligned}\mathbb{H}(\varkappa(z_1,z_2)) = \sum_{i=0}^{\infty}\sum_{j=0}^{\infty}\Bigg(&-\mathbb{H}(T_{ij})\frac{(\frac{1}{2}+\frac{\vartheta}{2}(1-\vartheta)\pi)t_1^{i\alpha_1}t_2^{j\alpha_2}}{\Gamma(i\alpha_1+1)\Gamma(i\alpha_2+1)} - \mathbb{H}(T_{ij})\mathbb{H}(B_1)\frac{t_1^{i\alpha_1}t_2^{(j+1)\alpha_2}}{\Gamma(i\alpha_1+1)\Gamma((j+1)\alpha_2)} \\ &-\mathbb{H}(T_{ij})\mathbb{H}(B_2)\frac{t_1^{(i+1)\alpha_1}t_2^{j\alpha_2}}{\Gamma(j\alpha_2+1)\Gamma((i+1)\alpha_1)} + \mathbb{H}(T_{i,j-1})\mathbb{H}(A_1)\frac{t_2^{j\alpha_2}}{\Gamma(j\alpha_2+1)}\frac{(1+\vartheta+2(1-\vartheta)\pi)t_1^{1+i\alpha_1}}{\Gamma(2+i\alpha_1)} \\ &+\mathbb{H}(T_{i-1,j})\mathbb{H}(A_2)\frac{t_1^{i\alpha_1}}{\Gamma(i\alpha_1+1)}(1+\vartheta+2(1-\vartheta)\pi)e^{z_2} + [\mathbb{H}(T_{i,j-1})\mathbb{H}(B_1)+\mathbb{H}(T_{i-1,j})\mathbb{H}(B_2)]\frac{t_1^{i\alpha_1}t_2^{j\alpha_2}}{\Gamma(i\alpha_1+1)\Gamma(j\alpha_2+1)}\Bigg). \end{aligned} \quad (57)$$

To validate the proposed fuzzy solution of the system (33), we compare it with the classical solution provided by Rogowski in [45]. The classical solution of system (33) is given as

$$\begin{aligned}\varkappa(z_1,z_2) = \sum_{i=0}^{\infty}\sum_{j=0}^{\infty}\Bigg(&-T_{ij}\frac{t_1^{i\alpha_1}}{\Gamma(i\alpha_1+1)}\frac{t_2^{j\alpha_2}}{\Gamma(i\alpha_2+1)}\varkappa(0,0) - T_{ij}B_1\frac{t_1^{i\alpha_1}}{\Gamma(i\alpha_1+1)}\frac{1}{\Gamma((j+1)\alpha_2)}\int_0^{z_2}(z_2-\tau_2)^{(j+1)\alpha_2-1}u(0,\tau_2)d\tau_2 \\ &- T_{ij}B_2\frac{t_2^{j\alpha_2}}{\Gamma(j\alpha_2+1)}\frac{1}{\Gamma((i+1)\alpha_1)}\int_0^{z_1}(z_1-\tau_1)^{(i+1)\alpha_1-1}u(\tau_1,0)d\tau_1 \\ &+ T_{i,j-1}A_1\frac{t_2^{j\alpha_2}}{\Gamma(j\alpha_2+1)}\frac{1}{\Gamma((i\alpha_1))}\int_0^{z_1}(z_1-\tau_1)^{i\alpha_1-1}\varkappa(\tau_1,0)d\tau_1 \\ &+ T_{i-1,j}A_2\frac{t_1^{i\alpha_1}}{\Gamma(i\alpha_1+1)}\frac{1}{\Gamma((j\alpha_2))}\int_0^{z_2}(z_2-\tau_2)^{j\alpha_2-1}\varkappa(0,\tau_2)d\tau_2 \\ &+[T_{i,j-1}B_1+T_{i-1,j}B_2]\frac{1}{\Gamma(i\alpha_1)\Gamma(j\alpha_2)}\int_0^{z_1}\int_0^{z_2}(z_1-\tau_1)^{i\alpha_1-1}(z_2-\tau_2)^{j\alpha_2-1}u(\tau_1,\tau_2)d\tau_1 d\tau_2\Bigg). \end{aligned} \quad (58)$$

Here, the coefficient matrices are defined as

$$A_1 = \begin{bmatrix} 1 & 2 \\ 0 & 1 \end{bmatrix}, \text{ and } B_1 = \begin{bmatrix} 1 \\ 2 \end{bmatrix}, \quad (59)$$

with the initial condition $\varkappa(0,0) = 1$, and boundary conditions $\varkappa(z_1,0) = 2z_1$ and $\varkappa(0,z_2) = 2e^{z_2}$. This classical solution coincides with the fuzzy solution in Equation (57) when the fuzzification parameter is $\vartheta = 1$. To illustrate the impact of fuzzification, we modify the initial condition to $\varkappa(0,0) = 1.1$ and the boundary conditions to $\varkappa(z_1,0) = 2.1z_1$ and $\varkappa(0,z_2) = 2.1e^{z_2}$. With these changes, the classical solution in Equation (58) corresponds to the fuzzy solution with $\vartheta = 0.99$. This comparative analysis demonstrates that the fuzzy analytical solution generalizes the crisp solution and allows a tolerance-based interpretation of the model. Therefore, the fuzzification of this system offers greater flexibility in modeling uncertainty and enhances its practical applicability.

Figure 7 illustrates the graphical representations of the fuzzy solution in terms of HMFs of fused sensor states $\varkappa_1$ and $\varkappa_2$ under the granular FFTDCT linear system for fixed spatial coordinates $z_1 = 1$ and $z_2 = 1$. The graph explores the dynamic behavior of the HMF as a solution function of two important parameters, ϑ and π. The ϑ-level represents the confidence level in the fuzzy measurement, with values ranging from 0 to 1. Moreover, π represents the RDM that captures the spatial or environmental variations that affect the sensor data. The parameter π governs the influence of environmental effects, which means that a higher value of π can represent conditions where sensors are deployed in large areas or highly variable surroundings. Figure 8 illustrates the graphical representations of the fuzzy solutions of $\varkappa_1(z_1,1,\vartheta)$ and $\varkappa_2(z_1,1,\vartheta)$. The graphs perfectly represent the triangular fuzzy nature of the FSD.

Figure 8 captures the degree of fuzziness in the fused sensor state at a specific location z_1 for a fixed z_2. For every ϑ-level value, the plot shows the confidence interval in the fusion output. At $\vartheta = 0$, the solution exhibits the widest uncertainty bounds, capturing the maximum fuzziness in the fused state. As ϑ-level values increase, the endpoints narrow, indicating greater confidence with reduced uncertainty. The system converges to the deterministic solution at $\vartheta = 1$, where the fuzzy bounds collapse with single crisp values. This visualization illustrates how a WSN system enhances its fusion output by reducing uncertainty. Figure 9 presents the graphical representations of the fuzzy fusion solutions $\varkappa_1(z_1, z_2, \vartheta)$ and $\varkappa_2(z_1, z_2, \vartheta)$ for WSN data fusion under uncertainty. Each point represents the potential state of the FSD corresponding to the different values of the ϑ-cut levels. The red points represent the lower bound of the sensor fusion outcome, and the blue points indicate the upper end of the *vartheta*-cut. This four-dimensional graph illustrates how the fused sensor output varies across the spatial positions (z_1, z_2) and the confidence level, highlighting the presence of environmental and sensor-induced uncertainty on the system behavior. This visualization allows the decision-makers in WSN-based systems, including environmental sensing and industrial monitoring, to understand the range of possible fused sensor outputs and sensor confidence.

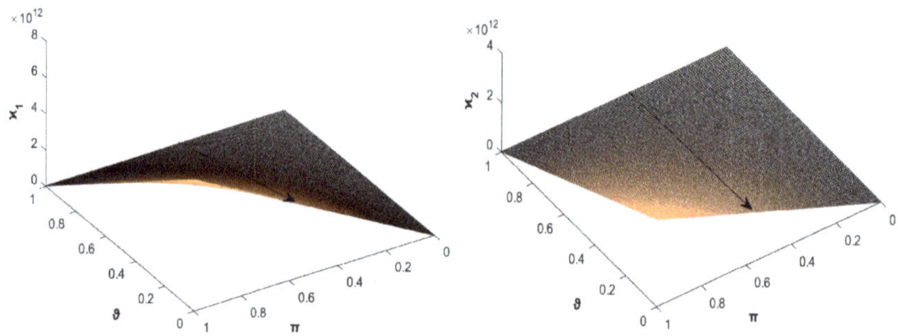

Figure 7. The graphical representation of HMFs of $\varkappa_1$ and $\varkappa_2$ for fixing the values $z_1 = 1$ and $z_2 = 1$ (left to right), respectively.

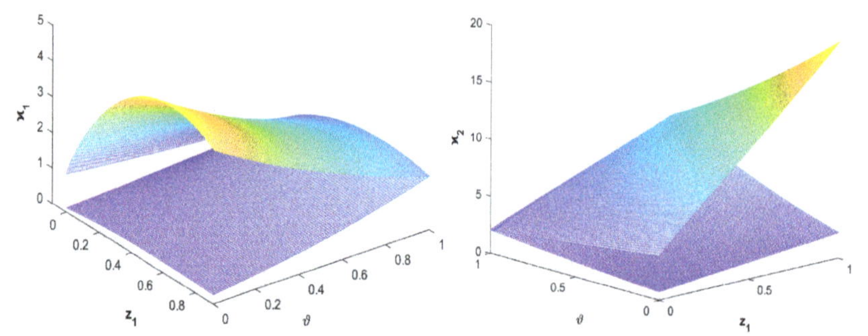

Figure 8. Graphical representations of fuzzy solutions $\varkappa_1(z_1, 1, \vartheta)$ and $\varkappa_2(z_1, 1, \vartheta)$, respectively.

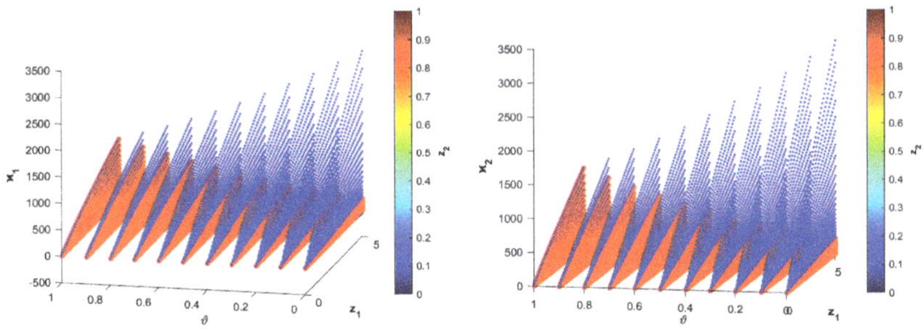

Figure 9. The left and right figures show the four-dimensional scatter plots of fuzzy solutions $\varkappa_1(z_1, z_2, \vartheta)$ and $\varkappa_2(z_1, z_2, \vartheta)$, respectively. The red points represent the left bound, and the blue points represent the right bound of the ϑ-cut of the FVF.

6. Conclusions

In this article, two classes of FFTDCT linear systems were introduced and investigated to address uncertainty and fuzziness in the system parameters. Firstly, the FFTDCT linear systems described by the Roesser model were analyzed. The potential solution of the fuzzy fractional system was extracted using a 2D granular Laplace transform approach. Secondly, the FFTDCT linear systems described by the second FM model structure were investigated, where the state-space equations contain two-dimensional and one-dimensional partial fractional-order Caputo derivatives. The fuzzy solution of the proposed models was obtained by using the 2D granular Laplace transform. The numerical examples were solved to support the theoretical developments.

The proposed study provides a structured approach for analyzing fuzzy fractional-order TDLSs under uncertainty, bridging the gap between traditional deterministic models and real-world applications where uncertainty is inherent.

Author Contributions: Concept, design, analysis, writing (original draft, review and editing), and revision of the manuscript: G.M., M.A., H.A., and N.H. All authors have read and agreed to the published version of the manuscript.

Funding: This research received no external funding.

Data Availability Statement: The original contributions presented in this study are included in the article. Further inquiries can be directed to the corresponding author(s).

Conflicts of Interest: The authors declare no conflicts of interest.

References

1. Zeng, G.; Chen, S.; Wu, H.; Yang, M. Continuous-discrete extended Kalman filtering based on the neural ordinary differential equations method. *Eng. Appl. Artif. Intell.* **2024**, *133*, 108611. [CrossRef]
2. Dubois, D.; Prade, H. Towards fuzzy differential calculus part 3: Differentiation. *Fuzzy Sets Syst.* **1982**, *8*, 225–233. [CrossRef]
3. Akram, M.; Muhammad, G.; Allahviranloo, T.; Pedrycz, W. Solution of initial-value problem for linear third-order fuzzy differential equations. *Comput. Appl. Math.* **2022**, *41*, 398. [CrossRef]
4. Muhammad, G.; Akram, M. Fuzzy fractional epidemiological model for Middle East respiratory syndrome coronavirus on complex heterogeneous network using Caputo derivative. *Inf. Sci.* **2024**, *659*, 120046. [CrossRef]
5. Muhammad, G.; Akram, M. Fuzzy fractional generalized Bagley-Torvik equation with fuzzy Caputo gH-differentiability. *Eng. Appl. Artif. Intell.* **2024**, *133*, 108265. [CrossRef]
6. Akram, M.; Muhammad, G.; Allahviranloo, T. Explicit analytical solutions of an incommensurate system of fractional differential equations in a fuzzy environment. *Inf. Sci.* **2023**, *645*, 119372. [CrossRef]
7. Akram, M.; Muhammad, G.; Allahviranloo, T.; Pedrycz, W. Incommensurate non-homogeneous system of fuzzy linear fractional differential equations using the fuzzy bunch of real functions. *Fuzzy Sets Syst.* **2023**, *473*, 108725. [CrossRef]

8. Mazandarani, M.; Pan, J. The challenges of modeling using fuzzy standard interval arithmetic: A case study in electrical engineering. *Inf. Sci.* **2024**, *653*, 119774. [CrossRef]
9. Mazarani, M.; Pariz, N.; Kamyad, A.V. Granular differentiability of fuzzy-number-valued functions. *IEEE Trans. Fuzzy Syst.* **2017**, *26*, 310–323. [CrossRef]
10. Cano, Y.C.; Flores, H.R. On new solutions of fuzzy differential equations. *Chaos Solitons Fractals* **2008**, *38*, 112–119. [CrossRef]
11. Roesser, R. A discrete state-space model for linear image processing. *IEEE Trans. Autom. Control* **1975**, *20*, 1–10. [CrossRef]
12. Fornasini, E.; Marchesini, G. State-space realization theory of two-dimensional filters. *IEEE Trans. Autom. Control* **1976**, *21*, 484–491. [CrossRef]
13. Kurek, J. The general state-space model for two-dimensional linear digital systems. *IEEE Trans. Autom. Control* **1985**, *30*, 600–602. [CrossRef]
14. Bose, N.K. *Applied Multidimensional Systems Theory*; Van Nostrand Reinhold Co.: New York, NY, USA, 1982.
15. Kaczorek, T. *Two-Dimensional Linear Systems*; Springer-Verlag: London, UK, 1985.
16. Galkowski, K. *State-Space Realizations of Linear 2-D Systems with Extensions to the General nD (n > 2) Case*; Springer-Verlag: London, UK, 2001.
17. Farina, L.; Rinaldi, S. *Positive Linear Systems: Theory and Applications*; John Wiley & Sons: New York, NY, USA, 2000.
18. Oldham, K.B.; Spanier, J. *The Fractional Calculus*; Academic Press: New York, NY, USA, 1974.
19. Miller, K.S.; Ross, B. *An Introduction to the Fractional Calculus and Fractional Differential Equations*; John Wiley & Sons: New York, NY, USA, 1993.
20. Podlubny, I. *Fractional Differential Equations*; Academic Press: London, UK, 1999.
21. Kaczorek, T. Fractional 2D linear systems. *J. Autom. Mob. Robot. Intell. Syst.* **2008**, *2*, 5–9.
22. Rogowski, K. General response formula for fractional 2D continuous-time linear systems described by the Roesser model. *Acta Mech. Autom.* **2011**, *5*, 112–116.
23. Kaczorek, T.; Rogowski, K. *Fractional Linear Systems and Electrical Circuits*; Springer International Publishing: Cham, Switzerland, 2015; pp. 49–80.
24. Rogowski, K. Selected Problems of Theory of 2D Non-Integer Order Systems Described by the Roesser Model. Ph.D. Thesis, Bialystok University of Technology, Bialystok, Poland, 2011. (In Polish)
25. Idczak, M.; Kamocki, T.; Majewski, M. On a fractional continuous counterpart of Fornasini-Marchesini model. In Proceedings of the International Conference on Multidimensional Systems, Erlangen, Germany, 9–11 September 2013; pp. 1–5.
26. Rogowski, K. Positivity analysis of continuous Fornasini-Marchesini fractional model. In Proceedings of the 5th International Symposium on Positive Systems, Rome, Italy, 14–16 September 2016.
27. Hu, H.; Meng, Y.; Huang, S. Dynamic event-triggered control of 2-D continuous systems in Roesser model. *Asian J. Control* **2025**, *27*, 646–660. [CrossRef]
28. Huang, Y.; Wu, B.; Wang, Y.E.; Liu, L. Practical exponential stability of switched generalized homogeneous positive nonlinear systems with bounded disturbances. *Circuits Syst. Signal Process.* **2025**, *44*, 3793–3809. [CrossRef]
29. Ma, H.; Tian, D.; Li, M.; Zhang, C. Reachable set estimation for 2-D switched nonlinear positive systems with impulsive effects and bounded disturbances described by the Roesser model. *Math. Model. Control* **2024**, *4*, 152–162. [CrossRef]
30. Dami, L.; Benzaouia, A. Stabilization of switched two dimensional fractional order positive systems modeled by the Roesser model. *J. Control. Autom. Electr. Syst.* **2023**, *34*, 1136–1144. [CrossRef]
31. Huang, S.; Yan, Z.; Zhang, Z.; Zeng, G. Finite-time boundedness of two-dimensional positive continuous-discrete systems in Roesser model. *Trans. Inst. Meas. Control* **2021**, *43*, 1452–1463. [CrossRef]
32. Gao, J.; Wang, W.; Zhang, G. Finite-time stability and control of 2D continuous–discrete systems in Roesser model. *Circuits Syst. Signal Process.* **2018**, *37*, 4789–4809. [CrossRef]
33. Ahn, C.K.; Shi, P.; Wu, L. l_∞-gain performance analysis for two-dimensional Roesser systems with persistent bounded disturbance and saturation nonlinearity. *Inf. Sci.* **2016**, *333*, 126–139. [CrossRef]
34. Nemati, A.; Mamehrashi, K. The use of the Ritz method and Laplace transform for solving 2D fractional-order optimal control problems described by the Roesser model. *Asian J. Control* **2019**, *21*, 1189–1201. [CrossRef]
35. Zhang, J.R.; Lu, J.G.; Zhu, Z. Stability analysis and stabilisation of continuous-discrete fractional-order 2D Fornasini-Marchesini first model. *Int. J. Syst. Sci.* **2023**, *54*, 333–344. [CrossRef]
36. Zhu, Z.; Lu, J.G. Robust stability and stabilization of continuous-discrete fractional-order 2D Fornasini-Marchesini second model with interval uncertainties. *Asian J. Control* **2024**, *26*, 3054–3066. [CrossRef]
37. Zhang, G.; Wang, W. Finite-region stability and boundedness for discrete 2D Fornasini-Marchesini second models. *Int. J. Syst. Sci.* **2017**, *48*, 778–787. [CrossRef]
38. Benyettou, K.; Bouagada, D.; Ghezzar, M.A. Solution of 2D state space continuous-time conformable fractional linear system using Laplace and Sumudu transform. *Comput. Math. Model.* **2021**, *32*, 94–109. [CrossRef]

39. Benyettou, K.; Bouagada, D.; Benamar, M.N. Controllability and minimum energy control problem of two-dimensional continuous-time fractional linear systems. *Int. J. Syst. Sci.* **2024**, *56*, 966–981. [CrossRef]
40. Yan, S.; Sun, L.; Xu, L.; Cai, Y.; Zhao, Q. State-space formulation of 2-D frequency transformation in Fornasini-Marchesini second model. *Multidimens. Syst. Signal Process.* **2018**, *29*, 361–383. [CrossRef]
41. Li, X.; Hou, X. Design of parametric controller for two-dimensional polynomial systems described by the Fornasini-Marchesini second model. *IEEE Access* **2019**, *7*, 44070–44079. [CrossRef]
42. Bede, B.; Stefanini, L. Generalized differentiability of fuzzy-valued functions. *Fuzzy Sets Syst.* **2013**, *230*, 119–141. [CrossRef]
43. Son, N.T.K.; Long, H.V.; Dong, N.P. Fuzzy delay differential equations under granular differentiability with applications. *Comput. Appl. Math.* **2019**, *38*, 107. [CrossRef]
44. Kaczorek, T. *Selected Problems in Fractional Systems Theory*; Springer: London, UK, 2011.
45. Rogowski, K. Solution to the fractional-order 2D continuous systems described by the second Fornasini-Marchesini model. *IFAC-PapersOnLine* **2017**, *50*, 9748–9752. [CrossRef]

fractal and fractional

MDPI

Article

Controllability of Mild Solution to Hilfer Fuzzy Fractional Differential Inclusion with Infinite Continuous Delay

Aeshah Abdullah Muhammad Al-Dosari

Department of Mathematics, Faculty of Science, Prince Sattam University, Al-Kharj 16273, Saudi Arabia; aa.aldosari@psau.edu.sa

Abstract: This work investigates the solvability of the generalized Hilfer fractional inclusion associated with the solution set of a controlled system of minty type–fuzzy mixed quasi-hemivariational inequality (FMQHI). We explore the assumed inclusion via the infinite delay and the semi-group arguments in the area of solid continuity that sculpts the compactness area. The conformable Hilfer fractional time derivative, the theory of fuzzy sets, and the infinite delay arguments support the solution set's controllability. We explain the existence due to the convergence properties of Mittage–Leffler functions ($\mathbb{E}_{\alpha,\beta}$), that is, hatching the existing arguments according to FMQHI and the continuity of infinite delay, which has not been presented before. To prove the main results, we apply the Leray–Schauder nonlinear alternative thereom in the interpolation of Banach spaces. This problem seems to draw new extents on the controllability field of stochastic dynamic models.

Keywords: Hilfer fuzzy multi-valued operator; existence and uniqueness; controllability; infinite continuous delay; mild solution

MSC: 26A33; 34A08; 34A12

1. Introduction

Strong theoretical visions via fractional calculus are some of the most significant ways to describe natural models. To our knowledge, fractional calculus is a vast field with many kinds of fractional differential operators and corresponding integrals. For examples, see [1–3]. One way to explain the importance of fractional calculus is by generating classical calculus, which is insufficient for modeling natural phenomena. The time-fractional operators substantially draw some fantastic results in the fractal topics field for modelings with memory. Here, we are interested in representing some medical and physical studies in [4–7]. In particular, see the usefulness of Hilfer fractional operators in papers on some different diseases [8–10].

The importance of controlled systems has arisen from Zadeh's work [11] with fuzzy sets used to understand the behavior of objects with a fractional grade of membership between zero and one. On the other hand, the controllability of fractional operators through the solvability region of mixed quasi-hemivariational inequalities has attracted attention to investigating and updating more results (in particular, with fuzzy sets). Here, we refer to [12,13]. In 2021, N. V. Hung [14] gave us strong and more worthwhile results on the generalization of Levitin–Polyak well-posedness for controlled systems of minty type–fuzzy mixed quasi-hemivariational inequalities (FMQHI). For more readings, it is worth looking into the engineering, mechanics, and economics literature as well, for example, [15–20].

Among the most robust theories that support stochastic modeling are differential inclusion theories and the continuous infinite delay ones. Many scientific teams have been conducting research on this topic in many different scientific fields. For examples, see [21,22].

Some researchers have presented several results by modeling with control, stochastic, delay, and memory systems. Many kinds are found in [12,23,24] and the references therein.

Y. Jiang et al. [13] prove the solvability theory of mild solution sets for multi-valued Caputo fractional differential initial problems with hemivariational inequality (HVI) with Clarke generalized directional derivatives.

$$\begin{aligned}
&D_c^{\alpha}x(t) \in Ax(t) + F(x(t), u(t)),\ t \in [0,b],\ \alpha \in [0,1]\\
&u(t) \in Solu(HVI),\\
&x(0) = \psi,
\end{aligned}$$

where A is the infinitesimal generator of a norm-continuous and uniformly bounded C_0 semi-group $\{K(\rho)\}_{\rho\geq 0}$ and F is a multi-valued map.

X. Pang et al. [25] presented the mild solution of Hilfer differential inclusion under the solvability constraints of variational–hemivariational inequality (VHVI).

$$\begin{aligned}
&D^{\nu,\mu}x(t) \in Ax(t) + (Rx)(t) + F(x(t), u(t)),\ t \in [0,b],\\
&u(t) \in Solu(VHVI),\\
&I_0^{(1-\nu)(1-\mu)} = x_0,\ \nu \in [0,1],\ \mu \in (0,1),
\end{aligned}$$

where A represents the infinitesimal generator of a norm-continuous and uniformly bounded C_0 semi-group $\{K(\rho)\}_{\rho\geq 0}$ and F is a multi-valued map. R is a history-dependent operator and for the order $(1-\nu)(1-\mu)$, I_0 defines the fractional order Riemann–Liouville integral.

N. T. V. Anh [26] focussed on the solvability of optimal control Caputo-fractional problems with HVI, Clarke-type subdifferentials and nonlocal initial conditions

$$\begin{aligned}
&D_c^{\alpha}z(\tau) \in Az(\tau) + F(z(\tau), w(\tau)) + \partial G(\tau,\ z(\tau),\ w(\tau)) + Bv(\tau),\\
&\tau \in [0,a],\ \alpha \in [0,1]\\
&w(t) \in Solu(HVI),\\
&z(0) = z_0 + \psi(z),\\
&v \in V_{ad},
\end{aligned}$$

where V_{ad} is an admissible control set of $v(.)$ and A denotes the infinitesimal generator of a norm-continuous and uniformly bounded C_0 semi-group $\{K(\tau)\}_{\tau\geq 0}$. $F,\ G$ are single-valued maps and ∂G represents the Clarke-type generalized subdifferential operator of G. B is a bounded linear operator.

The new work comes to define the area that produces the data of fractional order derivatives with orders between zero and one associated with the one of fuzzy sets with grades with the same property. We suggest the fractional differential inclusion concerned with the generalized conformable Hilfer fractional operator depending on $\tau \in \mathbb{R}$ and $\alpha \in (0,1]$ with $\tau + \alpha \neq 0$ [2,27]. That will be under the effect of infinite continuous delay. The reason for choosing this derivative is apparent if we know its benefits in describing control and diffusive systems and its decent iterating behavior in the order data $\alpha \in [0,1]$. This fact was explored in [27] as a conformable fractional derivative. This type has the ability as a measure to show different straight lines and planes drawing specific curves and surfaces. A. Has et al. [28] have produced an excellent study on the physical and geometric implications of the conformable type of derivatives talking about the attainability of approximating the tangent, which is not available with the classical type. We can overcome this limitation through the use of substitutional tangents. In addition, conformable derivatives are definable even if the tangent plane is undefined. For a general vision, the conformable tangent aircraft is available for all points containing points with undefined derivatives. On the other hand, the Hilfer derivative was presented as a generalization of Hilfer–Hadamard, Hilfer–Katugampola, Caputo–Hadamard, Riemann–Liouville, Hadamard, Hilfer, Caputo, etc., into single-form derivatives that draw a massive field of natural applications. For more details, see [3].

Furthermore, we consider the mild solution set of the suggested inclusion in the solvability region of FMQHI of minty type endowed with the Clarke-type generalized directional derivative.

The problem considered here will be helpful in modeling heterogeneous natural systems with memory.

2. Setting of the Problem

Let $\mathcal{F}(E) = \{\omega \in E | \omega : E \to [0,1]\}$ be the family of all fuzzy sets over a given Banach space E. Then,

(i) $\varpi : E \to \mathcal{F}(E)$ is called fuzzy mapping, for all ϖ.

(ii) $\varpi(r)$ is fuzzy set on E, $\forall r \in E$ and consequently $\omega_{\varpi(r)}(\rho)$ denotes the membership function of ρ in $\varpi(r)$.

(iii) Define by the set $M_\gamma = \{w \in E | \omega_M(w) \geq \gamma\}$, the $\gamma-$ cut set of M for all $M \in \mathcal{F}(E)$, $\gamma \in [0,1]$.

Let W, C be two reflexive Banach spaces, $K \subset W$ be a nonempty closed subset, and $L(W,C)$ be the space of all linear continuous functions. Let Z be the control reflexive Banach space and $U \subset Z$ be the set of all admissible controls which is nonempty and closed. Let $S : K \to \mathcal{F}(K)$ and $P : K \to \mathcal{F}(L(W,C))$ be fuzzy mappings and $\jmath : K \times K \to \mathbb{R}$ be a given locally Lipschitz function. Let $h : L(W,C) \times K \times K \to \mathbb{R}$, satisfying

(1) $h(v, w_2 - w_1, u) = -h(v, w_1 - w_2, u)$,

(2) $h(v, w - w, u) = 0$,

for all $w, w_1, w_2 \in K$, $v \in L(W,C)$, $u \in U$ and let $f : K \times K \to \mathbb{R}$ be a function satisfying

$$f(w,w) = 0, \; \forall w \in K.$$

We want to study Hilfer fuzzy-type fractional differential inclusion defined by

$$^{\delta}_{GH}D^{\beta,\theta}_{a^+} x(t) \in \mathcal{A}x(t) + \Pi(t, x(t), x_t, \mathbb{H}^u), \qquad t \in [a,T],\; a > 0\; \theta, \beta \in [0,1], \tag{1}$$

$$_{\delta}\mathcal{H}_a^{(1-\theta)(1-\beta)} x(a) = \frac{c\Gamma(\gamma)}{\Gamma(\omega+\gamma)} \left(\frac{t^\delta - a^\delta}{\delta}\right)^{\omega}, \tag{2}$$

$$0 < \omega < 1,\; \beta + \omega = 1,\; \gamma = \beta + \theta(1-\beta)$$

$$x(t) = \psi(t), \qquad t \in [a - \sigma, a], \tag{3}$$

where $\psi(a) = 0$, $\delta = \tau + \alpha$, $\tau \in \mathbb{R}$, $\alpha \in [0,1]$ and $\tau + \alpha \neq 0$,

$$x_t(r) = x(t+r), \qquad r \in [-\sigma, 0],\; \sigma \in [a,T),$$

$^{\delta}_{GH}D^{\beta,\theta}_{a^+}$, $_{\delta}\mathcal{H}_a^{\gamma}$ denote the generalized Hilfer-type fractional derivative and integral, respectively, that their definitions are given later, in Section 3.2. $\mathcal{A}$ denotes a generator of compact C_0 semi-groups and $\mathbb{H}^u$ defines solutions collection of the minty type FMQHI-controlled system written as follows.

FMQHI: Find $w_1 \in K \cap S(w_1)_\beta$ such that

$$h(v, w_2 - w_1, u) + \jmath^0(w_1, w_2 - w_1) + f(w_2, w_1) \geq 0, \qquad \forall v \in P(w_2)_\theta,\; \forall w_2 \in S(w_1)_\beta, \tag{4}$$

where $\jmath^0$ denotes the generalized directional derivative of Clarke type for the function $\jmath$ at the point $w_1 \in K$ in the direction of $w_2 - w_1$ given by the relation

$$\jmath^0(u,v) = \lim_{k \to u} \sup_{\lambda \to 0^+} \frac{\jmath(k + \lambda v) - \jmath(k)}{\lambda},\; u = w_1,\; v = w_2 - w_1.$$

$u(t)$ is a control function and $S(w_1)_\beta$, $P(w_2)_\theta$ are defined, respectively, by

a: $S(w_1)_\beta = \left\{ g \in K | \mu_{S(w_1)}(g) \geq \beta \right\}$,

b: $P(w_2)_\theta = \left\{ g \in K | \mu_{P(w_2)}(g) \geq \theta \right\}$.

3. Preliminaries and Auxiliary Statements

The main results depend on five important concepts: Hilfer fractional operators, C_0 semi-groups, infinite delay, multi-valued operators, and FMQHI. So, we must present some basic definitions and facts related to these concepts.

3.1. FMQH Inequalities

From [14], we can see the following

Lemma 1. *Let $u \in U$ and $w_1 \in K \cap S(w_1)_\beta$. Then,*

$$\mathbb{H}^u = \{w_1 \in K \cap S(w_1)_\beta \| h(v, w_2 - w_1, u) + \jmath^0(w_1, w_2 - w_1) + f(w_2, w_1) \geq 0 \\ , \forall w_2 \in S(w_1)_\beta, \ v \in P(w_2)_\theta\}$$

is a nonempty set.

Proof. Since $w_1 \in K \cap S(w_1)_\beta$, then $w_1 \in K$ and $w_1 \in S(w_1)_\beta$. Taking $w_2 = w_1 = w$ implies that $h(v, w - w, u) = 0$, *and* $f(w, w) = 0$. Since $\|\jmath^0(w, e)\| \leq L_e \|w\|$ if $e = 0$, then $\jmath^0(w, 0) = 0$. While $S(w_1)_\beta$ is nonempty and $w_2 = w_1 \in S(w_1)_\beta$ exists and satisfies (4), then $\mathbb{H}^u$ is a nonempty set. □

Definition 1. *Let $\mathbb{H}^u$ be the solution set of FMQHI. If*

(i) $\mathbb{H}^u$ *is nonempty,*

(ii) every ***LP*** *approximating sequence $\{x_n\}$ for FMQHI has a subsequence which converges to some points of $\mathbb{H}^u$,*

then we say that FMQHI is ***LP*** *well posed in the generalized sense.*

Let us define the approximate solution set of FMQHI by

$$\tilde{\mathbb{H}}^u(\epsilon) = \{x \in K \cap B(S(x)_\beta, \ \epsilon) | \ h(v, y - x, u) + \jmath^0(x, y - x) + f(y, x) + \epsilon \geq 0, \\ \forall y \in S(x)_\beta, \ \forall v \in P(y)_\theta\},$$

for arbitrary positive real numbers $\epsilon \geq 0$.

We can see clearly that $\forall \ \epsilon \geq 0$, $\tilde{\mathbb{H}}^u(0) = \mathbb{H}^u$ and $\mathbb{H}^u \subset \tilde{\mathbb{H}}^u(\epsilon)$.

The following Lemma has been proved in [29].

Lemma 2. *Consider that both Banach spaces W, O are reflexive. Let $K \subset W$ be a nonempty closed subset and*

$$L(W, \ O) = \{\eta | \eta : W \to O, \ \eta \text{ is linear continuous operator}\}.$$

Define the control–reflexive Banach space by Z and assume the nonempty closed subset $U \subset Z$ to be the collection of admissible controls. Suppose two fuzzy mappings $S : K \to \mathcal{F}(K)$ and $P : K \to \mathcal{F}(L(W, \ O))$ and a locally Lipschitz function $\jmath$. Let both functions $h : L(W, \ O) \times K \times U \to \mathbb{R}$ and $f : K \times K \to \mathbb{R}$ be given. If

(i) S is topologically closed on K and $w \to S(w)_\beta$ is l.s.c set-valued mapping with nonempty compact values on K;

(ii) P is l.s.c;

(iii) $\jmath$ is a locally Lipschitz function and f is u.s.c;

(iv) $\forall u \in U$, $h(,, \ u)$ is u.s.c.

then, $\mathbb{H}^u$ is a compact set for all $u \in U$. Furthermore, $\tilde{\mathbb{H}}^u$ is u.s.c at 0 and for all $\epsilon > 0$, $\tilde{\mathbb{H}}^u(\epsilon)$ is compact.

Let $\tilde{S}$, $\tilde{P}$ both be set-valued mappings defined, respectively, as follows

(i) $\tilde{S} : K \to \mathcal{F}(K)$ formed by

$$\tilde{S}(w) = S(w)_\beta, \ \forall w \in K, \tag{5}$$

(ii) $\tilde{P} : K \to \mathcal{F}(L(W, O))$ formed by

$$\tilde{P}(r) = P(r)_\theta, \ \forall r \in K. \tag{6}$$

Consequently, we have the following Lemma

Lemma 3. *Consider that both Banach spaces W, O are reflexive. Let $K \subset W$ be a nonempty closed subset and*

$$L(W,\ O) = \{\eta | \eta : W \to O,\ \eta \text{ is linear continuous operator}\}.$$

Define the control reflexive Banach space by Z and assume the nonempty closed subset $U \subset Z$ to be the collection of admissible controls. Suppose two fuzzy mappings $S : K \to \mathcal{F}(K)$ and $P : K \to \mathcal{F}(L(W,\ O))$ and a locally Lipschitz function $\jmath$. Let both functions $h : L(W,\ O) \times K \times U \to \mathbb{R}$ and $f : K \times K \to \mathbb{R}$ be given. Suppose the following conditions

(i) $\tilde{S} : K \to \mathcal{F}(K)$ *is a compact continuous set-valued mapping defined by (5);*
(ii) $\tilde{P} : K \to \mathcal{F}(L(W, O))$ *is an l.s.c set-valued mapping defined by (6);*
(iii) $\jmath$ *and* f *are, respectively, locally Lipschitz and u.s.c functions;*
(iv) $h(,, u)$ *is u.s.c for each* $u \in U$.

Then, the sufficient and necessary condition for FMQHI to be **LP** *well-posed in the generalized sense is that $\mathbb{H}^u$ is a nonempty set.*

Proof. See [14]. □

Definition 2. *For FMQHI-controlled systems, we say that $g : K \to \mathbb{R}$ is a gap function if*

(i) $g(w) \geq 0,\ \forall w \in \tilde{S}(w)$;
(ii) *The two sentences $g(w) = 0$ and $w \in \mathbb{H}^u$ are equivalent.*

Lemma 4. *Suppose that $\tilde{S}$ and $\tilde{P}$ have compact values in a neighborhood of the reference point. The function $g : D(K) \to \mathbb{R}$, where $D(K) = \bigcup_{w \in K} D(w) = \bigcup_{w \in K}\{w \in K : w \in \tilde{S}(w)\}$ defined by*

$$g(w) = \max_{r \in \tilde{S}(r)} \max_{v \in \tilde{P}(r)} \{h(v,\ w - r, u) - \jmath^0(w,\ r - w) - f(r,\ w)\}. \tag{7}$$

is a gap function for FMQHI-controlled systems. Moreover, the sentences $g(w^*) = 0$ and $w^* \in \mathbb{H}^u$ are equivalent.

Proof. See [14]. □

Lemma 5. *For FMQHI, g is continuous in K if*

(i) $\tilde{S}$ *and* $\tilde{P}$ *are compact continuous set-valued maps;*
(ii) f *is continuous;*
(iii) J *is a locally Lipschitz function;*
(iv) h *is continuous,* $\forall u \in U$.

Proof. See [14]. □

Lemma 6. *Assume that $\phi : \mathbb{R}_+ \times \mathbb{R}_+ \to \mathbb{R}$ is a real-valued function satisfying*

$$\phi(r,s) \geq 0,\ \forall r,\ s \geq 0, \phi(0,0) = 0; \tag{8}$$

$$s_n \to 0,\ r_n \geq 0,\ \phi(r_n,\ s_n) \to 0 \ imply\ r_n \to 0. \tag{9}$$

We can find a function ϕ satisfying (8) and (9) for which

$$|g(x)| \geq \phi(d(x, \mathbb{H}^u), d(x, \tilde{S}(x))), \forall x \in K. \tag{10}$$

*if $\mathbb{H}^u$ is **LP** well-posed in the generalized sense.*

Proof. See [14]. □

3.2. Fractional Calculus

Definition 3 (Conformable Integrable Function). *Let $[a_1, a_2] \subset [0, \infty)$, $0 < \alpha \leq 1$ and $\tau \in \mathbb{R}$ with $\tau + \alpha \neq 0$. Let $x \in L_\alpha[a_1, a_2] = \{x(t) : \int_{a_1}^{a_2} x(\rho) d_\alpha \rho < \infty\}$ where $d_\alpha \rho = d(\rho^\alpha)$. Then, the operator $K_{a_1}^{\tau,\alpha} : L_\alpha[a_1, a_2] \to \mathbb{R}$ given by*

$$K_{a_1}^{\tau,\alpha} = \int_{a_1}^{t} x(\rho) \rho^\tau d_\alpha \rho$$

represents a conformable fractional integral.

Definition 4 (Generalized Conformable (GC) Integrable Function). *For an order $\beta > 0$, the left-side GC fractional integral ${}_\delta\mathcal{H}_{a_1^+}^{\beta}$ with $0 < \alpha \leq 1$, $\tau \in \mathbb{R}$ and $\delta = \tau + \alpha \neq 0$ is defined by*

$${}_\delta\mathcal{H}_{a_1^+}^{\beta}(x)(t) = \frac{1}{\Gamma(\beta)} \int_{a_1}^{t} \left(\frac{t^\delta - \rho^\delta}{\delta} \right)^{\beta - 1} \rho^{\delta - 1} x(\rho) d\rho,$$

for all conformable type integrable functions x on the interval $[a_1, a_2] \subset [0, \infty)$.

Definition 5 (Generalized Hilfer-type (GH) fractional derivative). *Let $\beta \in (0,1)$, $\theta \in [0,1]$, $\tau \in \mathbb{R}$ and $0 < \alpha \leq 1$ such that $\delta = \tau + \alpha \neq 0$. For a conformable integrable function x on the interval $[a_1, a_2] \subset [0, \infty]$, the left-side GH fractional derivative operator of order β and type θ is defined by*

$${}_{GH}^{\delta}D_{a_1^+}^{\beta,\theta}(x)(t) = \left[{}_\delta\mathcal{H}_{a_1^+}^{\theta(1-\beta)} \left(t^{1-\delta} \frac{d}{dt} \right) {}_\delta\mathcal{H}_{a_1^+}^{(1-\theta)(1-\beta)} \right](x)(t).$$

Lemma 7. *Let β, θ, τ, α, δ, and x all be defined as in Definition 5. Then, we have the following statements*

(1) *For all $\nu > 0$,*

$${}_\delta\mathcal{H}_{a_1^+}^{\beta} \left(\frac{t^\delta - a^\delta}{\delta} \right)^{\nu - 1} = \frac{\Gamma(\nu)}{\Gamma(\nu + \beta)} \left(\frac{t^\delta - a^\delta}{\delta} \right)^{\nu + \beta - 1};$$

(2) *for $x \in C^1[a_1, a_2]$,*

$${}_{GH}^{\delta}D_{a_1^+}^{\beta,\theta} \, {}_\delta\mathcal{H}_{a_1^+}^{\beta}(x)(t) = x(t)$$

(3) *for $x \in C^1[a_1, a_2]$,*

$${}_\delta\mathcal{H}_{a_1^+}^{\beta} \, {}_{GH}^{\delta}D_{a_1^+}^{\beta,\theta}(x)(t) = x(t) - \left(\frac{t^\delta - a^\delta}{\delta} \right)^{\gamma - 1} {}_\delta\mathcal{H}_{a}^{(1-\theta)(1-\beta)} x(a),$$

where $\gamma = \beta + \theta(1 - \beta)$

Proof. In [1]: Lemma 2 and Theorems 5 and 7, take $\psi(t) = \frac{t^{(\alpha+\tau)}}{\alpha+\tau}$, $n = 1$. Then, we obtain the statements above. □

For more details, see [1–3,27,30].

3.3. Banach and Phase Banach Spaces

Here, we give some properties of Banach and phase spaces that help explore the solvability of the inclusion problem (1)–(3) with infinite delay.

3.3.1. Processes on Banach Spaces

According to both articles [31,32], the space

$$L^p[a,b] = \left\{ \omega(t) | \int_a^b |\omega(s)|^p ds < \infty \right\}, \quad 1 \le p < \infty$$

is a Banach space introduced with the norm

$$\|\omega\|_p = \left(\int_a^b |\omega(s)|^p ds \right)^{\frac{1}{p}}.$$

and $C[a,b] = \{\omega(t) |\ \omega(t) : [a,b] \to \mathbb{R}, |\omega(t)| \le M,\ for\ some\ M\}$ is endowed with the norm

$$\|\omega\|_C = \sup_{a<s<b} |\omega(s)| < \infty.$$

Accordingly, we have the next theorem

Theorem 1 ([31]). *Consider $1 \le p, q < \infty$ such that $\frac{1}{p} + \frac{1}{q} = 1$, then*

(i) Holder Inequality. *If $\omega \in L^p$ and $\omega^* \in L^q$. Then, $\omega\omega^* \in L^1$ and*

$$\|\omega\omega^*\|_{L^1} \le \|\omega\|_{L^p} \|\omega^*\|_{L^q}.$$

(ii) Minkowski Inequality. *If ω, $\omega^* \in L^p$. Then, $\omega + \omega^* \in L^p$ and*

$$\|\omega + \omega^*\|_{L^p} \le \|\omega\|_{L^p} + \|\omega^*\|_{L^p}.$$

(iii) Embedding Theorem. *If Ω has a finite positive measure and $q \le p$. Then, $L_P(\Omega) \subseteq L_q(\Omega)$ and*

$$\|\omega\|_{L^q} \le [\mu(\Omega)]^{\frac{1}{r}} \|\omega\|_{L^p},\ r > 0\ for\ which\ \frac{1}{q} - \frac{1}{p} = \frac{1}{r}.$$

(iv) $\lim_{p\to\infty} \|\omega\|_{L^p} = \|\omega\|_{L^\infty} = \|\omega\|_\infty = \sup_{t\in\Omega} |\omega(t)| = \|\omega\|_{C(\Omega)}.$

Definition 6. *Let W, W_0, and W_1 be given Banach spaces. Then,*

(a) Compatible couple of Banach Spaces *consists of two Banach spaces W_0 and W_1 continuously embedded in the same Housdroff topological vector space V. The spaces $W_0 \cap W_1$ and $W_0 + W_1$ are both Banach spaces equipped, respectively, with norms*

- $\|x\|_{W_0 \cap W_1} = \max(\|x\|_{W_0}, \|x\|_{W_1})$
- $\|x\|_{W_0+W_1} = \inf\{\|x_0\|_{W_0} + \|x_1\|_{W_1},\ x = x_0 + x_1,\ x_0 \in W_0,\ and\ x_1 \in W_1\}$

(b) Interpolation *is the family of all intermediate spaces W between W_0 and W_1 in the sense that*

$$W_0 \cap W_1 \subset W \subset W_0 + W_1,$$

where the two included maps are continuous.

Remark 1. *We can understand that:*

- *The couple $(L^\infty, L^1)(\mathbb{R})$ is a compatible couple since L^∞ and L^1 are both embedded in the space of measurable functions on the real line, equipped with topology convergence in measure;*

- *For all* $1 < p < \infty$, *the spaces* $L^p(\mathbb{R})$ *are intermediate spaces between* $L^\infty(\mathbb{R})$ *and* $L^1(\mathbb{R})$. *Hence,*
$$L^{1,\infty}(\mathbb{R}) = L^\infty(\mathbb{R}) \cap L^1(\mathbb{R}) \subset L^p(\mathbb{R}) \subset L^\infty(\mathbb{R}) + L^1(\mathbb{R}).$$

3.3.2. Phase Banach Space

From [33], denote by $\mathcal{B}$ the space of all continuous function mapping $[-\sigma, 0]$ to $\mathbb{R}$. For $-\infty < a < T$, let $x : [a-\sigma, T] \to \mathbb{R}$ be defined in $(a-\sigma, T)$ and continuous on $[a, T]$. For all $r \in [-\sigma, 0]$, $t \in [a, T]$, define $x_t : C[-\sigma, 0] \to \mathbb{R}$ by $x_t(r) = x(t+r)$, $\forall$. Note that x_t translates x from $[t-\sigma, t]$ back to $[-\sigma, 0]$ and $x_a = x|_{[a-\sigma,a]}$.

Definition 7. *The set* $\mathcal{B}$ *is said to be admissible whenever there exist two constants* A_1, $A_2 \geq 0$ *and a continuous function* $N : [0, \infty) \to [0, \infty)$ *such that if* $x : [a-\sigma, T] \to \mathbb{R}$ *is defined in* $(a-\sigma, T)$ *and continuous on* $[a, T)$ *with* $x_a \in \mathcal{B}$, *then for all* $t \in [a, T]$ *the following statements all hold:*

(a_1) $x_t \in \mathcal{B}$;

(a_2) x_t *is continuous in* t *with respect to* $\|.\|_{\mathcal{B}}$;

(a_3) $\|x_t\|_{\mathcal{B}} \leq A_1 \max_{s\in[a,t]} |x(s)| + N(t-a)\|x_a\|_{\mathcal{B}}$, *and* $N(t) \to 0$ *as* $t \to \infty$;

(a_4) $|v(0)| \leq A_2\|v\|_{\mathcal{B}}$ *for all* $v \in \mathcal{B}$.

Remark 2. *In* (a_2) *let* $A_3 > 0$ *be given. We can see for all* $r \in [-\sigma, 0]$, $A_3 > 0$, *and* $t \in [a-\sigma, T]$ *that* $s = t - r \in [a, T]$, *which implies the following:*

$$\begin{aligned} &x(t) = x((t-r)+r) = x_{t-r}(r), \\ &|x(t)| = |x_{t-r}(r)| \leq A_3\|x_s\|_{\mathcal{B}}, \qquad s = t-r \in [a, T] \\ &\|x(s)\|_{[a,T]} \leq \|x(t)\|_{[a-\sigma,T]} \leq A_3\|x_s\|_{\mathcal{B}} \end{aligned}$$

3.4. *Multi-Valued Mappings*

Here, we introduce some facts about multi-valued mappings and their properties. These facts are confirmed in [34–38].

Consider that we have two Banach spaces $(W, \|.\|)$ and $(O, \|.\|)$. We say that $\phi : W \to P_{cl}(W)$ is convex (closed) multi-valued mapping if $\phi(w)$ is convex (closed) for all $w \in W$. If $\phi(B)$ is relatively compact for every $B \in P_b(W)$, then ϕ is completely continuous.

ϕ is said to be upper semi-continuous if $E \subset W; \phi^{-1}(E)$ is a closed subset of W for each closed subset (i.e., the set $\{w \in W : \phi(w) \subseteq H\}$ is open whenever $H \subset W$ is open). In contrast, it is lower semi-continuous if $\forall Z \subset W; \phi^{-1}(Z)$ is an open subset of W. By another meaning, ϕ is lower semi-continuous whenever the set $\{w \in W : \phi(w) \cap H \neq \emptyset\}$ is open for all open sets $H \subset W$.

We say that a multi-valued map $\phi : [0, \tau] \to P_{cl}(W)$ is measurable if for every $w \in W$, the function $s \to d(w, A(s)) = \inf\{d(w, a) : a \in \phi(s)\}$ is an $\mathcal{L}-$measurable function.

Given $U, V \in P_{cl}(W)$, the Pompeiu–Housdorff distance of U, V is defined by

$$h(U, V) = H_d(U, V) = d_H(U, V) = \max\left\{\sup_{u\in U} d(u, V), \sup_{v\in V} d(U, v)\right\}.$$

Moreover, the diameter distance of V is given by

$$\hat{\delta}(V) = \sup_{v_1, v_2 \in V} d(v_1, v_2).$$

Note that there exists $M > 0$ such that $\hat{\delta}(V) \leq M$ if V is bounded.

Suppose we adopt ϕ as a nonempty compact valued completely continuous function. In that case, [ϕ is upper semi-continuous] is equivalent to [ϕ has a closed graph (i.e., if $v_n \to v_*$ *and* $y_n \to y_*$, then $y_n \in \phi(v_n)$ implies $y_* \in \phi(v_*)$)].

Definition 8. *Consider a multi-valued map $\Theta : [a,b] \times \mathbb{R}^n \to P(\mathbb{R})$. Then, Θ is said to be a Caratheodory if*

(1) $\tau \to \Theta(\tau, \{v_i\})$ is measurable, $\forall v_i \in \mathbb{R}, n \in \mathbb{N}$.
(2) $(\{v_i\}) \to \Theta(\tau, \{v_i\})$ a.e $\tau \in [a,b]$ is upper semi-continuous.

Adding to the assumptions (1) and (2), the map Θ is L^1- Caratheodory if for each $k > 0$, there exists $\phi_k \in L^\infty[a,b]$ satisfying $\sup_{\tau \geq 0}|\phi_k(\tau)| < +\infty$ and $\phi_k > 0$ and a nondecreasing map $Ł \in L^1[a,b]$ for which

$$\|\Theta(\tau, \{v_i\})\| = \sup\{|\theta| : \theta(\tau) \in \Theta(\tau, \{v_i\})\} \leq \phi_k(\tau)Ł(\{|v_i\|\}),$$

for all $\|v_i\| < k$, $i = 1, \ldots, n$, $n \in \mathbb{N}$, $\tau \in [a,b]$.

Lemma 8 ([39] (pp. 781–786)). *Let Ω be a Banach space,*

$$\Theta : [0,L] \times \Omega \to P_{cp,cv}(\Omega)$$

be a L^1-Caratheodory multi-valued map and P be a continuous and linear map from $L^1([0,L]\Omega)$ to $C([0,L],\Omega)$. Then, the operator:

$$P \circ S_\Theta : C([0,L],\Omega) \to P_{cp,cv}(C([0,L],\Omega)),$$

such that:

$$y \mapsto (P \circ S_\Theta)(y) = P(S_{\Theta,y})$$

is an operator with closed graph in $C([0,L],\Omega) \times C([0,L],\Omega)$.

Here,

$$S_{\Theta,y} = \left\{\theta \in L^1([0,L],\mathbb{R}) : \theta(\tau) \in \Theta(\tau, y(\tau))\right\}.$$

Theorem 2 (Leray–Schauder Nonlinear Alternative Type [40] (p. 169), [41] (p. 188)**).** *Assuming that Σ is Banach space, E is a convex closed subset of Σ, and Ω is an open subset of E with $0 \in \Omega$. If $\Psi : \overline{\Omega} \to P_{cp,cv}(E)$ is an upper semi-continuous multi-compact map, then either*

(i) there exists $\omega \in \partial\Omega$, $\rho \in (0,1)$ such that $\omega \in \rho\Psi(\omega)$, or
(ii) there exists a fixed point $\omega \in \overline{\Omega}$.

3.5. Auxiliary Statements

Lemma 9. *Take the function $\eta(t) \in \Pi(t, x(t), x_t, \mathbb{H}^u)$ for which we have*

$$\begin{aligned} &{}^{\delta}_{GH}D^{\beta,\theta}_{a^+}x(t) = \mathcal{A}x(t) + \eta(t), \qquad t \in [a,T],\ a > 0\ \alpha, \beta \in [0,1], &(11)\\ &{}_{\delta}\mathcal{H}_a^{(1-\theta)(1-\beta)}x(a) = \frac{c\Gamma(\gamma)}{\Gamma(\omega+\gamma)}\left(\frac{t^\delta - a^\delta}{\delta}\right)^{\omega}, &(12)\\ &\omega \in (0,1),\ \omega + \beta = 1. \end{aligned}$$

Then, the unique conformable solution is given by

$$\begin{aligned} x(t) &= \Gamma(\xi)x_0(t)\mathbb{E}_{\beta,\xi}\left(\mathcal{A}\left(\frac{t^\delta - a^\delta}{\delta}\right)^{\beta}\right) \\ &+ \int_0^t \left(\frac{t^\delta - \rho^\delta}{\delta}\right)^{\beta-1} \mathbb{E}_{\beta,\beta}\left(\mathcal{A}\left(\frac{t^\delta - \rho^\delta}{\delta}\right)^{\beta}\right)\eta(\rho)d\rho^\delta, \qquad (13) \end{aligned}$$

where

$$\mathbb{E}_{\alpha,\beta}(z) = \sum_{j=0}^{\infty} \frac{z^j}{\Gamma(\alpha j + \beta)}$$

and

$$x_0(t) = \frac{c}{\Gamma(\xi)}\left(\frac{t^\delta - a^\delta}{\delta}\right)^{\xi-1}, \ \xi = \gamma + \omega.$$

Proof. By applying ${}_\delta\mathcal{H}_a^\beta$ to both sides of (11) and applying condition (12), one has

$$x(t) = \frac{c}{\Gamma(\xi)}\left(\frac{t^\delta - a^\delta}{\delta}\right)^{\xi-1} + {}_\delta\mathcal{H}_a^\beta[\mathcal{A}x(t) + \eta(t)]$$

Take

$$x_0(t) = \frac{c}{\Gamma(\xi)}\left(\frac{t^\delta - a^\delta}{\delta}\right)^{\xi-1}.$$

So, we obtain

$$x(t) = x_0(t) + {}_\delta\mathcal{H}_a^\beta[\mathcal{A}x](t) + {}_\delta\mathcal{H}_a^\beta\eta(t).$$

The proof is similar to the proof of the solution in [30]: Theorem 4.

Now, to obtain the conformable solution, define the operator $\Im$ by

$$\Im(x)(t) = x_0(t) + {}_\delta\mathcal{H}_a^\beta[\mathcal{A}x](t) + {}_\delta\mathcal{H}_a^\beta\eta(t).$$

Accordingly, define the sequence $(x_k)_{k\geq 1}$ by

$$x_k(t) = \Im x_{k-1}(t).$$

Hence, we obtain the general formula

$$\begin{aligned} x_k(t) =& c\sum_{j=1}^{k+1}\frac{\mathcal{A}^{j-1}}{\Gamma(\beta j + \omega + \theta(1-\beta))}\left(\frac{t^\delta - a^\delta}{\delta}\right)^{\beta j + \omega + \theta(1-\beta) - 1} \\ &+ \int_a^t \sum_{j=1}^{k}\frac{\mathcal{A}^{j-1}}{\Gamma(\beta j)}\left(\frac{t^\delta - \rho^\delta}{\delta}\right)^{\beta j - 1}\eta(\rho)d\rho^\delta. \end{aligned}$$

Take the limit as $k \to \infty$ and apply the changing $j \to j+1$; we have

$$\begin{aligned} x(t) =& c\sum_{j=0}^{\infty}\frac{\mathcal{A}^{j}}{\Gamma(\beta j + \xi)}\left(\frac{t^\delta - a^\delta}{\delta}\right)^{\beta j + \xi - 1} \\ &+ \int_a^t \sum_{j=0}^{\infty}\frac{\mathcal{A}^{j}}{\Gamma(\beta j + \beta)}\left(\frac{t^\delta - \rho^\delta}{\delta}\right)^{\beta j + \beta - 1}\eta(\rho)d\rho^\delta \\ =& \Gamma(\xi)x_0(t)\mathbb{E}_{\beta,\xi}\left(\mathcal{A}\left(\frac{t^\delta - a^\delta}{\delta}\right)^{\beta}\right) \\ &+ \int_0^t \left(\frac{t^\delta - \rho^\delta}{\delta}\right)^{\beta-1}\mathbb{E}_{\beta,\beta}\left(\mathcal{A}\left(\frac{t^\delta - \rho^\delta}{\delta}\right)^{\beta}\right)\eta(\rho)d\rho^\delta. \end{aligned}$$

□

Now, define the set-valued map $\overline{S_{\Pi,x}^{u,(1,\infty)}}$ such as

$$\overline{S_{\Pi,x}^{u,(1,\infty)}} = \left\{\eta(t) \in L^{1,\infty}[a,T] \,|\, \eta(t) \in \Pi(t, x, x_t, \mathbb{H}^u)\right\},$$

and define the linear operator $\Delta_\eta : L^{1,\infty}[a,T] \to P(L^{1,\infty}[a,T])$ for all $\eta(t) \in \overline{S^{u,(1,\infty)}_{\Pi,x}}$ by

$$\Delta_\eta(t) = cQ^{\xi}_{\beta}\left(t^\delta - a^\delta\right) + \int_a^t \left(\frac{t^\delta - \rho^\delta}{\delta}\right)^{\beta-1} \hat{Q}_\beta\left(t^\delta - \rho^\delta\right)\eta(\rho)d\rho^\delta, \qquad \forall t \in [a,T], \tag{14}$$

$$Q^{\xi}_{\beta}\left(t^\delta - a^\delta\right) = \left(\frac{t^\delta - a^\delta}{\delta}\right)^{\xi-1} \mathbb{E}_{\beta,\xi}\left(\mathcal{A}(t)\left(\frac{t^\delta - a^\delta}{\delta}\right)^{\beta}\right), \tag{15}$$

$$\hat{Q}_\beta\left(t^\delta - \rho^\delta\right) = \mathbb{E}_{\beta,\beta}\left(\mathcal{A}(t)\left(\frac{t^\delta - \rho^\delta}{\delta}\right)^{\beta}\right). \tag{16}$$

After that, define the operator $\underline{\Delta}^{\psi}_{\eta} : L^{1,\infty}[a-\sigma,T] \to P(L^{1,\infty}[a-\sigma,T])$ by

$$\underline{\Delta}^{\psi}_{\eta}(t) = \begin{cases} \psi(t), & t \in [a-\sigma, a], \\ \Delta_\eta(t), & t \in [a,T] \end{cases} \tag{17}$$

where $\eta(t) \in \overline{S^{u,(1,\infty)}_{\Pi,x}}$ and then define the operator $\aleph : K \to P(L^{1,\infty}[a-\sigma,T])$ such as

$$\aleph(x)(t) = \left\{e(t) \in L^{1,\infty}[a-\sigma,T] \middle| e(t) = \Delta^{\psi}_{\eta}(t),\ \eta(t) \in \overline{S^{u,(1,\infty)}_{\Pi,x}},\ \psi \in L^{1,\infty}[a-\sigma,a]\right\}. \tag{18}$$

Hence,

$$\aleph_J(x)(t) = \left\{e_J(t) \in L^{1,\infty}[a,T] \middle| e_J(t) = \Delta_\eta(t),\ \eta(t) \in \overline{S^{u,(1,\infty)}_{\Pi,x}}\right\}. \tag{19}$$

Proposition 1. *Let $0 < \beta < 1$, $0 \le \theta$, $\alpha \le 1$, $\tau \in \mathbb{R}$ be given and define γ, ν, δ, respectively, by $\gamma = \beta + \theta(1-\beta)$, $\xi = \omega + \gamma$, $\nu = \xi - \beta$ and $\delta = \alpha + \tau \neq 0$. Then, the following statement is satisfied*

$$_{\delta}\mathcal{H}^{\nu}_{a^+}\left[\left(\frac{t^\delta - a^\delta}{\delta}\right)^{\beta-1} \hat{Q}_\beta\left(t^\delta - a^\delta\right)\right] = Q^{\xi}_{\beta}\left(t^\delta - a^\delta\right)$$

Proof.

$$\begin{aligned}
L.H.S &= {}_{\delta}\mathcal{H}^{\nu}_{a^+}\left[\left(\frac{t^\delta - a^\delta}{\delta}\right)^{\beta-1} \hat{Q}_\beta\left(t^\delta - a^\delta\right)\right] \\
&= {}_{\delta}\mathcal{H}^{\nu}_{a^+}\left[\left(\frac{t^\delta - a^\delta}{\delta}\right)^{\beta-1} \mathbb{E}_{\beta,\beta}\left(\mathcal{A}(t)\left(\frac{t^\delta - a^\delta}{\delta}\right)^{\beta}\right)\right] \\
&= \frac{1}{\Gamma(\nu)} \sum_{j=0}^{\infty} \frac{\mathcal{A}^j}{\Gamma(\beta j + \beta)} \int_a^t \left(\frac{t^\delta - \rho^\delta}{\delta}\right)^{\nu-1} \left(\frac{t^\delta - a^\delta}{\delta}\right)^{\beta j + \beta - 1} \rho^{\delta-1} d\rho \\
&= \sum_{j=0}^{\infty} \frac{\mathcal{A}^j}{\Gamma(\beta j + \beta)} \frac{\Gamma(\beta j + \beta)}{\Gamma(\beta j + \beta + \nu)} \left(\frac{t^\delta - a^\delta}{\delta}\right)^{\beta j + \beta + \nu - 1} \\
&= \left(\frac{t^\delta - a^\delta}{\delta}\right)^{\xi-1} \sum_{j=0}^{\infty} \frac{\left[\mathcal{A}\left(\frac{t^\delta - a^\delta}{\delta}\right)^{\beta}\right]^j}{\Gamma(\beta j + \xi)} \\
&= R.H.S
\end{aligned}$$

□

Now, since $\mathcal{A}$ is a generator of compact C_0 semi-groups, there exists $M_\beta > 0$ such that $\|\mathbb{E}_{\beta,\beta}\| \leq M_\beta$ and consequently we have the following proposition.

Proposition 2. *Let $0 < \beta < 1$, $0 \leq \theta$, $\alpha \leq 1$, $\tau \in \mathbb{R}$ be given and define γ, ν, δ, respectively, by $\gamma = \beta + \theta(1-\beta)$, $\xi = \omega + \gamma$, $\nu = \xi - \beta$ and $\delta = \alpha + \tau \neq 0$. Then, the following statement is valid.*

$$\left\|\mathcal{Q}_\beta^\xi\left(t^\delta - a^\delta\right)\right\| \leq \frac{M_\beta\Gamma(\beta)}{\Gamma(\xi)} \sup_{t\in[a,T]}\left|\left(\frac{t^\delta - a^\delta}{\delta}\right)^{\xi-1}\right|$$

Proof.

$$\begin{aligned}\left\|\mathcal{Q}_\beta^\xi\left(t^\delta - a^\delta\right)\right\| &\leq {}_\delta\mathcal{H}_{a^+}^\nu\left[\left(\frac{t^\delta - a^\delta}{\delta}\right)^{\beta-1}\left|\hat{\mathcal{Q}}_\beta\left(t^\delta - a^\delta\right)\right|\right] \\ &\leq M_\beta\, {}_\delta\mathcal{H}_{a^+}^\nu\left[\left(\frac{t^\delta - a^\delta}{\delta}\right)^{\beta-1}\right]\end{aligned}$$

Using [Lemma 7: (1)], one has

$$\left\|\mathcal{Q}_\beta^\xi\left(t^\delta - a^\delta\right)\right\| \leq \frac{M_\beta\Gamma(\beta)}{\Gamma(\xi)} \sup_{t\in[a,T]}\left|\left(\frac{t^\delta - a^\delta}{\delta}\right)^{\xi-1}\right|.$$

□

Define the statement
(P_R): For some $x \in L^p[a-\sigma, T]$, we have

$$\max\left\{\|x\|_{[a,T]}^{1,\infty},\ \|\psi\|_{\mathcal{B}}\right\} \leq R,$$

where

$$\|x\|_{[a-\sigma,T]}^{1,\infty} = \max\{\|x\|_{[a-\sigma,a]}^{1,\infty},\ \|x\|_{[a,T]}^{1,\infty}\}.$$

Then, define the set K by

$$K = \{x \in \mathcal{B} \cap L^p[a-\sigma, T] \,|\, x\ satisfies\ (P_R)\}.$$

It is clear that K is closed in $L^{1,\infty}[a-\sigma, T] \preceq L^p[a-\sigma, T]$ and in the phase Banach space $\mathcal{B}$.
Consider the following hypotheses.

($\mathcal{J}_1$) The mappings $\tilde{S}$, $\tilde{P}$, $\jmath$ and f satisfy all conditions given in Lemmas 2 and 3;

($\mathcal{J}_2$) $\Pi : [a,T] \times K \times \mathcal{B} \times \mathbb{H}^u \to P_{cp,cv}(\mathbb{R})$ is L^p- Caratheodory multi-valued mapping satisfying the below condition;
For each $R > 0$ there exist ϕ_R, $\hat{\phi}_R \in L^\infty([a,T], \mathbb{R}_+)$ and non-decreasing functions Ł$_1$, Ł$_2$, *and* Ł$_3 \in L^1([a,T], \mathbb{R})$ such that

$$\|\Pi\|^{1,\infty} \leq \phi_R(t)\left[Ł_1\left(\|x\|^{1,\infty}\right) + Ł_2(\|x_t\|_{\mathcal{B}})\right] + \hat{\phi}_R(t)Ł_3(\hat{\delta}(\mathbb{H}^u)),$$

for all $\|x\| \leq R$ and $\mathbb{H}^u$ is compact;

($\mathcal{J}_3$) The mappings $\tilde{S}$, $\tilde{P}$, $\jmath$ and f satisfy all conditions given in Lemmas 2, 4 and 5;

($\mathcal{J}_4$) $\Pi : [a,T] \times K \times \mathcal{B} \times \mathbb{H}^u \to P_{cp,cv}(\mathbb{R})$ is L^p- Caratheodory multi-valued mapping satisfying the below condition.
For each $R > 0$, there exist ϕ_R, $\hat{\phi}_R \in L^\infty([a,T], \mathbb{R}_+)$ and non-decreasing functions L_1, L_2, and $L_3 \in L^1([a,T], \mathbb{R})$ such that

$$\|\Pi\|^{1,\infty} \leq \phi_R(t)\left[L_1\left(\|x\|^{1,\infty}\right) + L_2(\|x_t\|_{\mathcal{B}})\right] + \hat{\phi}_R(t)L_3(\phi(\kappa_1,\kappa_2)),$$

for all $\|x\| \leq R$ and $\mathbb{H}^u$ is compact, where ϕ is defined by (8)–(10) in Lemma 6 with $\kappa_1 = d(x,\mathbb{H}^u)$ and $\kappa_2 = d(x,\tilde{S}(x))$.

Then, for all $t \in [a,T]$, $a > 0$ we have the following propositions

Proposition 3. *Let $x \in K$ be given. The operator $\aleph_J(x)(t)$ is convex if $(\mathcal{J}_2)$ holds.*

Proof. Let e_J^1, $e_J^2 \in \aleph_J(x)(t)$; then, there exist η_1, $\eta_2 \in \overline{S^{u,(1,\infty)}_{\Pi,x}}$ subject to

$$e_J^i = \Delta\eta_i, \qquad i = 1,2,$$

where Δ_η is defined by (14)–(16). Let $\lambda \in [0,1]$ be given. Then, by the linearty of Δ_η, we obtain

$$\begin{aligned}\lambda e_J^1 + (1-\lambda)e_J^2 =& \lambda\Delta_{\eta_1} + (1-\lambda)\Delta_{\eta_2}\\ =& \Delta(\lambda\eta_1 + (1-\lambda)\eta_2).\end{aligned}$$

By $(\mathcal{J}_2)$, $\lambda\eta_1 + (1-\lambda)\eta_2 \in \overline{S^{u,(1,\infty)}_{\Pi,x}}$ and then $\lambda e_J^1 + (1-\lambda)e_J^2 \in \aleph_J(x)(t)$ which completes the result. □

Proposition 4. *Let $x \in K$ with $x_a = \psi$ be given. The operator $\aleph_J(x)(t)$ is completely continuous if $(\mathcal{J}_1)$ and $(\mathcal{J}_2)$ are fulfilled and so are (a_1)–(a_4).*

Proof. To show that $\aleph_J(x)(t)$ is equicontinuous, we should prove that $\aleph_J(x)(t)$ is bounded and relatively compact on bounded subsets.

Step 1: Let $x \in K$ and $e_J \in \aleph_J(x)$; then,

$$\begin{aligned}|e_J(t)| =& |\Delta_\eta(t)|\\ \leq& |c|\left|Q_\beta^\xi\left(t^\delta - a^\delta\right)\right| + \left|\int_a^t \left(\frac{t^\delta-\rho^\delta}{\delta}\right)^{\beta-1} \hat{Q}_\beta\left(t^\delta-\rho^\delta\right)\eta(\rho)d\rho^\delta\right|.\end{aligned}$$

By using Propositions 1 and 2 and Lemma 7:(1) we have

$$\begin{aligned}|e_J(t)| \leq& |c|\frac{M_\beta\Gamma(\beta)}{\Gamma(\xi)}\sup_{t\in[a,T]}\left|\left(\frac{t^\delta-a^\delta}{\delta}\right)^{\xi-1}\right|\\
&+\int_a^t \left(\frac{t^\delta-\rho^\delta}{\delta}\right)^{\beta-1}\left|\hat{Q}_\beta\left(t^\delta-\rho^\delta\right)\eta(\rho)\right|d\rho^\delta\\
\leq& |c|\frac{M_\beta\Gamma(\beta)}{\Gamma(\xi)}\sup_{t\in[a,T]}\left|\left(\frac{t^\delta-a^\delta}{\delta}\right)^{\xi-1}\right|\\
&+\int_a^t \left(\frac{t^\delta-\rho^\delta}{\delta}\right)^{\beta-1}|\eta(\rho)|d\rho^\delta\\
\leq& |c|\frac{M_\beta\Gamma(\beta)}{\Gamma(\xi)}\sup_{t\in[a,T]}\left|\left(\frac{t^\delta-a^\delta}{\delta}\right)^{\xi-1}\right|\\
&+\frac{M_\beta\Gamma(\beta)}{\Gamma(\beta+1)}\left(\frac{T^\delta-a^\delta}{\delta}\right)^{\beta}G_0(R,\hat{\delta}(\mathbb{H}^u))\\
\leq& M_\beta\Gamma(\beta)G(\delta,\xi,\beta,R,\hat{\delta}(\mathbb{H}^u)),\end{aligned}$$

where

$$G_0(R,\hat{\delta}(\mathbb{H}^u)) = \|\phi_R\|[Ł_1(R) + Ł_2((A_1+N^*)R)] + \|\hat{\phi}_R\|Ł_3(\hat{\delta}(\mathbb{H}^u));$$

$$G(\delta,\xi,\beta,R,\hat{\delta}(\mathbb{H}^u)) = \frac{|c|}{\Gamma(\xi)}\sup_{t\in[a,T]}\left|\left(\frac{t^\delta - a^\delta}{\delta}\right)^{\xi-1}\right| + \frac{1}{\Gamma(\beta+1)}\left(\frac{T^\delta - a^\delta}{\delta}\right)^\beta G_0(R,\hat{\delta}(\mathbb{H}^u))$$

and $N^* = \sup_{t\in[a,T]}|N(t-a)|$.

Step 2: Suppose that $t_1,\ t_2 \in [a,T]$ such that $t_1 < t_2$ with $t_1 \to t_2$ and take $e_J \in \aleph_j(x),\ x \in K$

$$\begin{aligned}
|e_J(t_2) - e_J(t_1)| &= |\Delta_\eta(t_2) - \Delta_\eta(t_1)| \\
&\le |c|\left|Q_\beta^\xi\left(t_2^\delta - a^\delta\right) - Q_\beta^\xi\left(t_1^\delta - a^\delta\right)\right| \equiv (I_1) \\
&+ \left|\int_a^{t_1}\left(\frac{t_2^\delta - \rho^\delta}{\delta}\right)^{\beta-1}\hat{Q}_\beta\left(t_2^\delta - \rho^\delta\right)\eta(\rho)d\rho^\delta - I\right| \equiv (I_2) \\
&+ \left|I - \int_a^{t_1}\left(\frac{t_1^\delta - \rho^\delta}{\delta}\right)^{\beta-1}\hat{Q}_\beta\left(t_1^\delta - \rho^\delta\right)\eta(\rho)d\rho^\delta\right| \equiv (I_3) \\
&+ \left|\int_{t_1}^{t_2}\left(\frac{t_2^\delta - \rho^\delta}{\delta}\right)^{\beta-1}\hat{Q}_\beta\left(t_2^\delta - \rho^\delta\right)\eta(\rho)d\rho^\delta\right| \equiv (I_4),
\end{aligned}$$

where

$$I = \int_a^{t_1}\left(\frac{t_1^\delta - \rho^\delta}{\delta}\right)^{\beta-1}\hat{Q}_\beta\left(t_2^\delta - \rho^\delta\right)\eta(\rho)d\rho^\delta.$$

It is easy to understand that $I_1 \to 0$ as $t_1 \to t_2$ since Q_β^ξ is strongly continuous in $[a,T]$. For I_2, we have

$$\begin{aligned}
I_2 &= \left|\int_a^{t_1}\left[\left(\frac{t_2^\delta - \rho^\delta}{\delta}\right)^{\beta-1} - \left(\frac{t_1^\delta - \rho^\delta}{\delta}\right)^{\beta-1}\right]\hat{Q}_\beta\left(t_2^\delta - \rho^\delta\right)\eta(\rho)d\rho^\delta\right| \\
&\le \frac{M_\beta}{\beta}G_0(R,\hat{\delta}(\mathbb{H}^u))\left[\left(\frac{t_2^\delta - t_1^\delta}{\delta}\right)^\beta - \left(\frac{t_2^\delta - a^\delta}{\delta}\right)^\beta + \left(\frac{t_1^\delta - a^\delta}{\delta}\right)^\beta\right].
\end{aligned}$$

Hence, $I_2 \to 0$ as $t_1 \to t_2$

Since $\hat{Q}_\beta$ is also strongly continuous in $[a,T]$ and

$$I_3 \le \int_a^{t_1}\left(\frac{t_1^\delta - \rho^\delta}{\delta}\right)^{\beta-1}\left|\hat{Q}_\beta\left(t_2^\delta - \rho^\delta\right) - \hat{Q}_\beta\left(t_1^\delta - \rho^\delta\right)\right|\|\eta(\rho)\|d\rho^\delta,$$

then we can see that $I_3 \to 0$ as $t_1 \to t_2$.

Finally,

$$I_4 \le \frac{M_\beta}{\beta}G_0(R,\hat{\delta}(\mathbb{H}^u))\left[\left(\frac{t_2^\delta - a^\delta}{\delta}\right)^\beta - \left(\frac{t_1^\delta - a^\delta}{\delta}\right)^\beta\right],$$

which shows that $I_4 \to 0$ as $t_1 \to t_2$.

Because of that, $I_1,\ I_2,\ I_3$ and $I_4 \to 0$ as $t_1 \to t_2$, then we obtain the result $|e_J(t_2) - e_J(t_1)| \to 0$ as $t_1 \to t_2$.

According to Steps 1 and 2, we conclude that $\aleph_J(x)(t)$ is completely continuous. □

Proposition 5. *Let $x \in K$ with $x_a = \psi$ be given. The operator $\aleph_J(x)(t)$ is upper semi-continuous if $(\mathcal{J}_1)$, $(\mathcal{J}_2)$ and (a_1)–(a_4) are satisfied.*

Proof. Since $\aleph_J(x)(t)$ is completely continuous, it is enough to claim that it has a closed graph to obtain the upper semi-continuity of $\aleph_J(x)(t)$. Let $x_n \in K$, $x_n \to x^*$, $e_J^n \in \aleph_J(x_n)$ and $e_J^n \to e_J^*$. If $e_J^n \in \aleph_J(x_n)$, there exists $\eta_n \in \overline{S_{\Pi,x_n}^{u,(1,\infty)}}$ such that $e_J^n = \Delta_{\eta_n}$. Using the linearity of Δ and Lemma 8 shows that Δ has a closed graph. Thus, $e_J^n = \Delta_{\eta_n} \to \Delta_{\eta^*}$, $\eta^* \in \overline{S_{\Pi,x^*}^{u,(1,\infty)}}$. Take $e_J^* = \Delta_{\eta^*}$, then we obtain $e_J^* \in \aleph_J(x^*)$ which tends to the upper semi-continuity of $\aleph_J(x)(t)$. $\square$

4. Main Results

Theorem 3. *Consider that hypothesis $(\mathcal{J}_1)$, $(\mathcal{J}_2)$ and (a_1)–(a_4) are valid. Then, problem (1)–(3) has at least one solution in K if the following condition holds*

$$\frac{R}{\psi^* + M_\beta \Gamma(\beta) G\big(\delta, \xi, \beta, R, \hat{\delta}(\mathbb{H}^u)\big)} \geq 1,$$

where $x_a = \psi$

Proof. To obtain the suggested result, we follow all arguments given in Lemma 8 and Theorem 2 for the operator $\aleph(K)$ over the closed convex subset K.

Step 1: Let $x \in K$, $\lambda \in [0,1]$, e_1, $e_2 \in \aleph(x)(t)$ and $t \in [a-\sigma, T]$. We want to claim that $\lambda e_1 + (1-\lambda)e_2 \in \aleph(x)$. So, since e_1, $e_2 \in \aleph(x)(t)$ implies the existence of two elements, $\eta_i \in \overline{S_{\Pi,x}^{u,(1,\infty)}}$ such that

$$e_i = \underline{\Delta}_{\eta_i}^{\psi}(t), \; i = 1, 2,$$

where $\underline{\Delta}_{\eta_i}^{\psi}(t)$ is defined by (14)–(17). Due to the linearty of Δ, we can see the linearty of $\underline{\Delta}$ and by using Proposition 3 and the convexity of $\overline{S_{\Pi,x}^{u,(1,\infty)}}$, we have

$$\begin{aligned}
\lambda e_1 + (1-\lambda)e_2 &= \lambda \underline{\Delta}_{\eta_1}^{\psi}(t) + (1-\lambda)\underline{\Delta}_{\eta_2}^{\psi}(t) \\
&= \underline{\Delta}_{\lambda\eta_1 + (1-\lambda)\eta_2}^{(\lambda + (1-\lambda))\psi}(t) \\
&= \underline{\Delta}_{\lambda\eta_1 + (1-\lambda)\eta_2}^{\psi}(t) \in \aleph(x)(t),
\end{aligned}$$

We can understand the proof since Δ is convex due to Proposition 3.

Step 2: To show that that is completely continuous in K, we need to prove that $\aleph : K \to K$ and is equicontinuous.

(l_1) Let $x \in K$, $e(t) \in \aleph(x)(t)$. By using Proposition 4 Step 1, one has

$$\begin{aligned}
|e(t)| &= \left|\underline{\Delta}_{\eta}^{\psi}(t)\right| \\
&\leq \|\psi\|_{\mathcal{B}} + |\Delta_\eta(t)|_{[a,T]} \\
&\leq \psi^* + M_\beta \Gamma(\beta) G\big(\delta, \xi, \beta, R, \hat{\delta}(\mathbb{H}^u)\big) \leq R.
\end{aligned}$$

(l_2) Let t_1, $t_2 \in [a-\sigma, T]$, $t_1 < t_2$ with $t_1 \to t_2$

Case 1: If t_1, $t_2 \in [a-\sigma, a]$, then by continuity of ψ in $[a-\sigma, a]$ we obtain

$$|e(t_2) - e(t_1)| = |\psi(t_2) - \psi(t_1)| \to 0, \qquad as\ t_1 \to t_2.$$

Case 2: If t_1, $t_2 \in [a, T]$, then by using Proposition 4 Step 2, one has

$$|e(t_2) - e(t_1)| \leq |\aleph_J(x)(t_2) - \aleph_J(x)(t_1)| \to 0 \qquad as\ t_1 \to t_2.$$

Case 3: If $t_1 \in [a-\sigma, a]$, $t_2 \in [a, T]$ and $t_1 \to t_2$, then there exists $0 < \epsilon \to 0$ such that $t_1, t_2 \in (a-\epsilon, a+\epsilon)$ which implies that $t_1, t_2 \to a$. According to Case 1 and Case 2, we have

$$|e(t_2) - e(t_1)| \leq |e(t_2) - e(a)|_{(a,a+\epsilon)} + |e(a) - e(t_1)|_{(a-\epsilon,a)} \to 0$$

as $t_1, t_2 \to a$.

By (l_1) and (l_2), we conclude that $\aleph$ is completely continuous in K.

Step 3: We still need to explore that $\aleph$ has a closed graph to see the upper semi-continuity of $\aleph$. In the vision of Proposition 5 and the continuity of ψ, we understand the upper semi-continuity of $\aleph$.

Step 4: For the set K, we choose

$$R = \psi^* + M_\beta \Gamma(\beta) G(\delta, \xi, \beta, R, \delta(\mathbb{H}^u)) + 1.$$

By Theorem 2 and Step 1–Step 4, we conclude the solvability of problem (1)–(3). □

Theorem 4. *Consider that hypotheses $(\mathcal{J}_2)$–$(\mathcal{J}_4)$ and (a_1)–(a_4) are satisfied. Then, problem (1)–(3) has at least one solution in K if the following condition is valid.*

$$\frac{R}{\psi^* + M_\beta \Gamma(\beta) G(\delta, \xi, \beta, R, g^*)} \geq 1,$$

where $g^* = \|g\|$,

$$G_0(R, g^*) = \|\phi_R\|[L_1(R) + L_2((A_1 + N^*)R)] + \|\hat{\phi}_R\| L_3(g^*);$$

$$G(\delta, \xi, \beta, R, g^*) = \frac{|c|}{\Gamma(\xi)} \sup_{t \in [a,T]} \left| \left(\frac{t^\delta - a^\delta}{\delta} \right)^{\xi - 1} \right| + \frac{1}{\Gamma(\beta + 1)} \left(\frac{T^\delta - a^\delta}{\delta} \right)^\beta G_0(R, g^*)$$

and $x_a = \psi$.

Proof. Similarly to the proof of Theorem 3, we take

$$R = \psi^* + M_\beta \Gamma(\beta) G(\delta, \xi, \beta, R, g^*) + 1.$$

□

5. Applications

Example 1. *Consider that $\mathcal{J}_1$ holds and*

$$\Pi(t, x, x_t, \mathbb{H}^u) = \left[\int_{-\sigma}^{0} B_i(t, r) x_t(r) dr \right]_{i=1}^{\infty} + \chi_{\mathbb{H}^u}(x);$$

$$\sum_{i=1}^{\infty} |B_i(t, r)| x_t(r) dr \leq 1 \tag{20}$$

and

$$\chi_{\mathbb{H}^u}(x) = \begin{cases} 1, & x \in \mathbb{H}^u; \\ 0, & x \notin \mathbb{H}^u \end{cases} \tag{21}$$

Hence, if $\mathcal{B} = C[-\sigma, r]$*, one has*

$$\begin{aligned}|\Pi| &\leq \|x_t\|_{\mathcal{B}} \int_{-\sigma}^{0} |B_i(t,r)dr| + 1 \\ &\leq A_1\|x\|^{1,\infty} + N(t-a)\|x_a\|_{\mathcal{B}} + 1. \\ &\leq \|x\|^{1,\infty} + N^*\|\psi\|_{\mathcal{B}} + 1 \\ &\leq (A_1 + N^*)R + 1\end{aligned}$$

Take $\phi_R = \hat{\phi}_R = 1$, $Ł_1 = 0$, $Ł_2 = I$*(identity map) and* $Ł_3 = 1$*. So, we obtain* $\Gamma_0(R, \mathbb{H}^u) = (A_1 + N^*)R + 1$.

Furthermore, assume that $\beta = 1 \to \omega = 0$ *tends to* $\xi = \gamma = 1$*, which implies*

$$\mathbb{E}_{\beta,\xi}(z) = \mathbb{E}_{\beta,\beta}(z) = \mathbb{E}_{1,1}(z) = \exp(z).$$

If we take $z = \mathcal{A}(t)\left(\frac{t^\delta - \rho^\delta}{\delta}\right) = -\lambda\left(\frac{t^\delta - \rho^\delta}{\delta}\right)$, $\lambda \in \mathbb{R}^+$*, then we obtain*

$$\exp(z) \leq 1 = M_1, \ \forall \rho \in [a, t].$$

Moreover,

$$\begin{aligned}G(\delta, \xi, \beta, R, \hat{\delta}(\mathbb{H}^u)) &= G(\delta, 1, 1, R, \hat{\delta}(\mathbb{H}^u)) \\ &= |c| + \left(\frac{T^\delta - \rho^\delta}{\delta}\right) G_0(R, \hat{\delta}(\mathbb{H}^u))\end{aligned}$$

Take $R = \psi^* + G(\delta, 1, 1, R, \hat{\delta}(\mathbb{H}^u)) + 1$*; then, by Theorem 3 the problem (1)–(3) associated with (20) and (21) has at least one solution.*

Example 2. *Consider that* $\mathcal{J}_3$ *holds and*

$$\Pi(t, x, x_t, \mathbb{H}^u) = \left[\int_{-\sigma}^{0} B_i(t,r)x_t(r)dr\right]_{i=1}^{\infty} + W_{\mathbb{H}^u}(x);$$
$$\sum_{i=1}^{\infty} |B_i(t,r)|x_t(r)dr \leq 1 \tag{22}$$

and

$$W_{\mathbb{H}^u}(x) = \begin{cases} \inf |g(x)|, & x \in \mathbb{H}^u; \\ 0, & x \notin \mathbb{H}^u \end{cases} \tag{23}$$

and similarly β, z *in Example 1. Then, if* $\mathcal{B} = C[-\sigma, r]$*, one has*

$$\begin{aligned}|\Pi| &\leq \|x_t\|_{\mathcal{B}} \int_{-\sigma}^{0} |B_i(t,r)dr| + g^* \\ &\leq A_1\|x\|^{1,\infty} + N(t-a)\|x_a\|_{\mathcal{B}} + g^*. \\ &\leq \|x\|^{1,\infty} + N^*\|\psi\|_{\mathcal{B}} + g^* \\ &\leq (A_1 + N^*)R + g^*\end{aligned}$$

Take $\phi_R = \hat{\phi}_R = 1$, $L_1 = 0$, $L_2 = L_3 = I$*(identity map); we obtain*

$$\Gamma_0(R, g^*) = (A_1 + N^*)R + g^*.$$

Moreover,

$$G(\delta,\xi,\beta,R,g^*) = G(\delta,1,1,R,\hat{\delta}(\mathbb{H}^u)) \\ = |c| + \left(\frac{T^\delta - \rho^\delta}{\delta}\right) G_0(R,g^*)^{\cdot}$$

Take $R = \psi^* + G(\delta,1,1,R,g^*) + 1$; *then, by Theorem 4 the problem (1)–(3) associated with (22) and (23) has at least one solution.*

6. Conclusions

This article is devoted to the mild solution of Hilfer fractional inclusion with infinite delay. The solution set intersects with the solution set of FMQHI. We present two theorems according to Lemmas 1–6. We proved these theorems due to the compactness in interpolation of Banach spaces. We first look at the properties of the solution set in Propositions 1–5. After that, we apply the Leray–Schauder Nonlinear Alternative Theorem with phase Banach space rules to the suggested solution set. Finally, we presented some examples related to the proven theorems. We hope to study the stability of this model in subsequent work using the Ulam–Mittage–Lefller test.

Funding: The author extends her appreciation to the Deanship of Scientific Research (DSR), Prince Sattam bin Abdulaziz University for funding this research work through the project number (PSAU/2023/02/26683). Also, thanks to Prof. Ahmed El-Shreef ((DSR), King Abdulaziz university, Jeddah, Saudi Arabia) for sharing his opinions about the main idea.

Institutional Review Board Statement: Not applicable.

Informed Consent Statement: Not applicable.

Data Availability Statement: Data are contained within the article.

Conflicts of Interest: The authors declare no conflicts of interest.

References

1. Sousa, J.V.D.C.; De Oliveira, E.C. On ψ–Hilfer fractional derivative. *Commun. Nonlinear Sci. Numer. Simul.* **2018**, *60*, 72–91. [CrossRef]
2. Khan, T.U.; Khan, M.A.; Chu, Y.M. A new generalized Hilfer-type fractional derivative with applications to space-time diffusion equation. *Results Phys.* **2021**, *22*, 103953. [CrossRef]
3. Oliveira, D.S.; de Oliveira, E.C. Hilfer-Katugampola fractional derivative. *Comput. Appl. Math.* **2018**, *37*, 3672–3690. [CrossRef]
4. Aleen, M.; Caffarelli, L.; Vasseur, A. A Parabolic Problem with a Fractional Time Derivative. *Arch. Ration. Mech. Anal.* **2016**, *221*, 603–630. [CrossRef]
5. Singh, J.; Kumar, D.; Baleanu, D. New Aspects of Fractional Bloch Model Associated with Composite Fractional Derivative. *Math. Model. Nat. Phenom.* **2021**, *16*, 10. [CrossRef]
6. Hilfer, R. Fundation of Fractional Dynamics. *Fractals* **1995**, *3*, 549–556. [CrossRef]
7. Hilfer, R. Mathematical and physical interpretations of fractional derivatives and integrals. *Handb. Fract. Calc. Appl.* **2019**, *1*, 47–85.
8. Bahater, S.H.S.; Jangid, K.; Purohit, S.D. A Study of The Hepatitis B Virus Infection Using Hilfer Fractional Derivative. *Natl. Acad. Sci. Azerbaijan* **2022**, *48*, 100–117.
9. Joshi, H.; Jha, B.K. Chaos of Calcium Diffusion in Parkinson's Infectious Disease Model and Treatment Mechanism via Hilfer Fractional Derivative. *Math. Model. Numer. Simul. Appl.* **2021**, *1*, 84–94.
10. Al-Hdaibat, B.; Meetei, M.Z.; Ahmad, I.; Althobaiti, N.; Safi, M.A.; Khan, M.A.; Riaz, M.B. The Dynamics of Monkeypox Disease Under ψ–Hilfer Fractional Derivative: Application to Real Data. *Results Phys.* **2023**, *55*, 107–127. [CrossRef]
11. Zadeh, L.A. Fuzzy sets. *Inf. Control* **1965**, *8*, 338–353. [CrossRef]
12. Liu, Z.; Zeng, S.; Motreanu, D. Partial differential hemivariational inequalities. *Adv. Nonlinear Anal.* **2018**, *7*, 571–586. [CrossRef]
13. Jiang, Y.; Huang, N.; Wei, Z. Existence of a global attractor for fractional differential hemivariational inequalities. *Discret. Contin. Dyn. Syst.-Ser. B* **2020**, *25*, 1193–1212. [CrossRef]
14. Hung, N.V. Generalized Levitin–Polyak well–posedness for controlled systems of FMQHI–fuzzy mixed quasi–hemivariational inequalities of Minty type. *J. Comput. Appl. Math.* **2021**, *386*, 113–263. [CrossRef]
15. Hung, N.V.; Tam, V.M. Error Bound Analysis of The D-Gap Functions For a Class of Elliptic Variational Inequalities With Applications to Frictional Contact Mechanics. *Z. Angew. Math. Phys.* **2021**, *72*, 173. [CrossRef]

16. Hung, N.V.; Keller, A.A. Painlevé–Kuratowski Convergence of the Solution Sets for Controlled Systems of Fuzzy Vector Quasi-Optimization Problems with Application to Controlling Traffic Networks under Uncertainty. *Comput. Appl. Math.* **2021**, *40*, 28. [CrossRef]
17. Hung, N.V.; Keller, A.A. Existence and Generic Stability Conditions of Equilibrium Points to Controlled Systems for n-Player Multiobjective Generalized Games Using the Kakutani–Fan–Glicksberg Fixed-Point Theorem. *Optim. Lett.* **2022**, *16*, 1477–1493. [CrossRef]
18. Hung, N.V.; Migórski, S.; Tam, V.M.; Zeng, S.D. Gap Functions And Error Bounds For Variational– Hemivariational Inequalities. *Acta Appl. Math.* **2020**, *169*, 691–709. [CrossRef]
19. Hung, N.V.; Tam, V.M.; Liu, Z.; Yao, J.C. A Novel Approach to Hölder Continuity of a Class of Parametric Variational–Hemivariational Inequalities. *Oper. Res. Lett.* **2021**, *49*, 283–289. [CrossRef]
20. Migórski, S.; Ochal, A.; Sofonea, M. *Nonlinear Inclusions and Hemivariational Inequalities. Models and Analysis of Contact Problems*; Springer: New York, NY, USA, 2013.
21. Petrosyan, G.G. On antiperiodic boundary value problem for semilinear fractional differential inclusion with deviating argument Banach space. *Ufa Math. J.* **2020**, *12*, 69–80. [CrossRef]
22. L-Sarori, N.A.A.; Ghadle, K.P. Nonlocal fractional differential inclusion with impulse effects and delay. *J. Korean Soc. Ind. Appl. Math.* **2020**, *24*, 229–242.
23. Kavitha, K.; Vijayakumar, V.; Shukla, A.; Nissar, K.S.; Udhayakumar, R. Results on approximate Controllability Sobolve-Type Fractional Netural Differential Inclusions of Clarck Subdifferential Type. *Chaos Soliton Fractal* **2021**, *151*, 111264. [CrossRef]
24. Sedova, N.O. Development of the Direct Lyapunov Method for Functional-Differential Equations with Infinite Delay. *Math. Notes* **2008**, *84*, 826–841. [CrossRef]
25. Pang, X.; Li, X.; Liu, Z. Decay mild solutions of Hilfer fractional differential variational–hemivariational inequalities. *Nonlinear Anal. Real World Appl.* **2023**, *71*, 103834. [CrossRef]
26. Anh, N.T.V. Optimal control problem of fractional evolution inclusions with Clarke subdifferential driven by quasi-hemivariational inequalities. *Commun. Nonlinear Sci. Numer. Simul.* **2024**, *128*, 107682. [CrossRef]
27. Khan, T.U.; Khan, M.A. Generalized conformable fractional operators. *J. Comput. Appl. Math.* **2019**, *346*, 378–389. [CrossRef]
28. Has, A.; Yılmaz, B.; Baleanu, D. On the Geometric and Physical Properties of Conformable Derivative. *Math. Sci. Appl. E-NOTES* **2024**, *12*, 60–70.
29. Aubin, J.P.; Ekeland, I. *Applied Nonlinear Analysis*; John Wiley and Sons: New York, NY, USA, 1984.
30. Sousa, J.; de Oliveira, E.C. Ulam–Hyers–Rassias stability for a class of fractional integro-differential equations. *Results Math.* **2018**, *73*, 111.
31. Adams, R.; Fournier, J. *Sobolev Space*, 2nd ed.; Academic Press: Cambridge, MA, USA, 2003.
32. Bergh, J.; Lofstrom, J. *Interpolation Spaces. An Introduction*; Grundlehren der Mathematischen Wissenschaften; Springer: Berlin/Heidelberg, Germany; New York, NY, USA, 1976; Volume 223.
33. Haddock, J.; Tergeki, J. On the location of positive limit sets for autonomous fractional-differential equations with infinite delay. *J. Differ. Equ.* **1990**, *86*, 1–32. [CrossRef]
34. Smirnov, G.V. *Introduction to the Theory of Differential Equations*; American Mathematical Society: Providence, RI, USA, 2002; Volume 41.
35. Aubin, J.P.; Cellina, A. *Differential Inclusion*; Spring: Berlin/Heidelberg, Germany, 1984.
36. Aubin, J.P.; Frankowska, H. *Set-Valued Analysis*; Birkhauser: Bosten, MA, USA, 1990.
37. Deimling, K. *Multi-Valued Differential Equations*; Walter de Gruyter: Berlin, Germany; New York, NY, USA, 2011.
38. Howard, P.E. Definiton of compact. *J. Symb. Log.* **1990**, *55*, 645–655. [CrossRef]
39. Lasota, A.; Opial, Z. An application of the Kakutani-Ky Fan theorem in the theory of ordinary differential equations. *Bull. Acad. Olon. Sci. Ser. Sci. Math. Astronom. Phys.* **1965**, *13*, 781–786.
40. Granas, A.; Dugundji, J. *Fixed Point Theory*; Springer: New York, NY, USA, 2003.
41. Singh, S.P. Nonlinear functional analysis and its application, Mathematical and Physical Sciences. *Nato Sci. Aff. Div.* **1985**, *173*, 187–194.

fractal and fractional

MDPI

Article

Modeling and Analysis of Caputo–Fabrizio Definition-Based Fractional-Order Boost Converter with Inductive Loads

Donghui Yu *, Xiaozhong Liao and Yong Wang

School of Automation, Beijing Institute of Technology, Beijing 100081, China; liaoxiaozhong@bit.edu.cn (X.L.); wangyong_ok_0@163.com (Y.W.)

* Correspondence: 3120205479@bit.edu.cn; Tel.: +86-133-4222-6096

Abstract: This paper proposes a modeling and analysis method for a Caputo–Fabrizio (C-F) definition-based fractional-order Boost converter with fractional-order inductive loads. The proposed method analyzes the system characteristics of a fractional-order circuit with three state variables. Firstly, this paper constructs a large signal model of a fractional-order Boost converter by taking advantage of the state space averaging method, providing accurate analytical solutions for the quiescent operating point and the ripple parameters of the circuit with three state variables. Secondly, this paper constructs a small signal model of the C-F definition-based fractional-order Boost converter by small signal linearization, providing the transfer function of the fractional-order system with three state variables. Finally, this paper conducts circuit-oriented simulation experiments where the steady-state parameters and the transfer function of the circuit are obtained, and then the effect of the order of capacitor, induced inductor, and load inductor on the quiescent operating point and ripple parameters is analyzed. The experimental results show that the simulation results are consistent with those obtained by the proposed mathematical model and that the three fractional orders in the fractional model with three state variables have a significant impact on the DC component and steady-state characteristics of the fractional-order Boost converter. In conclusion, the proposed mathematical model can more comprehensively analyze the system characteristics of the C-F definition-based fractional-order Boost converter with fractional-order inductive loads, benefiting the circuit design of Boost converters.

Keywords: fractional-order boost converter; Caputo–Fabrizio fractional derivative; fractional-order systems modeling

1. Introduction

Fractional-order calculus is a mathematical tool related to memory processes, fractal geometry, and other physical phenomena [1,2]. In recent years, many studies have studied the fractional-order models of complex circuit systems by combining fractional-order operators with circuit system modeling [3–5]. Fractional calculus operators increase the degrees of freedom of mathematical models. They enable a concise and accurate description of memory properties and spatial global correlations in mechanical and physical processes [6]. The DC–DC converter, characterized as a circuit with the capability of controllable transformation of DC voltage, has found extensive applications in various power electronic equipment and systems. However, the pronounced nonlinearity inherent in DC–DC converters poses significant challenges in the construction of their precise mathematical models [7,8]. Studies have shown that fractional-order models are superior in characterizing the electrical properties of components in the context of DC–DC converters [9–13]. Applying fractional-order operators to mathematical modeling of DC–DC converters can provide a more comprehensive and accurate description of the electrical characteristics of DC–DC converters [14,15].

Up to now, fractional-order calculus has no universally accepted definition [16]. When studying practical systems, the Caputo definition is often used [17]. However, there is a bias in describing the full memory effect because of the singular kernel of the Caputo definition [18,19]. To overcome this issue, Caputo and Fabrizio proposed the C-F definition [20]. Applying the C-F definition to system modeling can solve the singularity problem and simplify the calculation process. Over the past few years, the C-F definition has been widely used in various fields such as thermodynamics [21,22], medicine [23–25], and power electronics [26–29].

With the progress of society, the industrial field has higher requirements for the accuracy of DC–DC converter models. Therefore, scholars have proposed various fractional-order modeling methods to obtain fractional-order mathematical models of DC–DC converters in different modes, such as the state space averaging method and equivalent small parameter method [30,31]. Studies have shown that fractional order can affect the output performance of circuit systems, including DC components and ripple parameters of current and voltage. Fractional calculus not only increases the degrees of freedom in the DC–DC converter design but also improves the accuracy of circuit system control [32–35]. However, the above studies are mostly based on the Caputo definition. Compared with actual circuits, traditional models based on the Caputo definition may ignore certain non-ideal discontinuous characteristics of components [36,37]. Therefore, the circuit parameters such as induced current and output voltage obtained from the analysis based on traditional fractional-order models are continuous. Additionally, the obtained steady-state characteristics, such as voltage ratio, are independent of component order [38,39]. These results differ from actual circuits. To obtain a more accurate and comprehensive mathematical model, some scholars have introduced additional components to the model. However, this approach increases the complexity of the model and affects further analysis and control of the circuit [40,41].

To overcome these problems, the C-F definition has been applied to the modeling of DC–DC converter circuits in recent studies. The C-F definition-based system modeling method can characterize the properties that Caputo definition-based fractional-order models cannot accurately represent [42–45]. The results indicate that the C-F definition can accurately characterize the nonlinear characteristics of capacitor voltage and inductor current in DC–DC converters, simplify the circuit topology, and make the electrical characteristics of the models closer to the actual circuits [46–48]. However, these studies only consider the operating conditions of resistive loads. In practical applications, the subordinate circuits carried are mostly capacitive or inductive loads, such as inductor coils, inductor filters, and capacitor couplers. Their electrical characteristics can also be described by fractional-order models [49–55]. Similar to integer-order models, considering loads with energy storage characteristics during mathematical modeling can transform the model from a fractional-order model with two state variables to a fractional-order model with three state variables, which can provide a more comprehensive description of the system characteristics of circuits. Therefore, this paper establishes and analyzes the C-F definition-based mathematical model of Boost converters with fractional-order inductive loads. Overall, this paper makes contributions as follows:

(1) A large signal model of a fractional-order Boost converter with a fractional-order inductive load based on the C-F definition is constructed by using the state space averaging method. The accurate analytical solutions of the quiescent operating point and the ripple parameters of three state variables are derived. Moreover, simulation experiments are conducted where the results are consistent with the calculation results, verifying the correctness of the proposed model.

(2) The transfer functions of the fractional-order circuit with three state variables are derived by performing the small-signal linearization method. Simulation experiments are conducted where the results from frequency sweep analysis verify the correctness of the transfer function.

(3) According to the aforementioned results, the effect of the DC component of the state variables and ripple parameters on the order of energy storage components is analyzed.

2. Preliminaries

The C-F fractional derivative can be defined as follows [20]:

$$ {}_{a}^{\mathrm{CF}}\mathcal{D}_{t}^{\alpha} f(t) = \frac{1}{(1-\alpha)} \int_{a}^{t} \dot{f}(\tau) e^{-\frac{\alpha(t-\tau)}{1-\alpha}} \mathrm{d}\tau, \tag{1} $$

where ${}_{a}^{\mathrm{CF}}\mathcal{D}_{t}^{\alpha}$ denotes the α-order C-F fractional derivative. The Laplace transform is derived as follows:

$$ \mathcal{L}\left[{}_{a}^{\mathrm{CF}}\mathcal{D}_{t}^{\alpha} f(t)\right] = \frac{s\mathcal{L}[f(t)] - f(0)}{s + \alpha(1-s)}. \tag{2} $$

When applying the C-F definition to the electronic component modeling, the impedance expressions for capacitors and inductors are as follows:

$$ \begin{aligned} Z(C_{\alpha}, \alpha) &= \frac{(1-\alpha)s + \alpha}{sC_{\alpha}} = \frac{1-\alpha}{C_{\alpha}} + \frac{1}{s\frac{C_{\alpha}}{\alpha}}, \\ Z(L_{\beta}, \beta) &= \frac{sL_{\beta}}{s(1-\beta) + \beta} = \frac{L_{\beta}}{\beta}s // \frac{L_{\beta}}{1-\beta}, \end{aligned} \tag{3} $$

where α, β, L_{β}, and C_{α} are the order, the inductance, and the capacitance of components. // is the parallel symbol. The equivalent circuit topology of the fractional-order capacitor and inductor based on the C-F definition are shown in Figure 1.

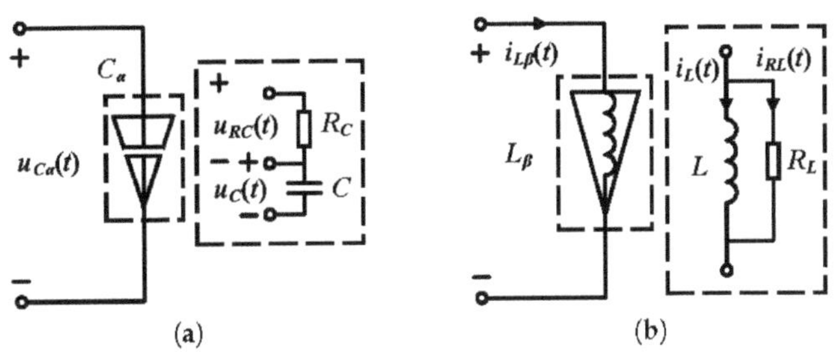

Figure 1. The equivalent circuit topology defined by the C-F derivative. (**a**) Capacitor. (**b**) Inductor.

As shown in Equation (2), when α and β are greater than 1, the equivalent resistance is negative, which means that the system requires external energy injection and does not match the actual electronic components [56]. Therefore the orders between 0 and 1 are considered only in this paper.

3. Modeling of the C-F Definition-Based Fractional-Order Boost Converter with Inductive Load

The fractional-order Boost converter with inductive load is shown in Figure 2. $u_{C_{\alpha}}(t)$ is the voltage of fractional-order capacitor C_{α} with order α. $i_{L_{\beta}}(t)$ is the current of fractional-order inductor L_{β} with order β. $i_{L_{\gamma}}(t)$ is the current of fractional-order inductive load L_{γ} with order γ and R is purely resistive load. $E(t)$ is the voltage of the power supply. According to Equation (2), the equivalent circuit parameters of the energy storage component in the circuit can be expressed by

$$ \begin{cases} R_{C} = \dfrac{1-\alpha}{C_{\alpha}}, C = \dfrac{C_{\alpha}}{\alpha} \\ R_{L} = \dfrac{L_{\beta}}{1-\beta}, L = \dfrac{L_{\beta}}{\beta} \\ R_{LR} = \dfrac{L_{\gamma}}{1-\gamma}, L_{R} = \dfrac{L_{\gamma}}{\gamma} \end{cases}, \tag{4} $$

where R_C, C, R_L, L, R_{LR}, and L_R are the equivalent resistance and capacitance. VT and VD are the ideal switch and diode, assuming that the circuit operates in continuous conduction mode, which means that $i_{L_\beta}(t)$ never equals 0. There are two states during the operation of the circuit. In State 1, VT is on and VD is off, for $nT < t \leq (n+d)T$. In State 2, VT is off and VD is on, for $(n+d)T < t \leq (n+1)T$. T is the switching period, d is the duty ratio, and n is the number of switching periods.

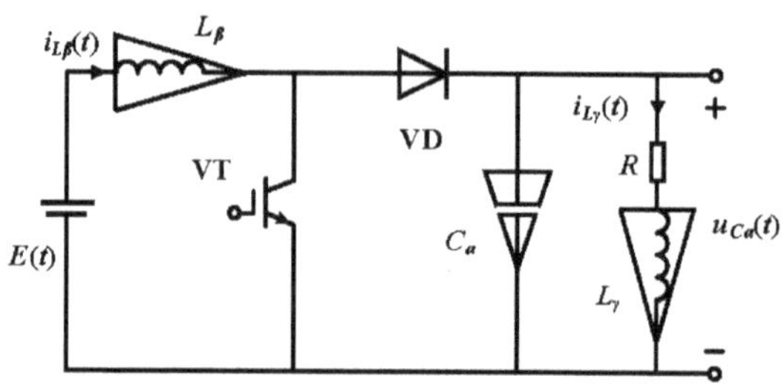

Figure 2. The fractional-order Boost converter circuit with inductive loads.

According to the equivalent circuits of capacitors and inductors, the equivalent circuits of Boost converters in different states are shown in Figure 3.

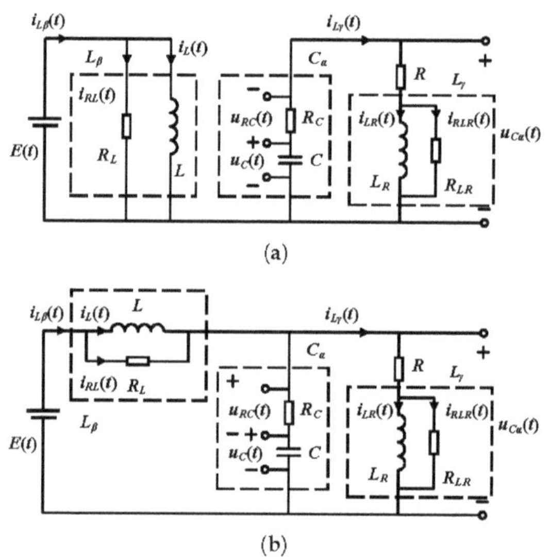

Figure 3. The equivalent circuit of the C-F definition-based Boost converter in different states. (**a**) State 1. (**b**) State 2.

3.1. Quiescent Operating Point

To analyze the system characteristics of the circuit in stable operating conditions, it is necessary to first solve the circuit parameters at the quiescent operating point. Normally, a small signal analysis of the circuit is required during the solving process. However, the fractional-order energy storage components in the circuit are based on the C-F definition, so there are resistive components in the equivalent circuit of fractional-order energy storage components that cannot store energy. This leads to discontinuity in the current and voltage in fractional-order Boost converters based on the C-F definition, which makes traditional small signal analysis methods unable to function properly. Therefore, this article sets the equivalent output voltage, induced current, and load inductor current as state variables, which satisfy continuity and exhibit continuous small ripple. Therefore, a small signal analysis of fractional-order Boost converters based on the C-F definition can be carried out. The state vector and output vector are set as follows:

$$\begin{cases} x(t) = \begin{bmatrix} i_L(t) \\ u_C(t) \\ i_{LR}(t) \end{bmatrix} \\ y(t) = \begin{bmatrix} i_{L_\beta}(t) \\ u_{C_\alpha}(t) \\ i_{L_\gamma}(t) \end{bmatrix} \end{cases}. \quad (5)$$

As shown in Figure 3a, for State 1, the state equation and output equation are derived as follows:

$$\begin{cases} L\frac{\mathrm{d}i_L(t)}{\mathrm{d}t} = E(t) \\ C\frac{\mathrm{d}u_C(t)}{\mathrm{d}t} = -\left[i_{LR}(t) + \frac{L_R}{R_{LR}}\frac{\mathrm{d}i_{LR}(t)}{\mathrm{d}t}\right] \\ L_R\frac{\mathrm{d}i_{LR}(t)}{\mathrm{d}t} = u_C(t) + C\frac{\mathrm{d}u_C(t)}{\mathrm{d}t}(R_C + R) \end{cases}, \quad (6)$$

$$\begin{cases} i_{L_\beta}(t) = i_L(t) + \frac{E(t)}{R_{LR}} \\ u_{C_\alpha}(t) = -R_C i_{L_\gamma}(t) + u_C(t) \\ i_{L_\gamma}(t) = i_{LR}(t) + \frac{u_{C_\alpha}(t) - R i_{L_\gamma}(t)}{R_{LR}} \end{cases}. \quad (7)$$

Then, Equations (6) and (7) can be simplified as follows:

$$\begin{cases} \boldsymbol{K}\frac{\mathrm{d}\boldsymbol{x}(t)}{\mathrm{d}t} = \boldsymbol{A_1}\boldsymbol{x}(t) + \boldsymbol{B_1}u(t) \\ y(t) = \boldsymbol{C_1}\boldsymbol{x}(t) + \boldsymbol{F_1}u(t) \end{cases}, \quad (8)$$

where

$$\boldsymbol{K} = \begin{bmatrix} L & 0 & 0 \\ 0 & C & 0 \\ 0 & 0 & L_R \end{bmatrix}, \boldsymbol{A_1} = \begin{bmatrix} 0 & 0 & 0 \\ 0 & -\frac{1}{R_C+R+R_{LR}} & -\frac{R_{LR}}{R_C+R+R_{LR}} \\ 0 & \frac{R_{LR}}{R_C+R+R_{LR}} & -\frac{R_{LR}(R_C+R)}{R_C+R+R_{LR}} \end{bmatrix}, \boldsymbol{B_1} = \begin{bmatrix} 1 \\ 0 \\ 0 \end{bmatrix},$$
$$\boldsymbol{C_1} = \begin{bmatrix} 1 & 0 & 0 \\ 0 & \frac{(R+R_{LR})}{R+R_{LR}+R_C} & -\frac{R_C R_{LR}}{R+R_{LR}+R_C} \\ 0 & \frac{1}{R+R_{LR}+R_C} & \frac{R_{LR}}{R+R_{LR}+R_C} \end{bmatrix}, \boldsymbol{F_1} = \begin{bmatrix} \frac{1}{R_L} \\ 0 \\ 0 \end{bmatrix}, u(t) = E(t). \quad (9)$$

As shown in Figure 3b, for State 2, the state equation is derived as follows:

$$\begin{cases} L\frac{\mathrm{d}i_L(t)}{\mathrm{d}t} = E(t) - u_C(t) - C\frac{\mathrm{d}u_C(t)}{\mathrm{d}t}R_C \\ C\frac{\mathrm{d}u_C(t)}{\mathrm{d}t} = i_L(t) + \frac{L}{R_L}\frac{\mathrm{d}i_L(t)}{\mathrm{d}t} - i_{LR}(t) - \frac{L_R}{R_{LR}}\frac{\mathrm{d}i_{LR}(t)}{\mathrm{d}t} \\ L_R\frac{\mathrm{d}i_{LR}(t)}{\mathrm{d}t} = E - L\frac{\mathrm{d}i_L(t)}{\mathrm{d}t} - R\left[i_{LR}(t) + \frac{L_R}{R_{LR}}\frac{\mathrm{d}i_{LR}(t)}{\mathrm{d}t}\right] \end{cases}, \quad (10)$$

$$\begin{cases} i_{L_\beta}(t) = i_L(t) + \frac{E(t) - u_{C_\alpha}(t)}{R_L} \\ u_{C_\alpha}(t) = R_C\left[i_{L_\beta}(t) - i_{L_\gamma}(t)\right] + u_C(t) \\ i_{L_\gamma}(t) = i_{LR}(t) + \frac{u_{C_\alpha}(t) - R i_{L_\gamma}(t)}{R_{LR}} \end{cases}. \quad (11)$$

Then, Equations (10) and (11) can be simplified as follows:

$$\begin{cases} \boldsymbol{K}\frac{\mathrm{d}\boldsymbol{x}(t)}{\mathrm{d}t} = \boldsymbol{A_2}\boldsymbol{x}(t) + \boldsymbol{B_2}u(t) \\ y(t) = \boldsymbol{C_2}\boldsymbol{x}(t) + \boldsymbol{F_2}u(t) \end{cases}, \quad (12)$$

where

$$\boldsymbol{A_2}=\begin{bmatrix} -\frac{R_C R_L (R+R_{LR})}{\delta} & -\frac{R_L (R+R_{LR})}{\delta} & \frac{R_C R_L R_{LR}}{\delta} \\ \frac{R_L (R+R_{LR})}{\delta} & -\frac{R_L+R+R_{LR}}{\delta} & -\frac{R_L R_{LR}}{\delta} \\ \frac{R_C R_L R_{LR}}{\delta} & \frac{R_L R_{LR}}{\delta} & -\frac{R_{LR}(RR_C+R_C R_L+RR_L)}{\delta} \end{bmatrix}, \boldsymbol{B_2}=\begin{bmatrix} \frac{R_L(R+R_{LR}+R_C)}{\delta} \\ \frac{R+R_{LR}}{\delta} \\ \frac{R_C R_{LR}}{\delta} \end{bmatrix},$$
$$\boldsymbol{C_2}=\begin{bmatrix} \frac{R_C R_L (R_{LR}+R)}{\delta} & \frac{R_L (R_{LR}+R)}{\delta} & -\frac{R_C R_L R_{LR}}{\delta} \\ \frac{R_C R_L}{\delta} & \frac{R_L}{\delta} & \frac{R_{LR}(R_L+R_C)}{\delta} \\ \frac{RR_L+R_L R_{LR}+R_C R_L}{\delta} & -\frac{(R_{LR}+R)}{\delta} & \frac{R_C R_{LR}}{\delta} \end{bmatrix}, \boldsymbol{F_2}=\begin{bmatrix} \frac{R_C(R_{LR}+R)}{\delta} \\ \frac{R_C}{\delta} \\ \frac{R+R_{LR}+R_C}{\delta} \end{bmatrix}, \tag{13}$$

where $\delta = RR_L + R_L R_{LR} + R_C R_L + RR_C + R_C R_{LR}$.

Then, the steady-state converter model can be expressed as follows:

$$\begin{cases} \boldsymbol{K}\frac{\mathrm{d}\boldsymbol{x}(t)}{\mathrm{d}t} = \boldsymbol{A}\boldsymbol{x}(t) + \boldsymbol{B}u(t) \\ \boldsymbol{y}(t) = \boldsymbol{C}\boldsymbol{x}(t) + \boldsymbol{F}u(t) \end{cases}, \tag{14}$$

where

$$\begin{cases} \boldsymbol{A} = d\boldsymbol{A_1} + (1-d)\boldsymbol{A_2} \\ \boldsymbol{B} = d\boldsymbol{B_1} + (1-d)\boldsymbol{B_2} \\ \boldsymbol{C} = d\boldsymbol{C_1} + (1-d)\boldsymbol{C_2} \\ \boldsymbol{F} = d\boldsymbol{F_1} + (1-d)\boldsymbol{F_2} \end{cases}. \tag{15}$$

Considering only the DC component of the system state variable, Equation (14) can be transformed as follows:

$$\begin{cases} \boldsymbol{0} = \boldsymbol{AX} + \boldsymbol{B}U \\ \boldsymbol{Y} = \boldsymbol{CX} + \boldsymbol{F}U' \end{cases} \tag{16}$$

where **0** is null vector $\begin{bmatrix} 0 \\ 0 \end{bmatrix}$.

By solving Equation (16), the quiescent operating point of the system can be obtained as follows:

$$\begin{cases} i_{L_\beta} = i_L = \dfrac{(R_L + Rd)(R_C + R + R_{LR}) + [R_C R_{LR} - R(R + R_{LR})]d^2}{R_L(1-d)\{(R_C + R + R_{LR})R + [R_C R_{LR} - R(R + R_{LR})]d\}}E \\ u_{C_\alpha} = u_C = \dfrac{(R_C + R + R_{LR})R}{(R_C + R + R_{LR})R + [R_C R_{LR} - R(R + R_{LR})]d}E \\ i_{L_\gamma} = i_{LR} = \dfrac{R_C + R + R_{LR}}{(R_C + R + R_{LR})R + [R_C R_{LR} - R(R + R_{LR})]d}E \end{cases}. \tag{17}$$

Substituting Equation (4) into Equation (17), the voltage ratio is derived as follows:

$$\frac{u_{C_\alpha}}{E} = \frac{RC_\alpha[(1-\gamma)R + L_\gamma] + R(1-\alpha)(1-\gamma)}{(1-d)RC_\alpha[(1-\gamma)R + L_\gamma] + R(1-\alpha)(1-\gamma) + d(1-\alpha)L_\gamma}. \tag{18}$$

3.2. Ripple Parameters

Ripple parameters are important in the design of DC–DC converters. In State 1, the expression for the change in equivalent current Δi_L is derived as follows:

$$\Delta i_L = \frac{E}{L}dT. \tag{19}$$

The expressions for u_C and i_{LR} are

$$\begin{cases} \frac{\mathrm{d}u_C}{\mathrm{d}t} = -\frac{1}{C(R_C+R+R_{LR})}u_C - \frac{R_{LR}}{C(R_C+R+R_{LR})}i_{LR} \\ \frac{\mathrm{d}i_{LR}}{\mathrm{d}t} = \frac{R_{LR}}{L_R(R_C+R+R_{LR})}u_C - \frac{R_{LR}(R_C+R)}{L_R(R_C+R+R_{LR})}i_{LR} \end{cases}. \tag{20}$$

After applying Laplace transform to Equation (20), the solution yields as follows:

$$\begin{cases} u_C(s) = \dfrac{\left[s+\frac{R_{LR}(R_C+R)}{L_R(R_C+R+R_{LR})}\right]u_C(0)-\frac{R_{LR}}{C(R_C+R+R_{LR})}i_{LR}(0)}{s^2+\frac{CR_{LR}(R_C+R)+L_R}{L_RC(R_C+R+R_{LR})}s+\frac{R_{LR}}{CL_R(R_C+R+R_{LR})}} \\ i_{LR}(s) = \dfrac{\frac{R_{LR}}{L_R(R_C+R+R_{LR})}u_C(0)+\left[s+\frac{1}{C(R_C+R+R_{LR})}\right]i_{LR}(0)}{s^2+\frac{CR_{LR}(R_C+R)+L_R}{CL_R(R_C+R+R_{LR})}s+\frac{R_{LR}}{L_RC(R_C+R+R_{LR})}} \end{cases}. \quad (21)$$

To solve Equation (21), it is necessary to discuss the denominator characteristic roots, and the judgment item is

$$\vartheta = \left[\frac{CR_{LR}(R_C+R)+L_R}{L_RC(R_C+R+R_{LR})}\right]^2 - 4\frac{R_{LR}}{CL_R(R_C+R+R_{LR})}. \quad (22)$$

When $\vartheta > 0$, the solution of the denominator is

$$\begin{cases} s_1 = \frac{1}{2}\left[-\frac{CR_{LR}(R_C+R)+L_R}{L_RC(R_C+R+R_{LR})} + \sqrt{\vartheta}\right] \\ s_2 = \frac{1}{2}\left[-\frac{CR_{LR}(R_C+R)+L_R}{L_RC(R_C+R+R_{LR})} - \sqrt{\vartheta}\right] \end{cases}. \quad (23)$$

Then, Equation (21) can be simplified as follows:

$$\begin{cases} u_C(s) =-\dfrac{s_1+a}{(s_2-s_1)(s-s_1)}u_C(0) + \dfrac{s_2+a}{(s_2-s_1)(s-s_2)}u_C(0) \\ \quad +\dfrac{b}{(s_2-s_1)(s-s_1)}i_{LR}(0) - \dfrac{b}{(s_2-s_1)(s-s_2)}i_{LR}(0) \\ i_{LR}(s) =-\dfrac{j}{(s_2-s_1)(s-s_1)}u_C(0) + \dfrac{j}{(s_2-s_1)(s-s_2)}u_C(0) \\ \quad -\dfrac{s_1+k}{(s_2-s_1)(s-s_1)}i_{LR}(0) + \dfrac{s_2+k}{(s_2-s_1)(s-s_2)}i_{LR}(0) \end{cases}, \quad (24)$$

where

$$\begin{aligned} a &= \frac{R_{LR}(R_C+R)}{L_R(R_C+R+R_{LR})}, b = \frac{R_{LR}}{C(R_C+R+R_{LR})}, \\ j &= \frac{R_{LR}}{L_R(R_C+R+R_{LR})}, k = \frac{1}{C(R_C+R+R_{LR})}. \end{aligned} \quad (25)$$

By inverse Laplace transform, Equation (24) can be rewritten as follows:

$$\begin{cases} u_C(t) = \left[-\dfrac{s_1+a}{s_2-s_1}\exp(s_1t) + \dfrac{s_2+a}{s_2-s_1}\exp(s_2t)\right]u_C(0) \\ \quad +\left[\dfrac{b}{s_2-s_1}\exp(s_1t) - \dfrac{b}{s_2-s_1}\exp(s_2t)\right]i_{LR}(0) \\ i_{LR}(t) = \left[-\dfrac{j}{s_2-s_1}\exp(s_1t) + \dfrac{j}{s_2-s_1}\exp(s_2t)\right]u_C(0) \\ \quad +\left[-\dfrac{s_1+k}{s_2-s_1}\exp(s_1t) + \dfrac{s_2+k}{s_2-s_1}\exp(s_2t)\right]i_{LR}(0) \end{cases}. \quad (26)$$

By inputting the time parameters of State 1, Equation (26) can be rewritten as follows:

$$\begin{cases} \Delta u_C = u_C(0) - u_C(dT) = (1+\chi+a\phi)u_C(0) - b\phi i_{LR}(0) \\ \Delta i_{LR} = i_{LR}(0) - i_{LR}(dT) = j\phi u_C(0) + (1+\chi+k\phi)i_{LR}(0) \end{cases}, \quad (27)$$

where

$$\begin{aligned} \phi &= \frac{1}{s_2 - s_1}\exp(s_1 dT) - \frac{1}{s_2 - s_1}\exp(s_2 dT), \\ \chi &= \frac{s_1}{s_2 - s_1}\exp(s_1 dT) - \frac{s_2}{s_2 - s_1}\exp(s_2 dT), \end{aligned} \tag{28}$$

and

$$\begin{cases} u_C(0) = u_C + \frac{1}{2}\Delta u_C \\ i_{LR}(0) = i_{LR} + \frac{1}{2}\Delta i_{LR} \end{cases}. \tag{29}$$

By Equations (27) and (29), the values of Δu_C and Δi_{LR} can be obtained as follows:

$$\begin{cases} \Delta u_C = 2\frac{[R(1+\chi)+Ra\phi-b\phi](1-\chi-k\phi)-b\phi[(1+\chi)+k\phi+Rj\phi]}{R(1-\chi-a\phi)(1-\chi-k\phi)+bjR\phi^2}u_C \\ \Delta i_{LR} = 2\frac{j\phi[R(1+\chi)+Ra\phi-b\phi]+(1-\chi-a\phi)[(1+\chi)+k\phi+Rj\phi]}{R(1-\chi-a\phi)(1-\chi-k\phi)+bjR\phi^2}u_C \end{cases}. \tag{30}$$

When $\vartheta = 0$, the solution of the denominator is

$$s_1 = s_2 = -\frac{CR_{LR}(R_C + R) + L_R}{2L_R C(R_C + R + R_{LR})}. \tag{31}$$

Then, Equation (21) can be simplified as follows:

$$\begin{cases} u_C(s) = \frac{1}{(s-s_1)}u_C(0) + \frac{s_1+a}{(s-s_1)^2}u_C(0) - \frac{b}{(s-s_1)^2}i_{LR}(0) \\ i_{LR}(s) = \frac{j}{(s-s_1)^2}u_C(0) + \frac{1}{(s-s_1)}i_{LR}(0) + \frac{s_1+k}{(s-s_1)^2}i_{LR}(0) \end{cases}. \tag{32}$$

The parameters are consistent with those in Equation (25). By inverse Laplace transform, Equation (32) can be rewritten as follows:

$$\begin{cases} u_C(t) = [1 + (s_1 + a)t]\exp(s_1 t)u_C(0) - bt\exp(s_1 t)i_{LR}(0) \\ i_{LR}(t) = jt\exp(s_1 t)u_C(0) + [1 + (s_1 + k)t]\exp(s_1 t)i_{LR}(0) \end{cases}. \tag{33}$$

By inputting the time parameters of State 1, Equation (33) can be rewritten as follows:

$$\begin{cases} \Delta u_C = u_C(0) - u_C(dT) = \{1 - [1 + (s_1 + a)dT]\exp(s_1 dT)\}u_C(0) + bdT\exp(s_1 dT)i_{LR}(0) \\ \Delta i_{LR} = i_{LR}(0) - i_{LR}(dT) = \{1 - [1 + (s_1 + k)dT]\exp(s_1 dT)\}i_{LR}(0) - jdT\exp(s_1 dT)u_C(0) \end{cases}. \tag{34}$$

By Equations (34) and (29), the values of Δu_C and Δi_{LR} can be obtained as follows:

$$\begin{cases} \Delta u_C = 2\left\{\frac{[R-R\delta-(aR-b)\varepsilon](1+\delta+k\varepsilon)+b\varepsilon[1-(k+Rj)\varepsilon-\delta]}{R[(1+\delta+a\varepsilon)(1+\delta+k\varepsilon)+bj\varepsilon^2]}\right\}u_C \\ \Delta i_{LR} = 2\left\{\frac{[1-\delta-(k+Rj)\varepsilon](1+\delta+a\varepsilon)-j\varepsilon[R-R\delta-(aR-b)\varepsilon]}{R[(1+\delta+a\varepsilon)(1+\delta+k\varepsilon)+bj\varepsilon^2]}\right\}u_C \end{cases}, \tag{35}$$

where

$$\varepsilon = dT\exp(s_1 dT); \delta = (1 + s_1 dT)\exp(s_1 dT). \tag{36}$$

When $\vartheta < 0$, Equation (21) can be simplified as follows:

$$\begin{cases} u_C(s) = \frac{s}{(s+\mu)^2 + \omega^2}u_C(0) + \frac{R_{LR}(R_C + R)}{L_R\omega(R_C + R + R_{LR})}\frac{\omega}{(s+\mu)^2 + \omega^2}u_C(0) \\ \qquad - \frac{R_{LR}}{C\omega(R_C + R + R_{LR})}\frac{\omega}{(s+\mu)^2 + \omega^2}i_{LR}(0) \\ i_{LR}(s) = \frac{R_{LR}}{L_R\omega(R_C + R + R_{LR})}\frac{\omega}{(s+\mu)^2 + \omega^2}u_C(0) + \frac{s}{(s+\mu)^2 + \omega^2}i_{LR}(0) \\ \qquad + \frac{1}{C\omega(R_C + R + R_{LR})}\frac{\omega}{(s+\mu)^2 + \omega^2}i_{LR}(0) \end{cases}, \tag{37}$$

where

$$\mu = \frac{CR_{LR}(R_C + R) + L_R}{2L_R C(R_C + R + R_{LR})}, \omega = \sqrt{\frac{R_{LR}}{CL_R(R_C + R + R_{LR})} - \mu^2}. \tag{38}$$

By inverse Laplace transform, Equation (38) can be rewritten as follows:

$$\begin{cases} u_C(t) = \exp(-\mu t)\cos(\omega t)u_C(0) + \dfrac{R_{LR}(R_C + R)}{L_R\omega(R_C + R + R_{LR})}\exp(-\mu t)\sin(\omega t)u_C(0) \\ \quad -\dfrac{R_{LR}}{C\omega(R_C + R + R_{LR})}\exp(-\mu t)\sin(\omega t)i_{LR}(0) \\ i_{LR}(t) = \dfrac{R_{LR}}{L_R\omega(R_C + R + R_{LR})}\exp(-\mu t)\sin(\omega t)u_C(0) + \exp(-\mu t)\cos(\omega t)i_{LR}(0) \\ \quad +\dfrac{1}{C\omega(R_C + R + R_{LR})}\exp(-\mu t)\sin(\omega t)i_{LR}(0) \end{cases}. \tag{39}$$

By inputting the time parameters of State 1, Equation (39) can be rewritten as follows:

$$\begin{cases} \Delta u_C = u_C(0) - u_C(dT) = (1 - q_1)u_C(0) + q_2 i_{LR}(0) \\ \Delta i_{LR} = i_{LR}(0) - i_{LR}(dT) = -q_3 u_C(0) + (1 - q_4)i_{LR}(0) \end{cases}, \tag{40}$$

where

$$\begin{aligned} q_1 &= \left[\cos(\omega dT) + \frac{R_{LR}(R_C + R)}{L_R\omega(R_C + R + R_{LR})}\sin(\omega dT)\right]\exp(-\mu dT), \\ q_2 &= \frac{R_{LR}}{C\omega(R_C + R + R_{LR})}\sin(\omega dT)\exp(-\mu dT), \\ q_3 &= \frac{R_{LR}}{L_R\omega(R_C + R + R_{LR})}\sin(\omega dT)\exp(-\mu dT), \\ q_4 &= \left[\cos(\omega dT) + \frac{1}{C\omega(R_C + R + R_{LR})}\sin(\omega dT)\right]\exp(-\mu dT). \end{aligned} \tag{41}$$

By Equations (41) and (29), the values of Δu_C and Δi_{LR} can be obtained as follows:

$$\begin{cases} \Delta u_C = 2\frac{(1-q_1)(1+q_4) + \frac{2}{R}q_2 - q_2 q_3}{(1+q_1)(1+q_4) + q_2 q_3}u_C \\ \Delta i_{LR} = 2\frac{\frac{1}{R}(1-q_4)(1+q_1) - 2q_3 - \frac{1}{R}q_2 q_3}{(1+q_1)(1+q_4) + q_2 q_3}u_C \end{cases}. \tag{42}$$

In summary, the extreme values of the voltages of the equivalent capacitor ($u_{C\max}$ and $u_{C\min}$) and the current of the equivalent inductances ($i_{L\max}$, $i_{L\min}$, $I_{LR\max}$ and $I_{LR\min}$) are as follows:

$$\begin{cases} u_{C\max} = u_C + \frac{1}{2}\Delta u_C; u_{C\min} = u_C - \frac{1}{2}\Delta u_C \\ i_{L\max} = i_L + \frac{E}{2L}dT; i_{L\min} = i_L - \frac{E}{2L}dT \\ i_{LR\max} = i_{LR} + \frac{1}{2}\Delta i_{LR}; i_{LR\min} = i_{LR} - \frac{1}{2}\Delta i_{LR} \end{cases}. \tag{43}$$

According to the circuit in Figure 3, the theoretical waveforms of a fractional-order Boost converter with inductive load based on the C-F are shown in Figure 4. Due to the short duration of a single cycle, the output voltage change can be regarded as a linear change.

In State 1, the induced current i_{L_β} continuously increases. The maximum value of the induced current $i_{L_\beta\max}$ is as follows:

$$i_{L_\beta\max} = i_{L_\beta}(dT) = i_{L\max} + \frac{E}{R_L}. \tag{44}$$

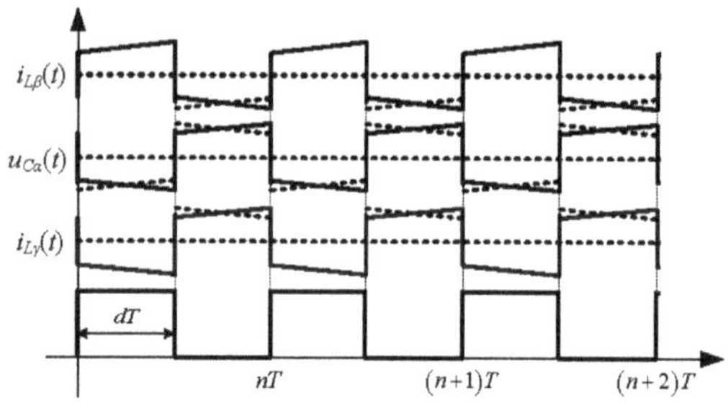

Figure 4. The theoretical waveforms.

There is a coupling relationship between the output voltage and the load current in state 1. So their changing trends are variable. The load current and output voltage at the beginning and the ending can be obtained as follows:

$$\begin{cases} u_{C\alpha}(dT) = -\frac{R_C R_{LR}}{(R+R_{LR}+R_C)} i_{LR\min} + \frac{(R+R_{LR})}{(R+R_{LR}+R_C)} u_{C\min} \\ i_{L\gamma}(dT) = \frac{R_{LR}}{(R+R_{LR}+R_C)} i_{LR\min} + \frac{1}{(R+R_{LR}+R_C)} u_{C\min} \\ u_{C\alpha}(0) = -\frac{R_C R_{LR}}{(R+R_{LR}+R_C)} i_{LR\max} + \frac{(R+R_{LR})}{(R+R_{LR}+R_C)} u_{C\max} \\ i_{L\gamma}(0) = \frac{R_{LR}}{(R+R_{LR}+R_C)} i_{LR\max} + \frac{1}{(R+R_{LR}+R_C)} u_{C\max} \end{cases}. \quad (45)$$

From Equation (45), $i_{L\gamma}(dT) < i_{L\gamma}(0)$. So, the minimum values of the load current $i_{L\gamma\min}$ and capacitor voltage $u_{C\alpha\min}$ are as follows:

$$i_{L\gamma\min} = i_{L\gamma}(dT), u_{C\alpha\min} = \min[u_{C\alpha}(0), u_{C\alpha}(dT)]. \quad (46)$$

In State 2, the induced current, output voltage, and load current are coupled, their changing trend is not fixed. The values at the beginning and the ending can be obtained as follows:

$$\begin{cases} u_{C\alpha}(T) = \frac{R_L(R_{LR}+R)}{\delta} u_{C\max} + \frac{R_C R_L(R_{LR}+R)}{\delta} i_{L\min} - \frac{R_C R_L R_{LR}}{\delta} i_{LR\max} + \frac{R_C(R_{LR}+R)}{\delta} E \\ i_{L\gamma}(T) = \frac{R_L}{\delta} u_{C\max} + \frac{R_C R_L}{\delta} i_{L\min} + \frac{R_{LR}(R_L+R_C)}{\delta} i_{LR\max} + \frac{R_C}{\delta} E \\ i_{L\beta}(T) = -\frac{(R_{LR}+R)}{\delta} u_{C\max} + \frac{RR_L+R_L R_{LR}+R_C R_L}{\delta} i_{L\min} + \frac{R_C R_{LR}}{\delta} i_{LR\max} + \frac{R+R_{LR}+R_C}{\delta} E \\ u_{C\alpha}(dT) = \frac{R_L(R_{LR}+R)}{\delta} u_{C\min} + \frac{R_C R_L(R_{LR}+R)}{\delta} i_{L\max} - \frac{R_C R_L R_{LR}}{\delta} i_{LR\min} + \frac{R_C(R_{LR}+R)}{\delta} E \\ i_{L\gamma}(dT) = \frac{R_L}{\delta} u_{C\min} + \frac{R_C R_L}{\delta} i_{L\max} + \frac{R_{LR}(R_L+R_C)}{\delta} i_{LR\min} + \frac{R_C}{\delta} E \\ i_{L\beta}(dT) = -\frac{(R_{LR}+R)}{\delta} u_{C\min} + \frac{RR_L+R_L R_{LR}+R_C R_L}{\delta} i_{L\max} + \frac{R_C R_{LR}}{\delta} i_{LR\min} + \frac{R+R_{LR}+R_C}{\delta} E \end{cases}. \quad (47)$$

So, the maximum values of the load current $i_{L\gamma\max}$ and output voltage $u_{C\alpha\max}$, as well as the minimum value of the induced current $i_{L_\beta\min}$ are as follows:

$$\begin{cases} i_{L\beta\min} = \min[i_{L\beta}(dT), i_{L\beta}(T)] \\ u_{C\alpha\max} = \max[u_{C\alpha}(dT), u_{C\alpha}(T)] \\ i_{L\gamma\max} = \max[i_{L\gamma}(dT), i_{L\gamma}(T)] \end{cases}. \quad (48)$$

3.3. Small-Signal Model

The state vector and output vector in Equation (5) are continuous with minimal ripple. To create a small-signal AC model, the converter waveform can be linearized as follows:

$$\begin{cases} \langle \boldsymbol{x}(t) \rangle = \boldsymbol{X} + \hat{\boldsymbol{x}}(t) \\ \langle \boldsymbol{u}(t) \rangle = \boldsymbol{U} + \hat{\boldsymbol{u}}(t) \\ \langle \boldsymbol{y}(t) \rangle = \boldsymbol{Y} + \hat{\boldsymbol{y}}(t) \\ \langle d(t) \rangle = d + \hat{d}(t) \end{cases}. \quad (49)$$

Substitute Equation (49) into Equation (14) and set $\hat{E}$ to 0. Then, neglecting DC components and second-order nonlinear terms, the small signal components in the equation can be sorted out as follows:

$$\begin{cases} \frac{\mathrm{d}\hat{\boldsymbol{x}}(t)}{\mathrm{d}t} = \boldsymbol{A}'\hat{\boldsymbol{x}}(t) + \boldsymbol{B}'\hat{d}(t) \\ \hat{\boldsymbol{y}}(t) = \boldsymbol{C}'\hat{\boldsymbol{x}}(t) + \boldsymbol{D}'\hat{d}(t) \end{cases}, \tag{50}$$

where

$$\begin{cases} \boldsymbol{A}' = \begin{bmatrix} A_{11} & A_{12} & A_{13} \\ A_{21} & A_{22} & A_{23} \\ A_{31} & A_{32} & A_{33} \end{bmatrix} \\ = \begin{bmatrix} -\frac{(1-d)R_C R_L (R+R_{LR})}{L\delta} & -\frac{(1-d)R_L(R+R_{LR})}{L\delta} & \frac{R_C R_L R_{LR}}{L\delta}(1-d) \\ \frac{(1-d)R_L(R+R_{LR})}{C\delta} & -\frac{R_L+R+R_{LR}}{C\delta} + \frac{d(R+R_{LR})^2}{C\delta(R_C+R+R_{LR})} & -\frac{R_L R_{LR}}{C\delta} - \frac{dR_C R_{LR}(R+R_{LR})}{C\delta(R_C+R+R_{LR})} \\ \frac{(1-d)R_C R_L R_{LR}}{L_R\delta} & \frac{R_L R_{LR}}{L_R\delta} + \frac{dR_C R_{LR}(R+R_{LR})}{L_R(R_C+R+R_{LR})\delta} & -\frac{R_{LR}(RR_C+R_C R_L+RR_L)}{L_R\delta} - \frac{dR_C{}^2 R_{LR}{}^2}{L_R(R_C+R+R_{LR})\delta} \end{bmatrix} \\ \boldsymbol{B}' = \begin{bmatrix} B_1 \\ B_2 \\ B_3 \end{bmatrix} = \begin{bmatrix} \frac{E}{(1-d)L} \\ -\frac{(R+R_{LR})E}{C(1-d)\{(R_C+R+R_{LR})R+[R_C R_{LR}-R(R+R_{LR})]d\}} \\ -\frac{R_C R_{LR} E}{L_R(1-d)\{(R_C+R+R_{LR})R+[R_C R_{LR}-R(R+R_{LR})]d\}} \end{bmatrix} \\ \boldsymbol{C}' = \begin{bmatrix} C_{11} & C_{12} & C_{13} \\ C_{21} & C_{22} & C_{23} \\ C_{31} & C_{32} & C_{33} \end{bmatrix} \\ = \begin{bmatrix} \frac{RR_L+R_L R_{LR}+R_C R_L}{\delta} + \frac{dR_C(R+R_{LR})}{\delta} & -\frac{(1-d)(R_{LR}+R)}{\delta} & \frac{(1-d)R_C R_{LR}}{\delta} \\ \frac{(1-d)R_C R_L(R_{LR}+R)}{\delta} & \frac{R_L(R_{LR}+R)}{\delta} + \frac{dR_C(R+R_{LR})(R+R_{LR})}{(R+R_{LR}+R_C)\delta} & -\frac{R_C R_L R_{LR}}{\delta} - \frac{dR_C{}^2 R_{LR}(R+R_{LR})}{\delta(R+R_{LR}+R_C)} \\ \frac{(1-d)R_C R_L}{\delta} & \frac{R_L}{\delta} + \frac{dR_C(R+R_{LR})}{\delta(R+R_{LR}+R_C)} & \frac{R_{LR}(R_L+R_C)}{\delta} - \frac{dR_C R_C R_{LR}}{\delta(R+R_{LR}+R_C)} \end{bmatrix} \\ \boldsymbol{D}' = \begin{bmatrix} D_1 \\ D_2 \\ D_3 \end{bmatrix} = \begin{bmatrix} \frac{E}{R_L(1-d)} \\ -\frac{R_C(R+R_{LR})E}{(1-d)\{(R_C+R+R_{LR})R+[R_C R_{LR}-R(R+R_{LR})]d\}} \\ -\frac{R_C E}{(1-d)\{(R_C+R+R_{LR})R+[R_C R_{LR}-R(R+R_{LR})]d\}} \end{bmatrix} \end{cases}. \tag{51}$$

By inverse Laplace transform, Equation (50) can be rewritten as follows:

$$\begin{cases} s\hat{\boldsymbol{x}}(s) = \boldsymbol{A}'\hat{\boldsymbol{x}}(s) + \boldsymbol{B}'\hat{d}(s) \\ \hat{\boldsymbol{y}}(s) = \boldsymbol{C}'\hat{\boldsymbol{x}}(s) + \boldsymbol{D}'\hat{d}(s) \end{cases}. \tag{52}$$

According to Equation (52), the transfer function $\boldsymbol{G}(s)$ of the circuit system is as follows:

$$\boldsymbol{G}(s) = \frac{\hat{\boldsymbol{y}}(s)}{\hat{d}(s)} = \boldsymbol{C}'(s\boldsymbol{I} - \boldsymbol{A}')^{-1}\boldsymbol{B}' + \boldsymbol{D}'. \tag{53}$$

Therefore, the transfer function from duty cycle $\hat{d}$ to induced current $\hat{i}_{L\beta}$ is

$$G_{id}(s) = \frac{\hat{i}_{L\beta}(s)}{\hat{d}(s)} = \frac{D_1 s^3 + X_1 s^2 + X_2 s + X_3}{s^3 + W_1 s^2 + W_2 s + W_3}, \tag{54}$$

where

$$\begin{cases} W_1 = -(A_{11} + A_{22} + A_{33}) \\ W_2 = A_{11}A_{33} + A_{11}A_{22} + A_{22}A_{33} - A_{12}A_{21} - A_{13}A_{31} - A_{23}A_{32} \\ W_3 = A_{11}A_{23}A_{32} + A_{22}A_{13}A_{31} + A_{33}A_{12}A_{21} - A_{11}A_{22}A_{33} - A_{12}A_{23}A_{31} - A_{13}A_{21}A_{32} \\ X_1 = B_1C_{11} + B_2C_{12} + B_3C_{13} - (A_{11} + A_{22} + A_{33})D_1 \\ X_2 = [A_{21}C_{12} + A_{31}C_{13} - (A_{22} + A_{33})C_{11}]B_1 + [A_{12}C_{11} + A_{32}C_{13} - (A_{11} + A_{33})C_{12}]B_2 \\ \quad +[A_{13}C_{11} + A_{23}C_{12} - (A_{11} + A_{22})C_{13}]B_3 \\ \quad +(A_{11}A_{33} + A_{11}A_{22} + A_{22}A_{33} - A_{12}A_{21} - A_{13}A_{31} - A_{23}A_{32})D_1 \\ X_3 = [(A_{22}A_{33} - A_{23}A_{32})C_{11} + (A_{23}A_{31} - A_{21}A_{33})C_{12} + (A_{21}A_{32} - A_{22}A_{31})C_{13}]B_1 \\ \quad +[(A_{13}A_{32} - A_{12}A_{33})C_{11} + (A_{11}A_{33} - A_{13}A_{31})C_{12} + (A_{12}A_{31} - A_{11}A_{32})C_{13}]B_2 \\ \quad +[(A_{12}A_{23} - A_{13}A_{22})C_{11} + (A_{13}A_{21} - A_{11}A_{23})C_{12} + (A_{11}A_{22} - A_{12}A_{21})C_{13}]B_3 \\ \quad +(A_{11}A_{23}A_{32} + A_{22}A_{13}A_{31} + A_{33}A_{12}A_{21} - A_{11}A_{22}A_{33} - A_{12}A_{23}A_{31} - A_{13}A_{21}A_{32})D_1 \end{cases}. \tag{55}$$

The transfer function from duty cycle $\hat{d}$ to output voltage $\hat{u}_{C\alpha}$ is

$$G_{ud}(s) = \frac{\hat{u}_{C\alpha}(s)}{\hat{d}(s)} = \frac{D_2s^3 + Y_1s^2 + Y_2s + Y_3}{s^3 + W_1s^2 + W_2s + W_3}, \tag{56}$$

where

$$\begin{cases} Y_1 = B_1C_{21} + B_2C_{22} + B_3C_{23} - (A_{11} + A_{22} + A_{33})D_2 \\ Y_2 = [A_{21}C_{22} + A_{31}C_{23} - (A_{22} + A_{33})C_{21}]B_1 + [A_{12}C_{21} + A_{32}C_{23} - (A_{11} + A_{33})C_{22}]B_2 \\ \quad +[A_{13}C_{21} + A_{23}C_{22} - (A_{11} + A_{22})C_{23}]B_3 \\ \quad +(A_{11}A_{33} + A_{11}A_{22} + A_{22}A_{33} - A_{12}A_{21} - A_{13}A_{31} - A_{23}A_{32})D_2 \\ Y_3 = [(A_{22}A_{33} - A_{23}A_{32})C_{21} + (A_{23}A_{31} - A_{21}A_{33})C_{22} + (A_{21}A_{32} - A_{22}A_{31})C_{23}]B_1 \\ \quad +[(A_{13}A_{32} - A_{12}A_{33})C_{21} + (A_{11}A_{33} - A_{13}A_{31})C_{22} + (A_{12}A_{31} - A_{11}A_{32})C_{23}]B_2 \\ \quad +[(A_{12}A_{23} - A_{13}A_{22})C_{21} + (A_{13}A_{21} - A_{11}A_{23})C_{22} + (A_{11}A_{22} - A_{12}A_{21})C_{23}]B_3 \\ \quad +(A_{11}A_{23}A_{32} + A_{22}A_{13}A_{31} + A_{33}A_{12}A_{21} - A_{11}A_{22}A_{33} - A_{12}A_{23}A_{31} - A_{13}A_{21}A_{32})D_2 \end{cases}. \tag{57}$$

The transfer function from duty cycle $\hat{d}$ to load current $\hat{i}_{L\gamma}$ is

$$G_{ird}(s) = \frac{\hat{i}_{L\gamma}(s)}{\hat{d}(s)} = \frac{D_3s^3 + Z_1s^2 + Z_2s + Z_3}{s^3 + W_1s^2 + W_2s + W_3}, \tag{58}$$

where

$$\begin{cases} Z_1 = B_1C_{31} + B_2C_{32} + B_3C_{33} - (A_{11} + A_{22} + A_{33})D_3 \\ Z_2 = [A_{21}C_{32} + A_{31}C_{33} - (A_{22} + A_{33})C_{31}]B_1 + [A_{12}C_{31} + A_{32}C_{33} - (A_{11} + A_{33})C_{32}]B_2 \\ \quad +[A_{13}C_{31} + A_{23}C_{32} - (A_{11} + A_{22})C_{33}]B_3 \\ \quad +(A_{11}A_{33} + A_{11}A_{22} + A_{22}A_{33} - A_{12}A_{21} - A_{13}A_{31} - A_{23}A_{32})D_3 \\ Z_3 = [(A_{22}A_{33} - A_{23}A_{32})C_{31} + (A_{23}A_{31} - A_{21}A_{33})C_{32} + (A_{21}A_{32} - A_{22}A_{31})C_{33}]B_1 \\ \quad +[(A_{13}A_{32} - A_{12}A_{33})C_{31} + (A_{11}A_{33} - A_{13}A_{31})C_{32} + (A_{12}A_{31} - A_{11}A_{32})C_{33}]B_2 \\ \quad +[(A_{12}A_{23} - A_{13}A_{22})C_{31} + (A_{13}A_{21} - A_{11}A_{23})C_{32} + (A_{11}A_{22} - A_{12}A_{21})C_{33}]B_3 \\ \quad +(A_{11}A_{23}A_{32} + A_{22}A_{13}A_{31} + A_{33}A_{12}A_{21} - A_{11}A_{22}A_{33} - A_{12}A_{23}A_{31} - A_{13}A_{21}A_{32})D_3 \end{cases}. \tag{59}$$

4. Simulation Experiment Results

4.1. Analysis of Circuit Parameters at the Quiescent Operating Point

To validate the correctness of derivation, the calculation values are compared with the circuit-oriented simulation results. The simulation circuit is constructed with Multisim regarding Figure 2, and the C-F derivative defines the fractional-order models of capacitors and inductors in circuit-oriented simulations. To make the simulation more convincing, the following two sets of parameters are set in this paper.

Set 1: R= 5 Ω, d= 0.5, E= 10 V, $C\alpha$= 680 μF/s$^{0.001}$, α= 0.999, $L\beta$= 20 mHs$^{0.005}$, β= 0.995, $L\gamma$= 1 mHs$^{0.05}$, γ= 0.95.
Set 2: R= 5 Ω, d= 0.5, E= 10 V, $C\alpha$= 3300 μF/s$^{0.01}$, α= 0.99, $L\beta$= 5 mHs$^{0.001}$, β= 0.999, $L\gamma$= 10 mHs$^{0.01}$, γ= 0.99.

The comparison results are shown in Table 1 and the circuit-oriented simulation results are shown in Figure 5. Due to software limitations, while ensuring data accuracy, circuit-oriented simulation results retain four significant digits and calculation results retain six significant digits. It can be seen from Table 1 that within the allowable error range, the calculated results are consistent with the simulation results. The waveforms in Figure 5 conform to the changing trend of the theoretical waveforms in Figure 4. These results demonstrate consistency between theoretical analysis and numerical simulation results. Further verified the accuracy of the previous derivation.

Table 1. The comparison results between circuit-oriented simulation results and calculation results.

		Simulation	Calculation			Simulation	Calculation
$U_{C_\alpha \max}$	Set1	20.04 V	20.0447 V	$U_{C_\alpha \min}$	Set1	12.52 V	12.5155 V
	Set2	20.06 V	20.0638 V		Set2	8.509 V	8.50889 V
$I_{L_\beta \max}$	Set1	11.53 A	11.5299 A	$I_{L_\beta \min}$	Set1	6.494 A	6.49380 A
	Set2	9.753 A	9.75330 A		Set2	5.666 A	5.66617 A
$I_{L_\gamma \max}$	Set1	4.006 A	4.00596 A	$I_{L_\gamma \min}$	Set1	2.506 A	2.50612 A
	Set2	3.819 A	3.81937 A		Set2	1.893 A	1.89264 A
U_{C_α}	Set1	16.29 V	16.2936 V	I_{L_β}	Set1	9.017 A	9.01742 A
	Set2	14.26 V	14.2583 V		Set2	7.703 A	7.70335 A
I_{L_γ}	Set1	3.259 A	3.25871 A				
	Set2	2.852 A	2.85167 A				

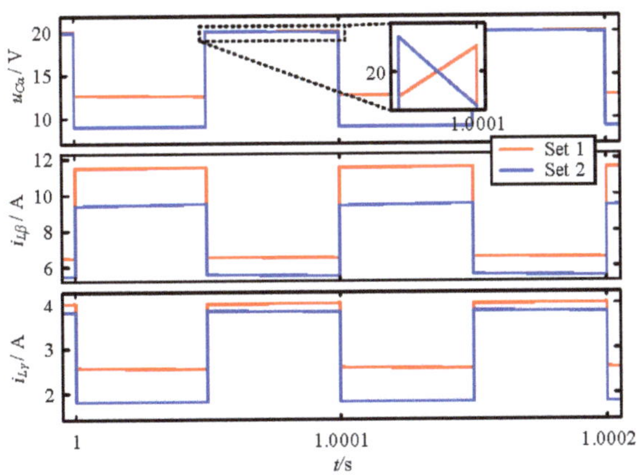

Figure 5. The circuit-oriented simulation results with different conditions.

To explore the effect of the order of components on the induced current, output voltage, and load current, the system performance is analyzed through simulation with MATLAB R2012a. According to [29,57], the fractional order of the real capacitor and inductor is close to 1. According to the simulation results, the order of the induced inductor has a much greater impact on the state variables of the circuit than the order of the capacitor and load inductor. Depending on the actual application conditions of the circuit, the analog components are analyzed in the range of orders $\alpha, \gamma \in [0.95, 1)$, $\beta \in [0.99, 1)$ for the characteristics of the converter. The remaining circuit parameters use the data from Set 2. It can be seen from Equation (17) that the output voltage and the load current are only related to α and γ as shown in Figure 6. Similarly, the induced current is related to α, β and γ as shown in Figure 7. According to the simulation results, the average value of capacitor voltage increases with the increase of α, and its rising slope also increases accordingly; The change is small with the increase of γ. When γ approaches 1, the average value of capacitor voltage decreases with the increase of γ, and its slope of decrease also increases. The variation trends of load current and induced current are consistent with the variation trends of capacitor voltage, with only numerical variations. The induced current decreases linearly with the increase of β, and the effect of β is much greater than that of α and γ.

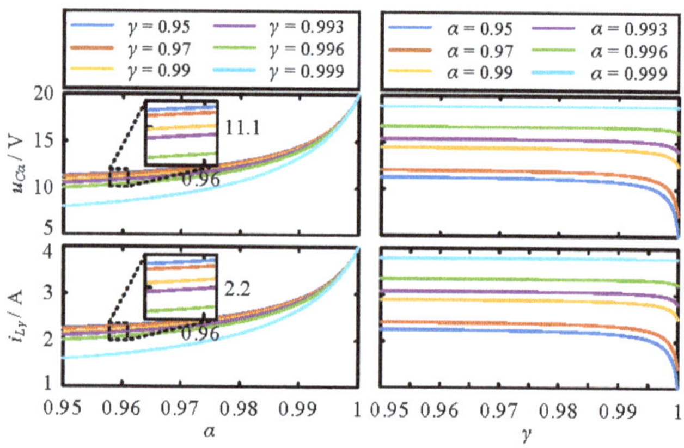

Figure 6. The effect of α and γ on the value of the output voltage and load current.

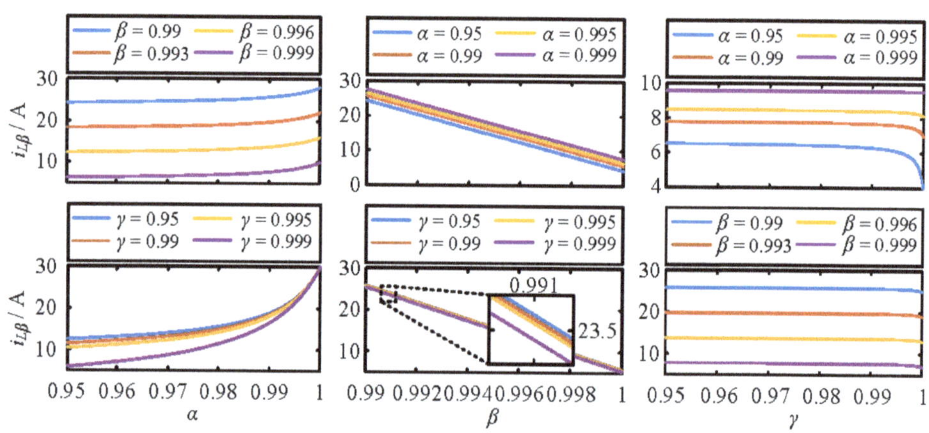

Figure 7. The effect of α, β, and γ on the value of the induced current.

The effect of α, β, and γ on ripple amplitude is shown in Figure 8. From the simulation results, as α increases, the ripple amplitude of the load current and output voltage decreases, while the ripple amplitude of the induced current increases, and the slope of the change also increases continuously. As β increases, the ripple amplitude of the output voltage and load current increases, and the slope of the rise also increases continuously, while the ripple amplitude of the induced current decreases linearly. As γ increases, the ripple amplitude of the induced current and output voltage increases, while the ripple amplitude of the load current decreases. The slope of the change increases significantly when γ

approaches 1. From a numerical perspective, α and γ have a significant effect on the ripple amplitude of the load current and output voltage, while β has a significant effect on the ripple amplitude of the induced current. It is worth noting that there are discontinuous points in the waveform of the ripple amplitude of the induced current, output voltage, and load current at point A in Figure 8. This is because $\vartheta|_{\gamma=0.9644} = 0$, meaning the judgment item Equation (22) has changed from negative to positive, that the calculation method for the extreme value of the state variable has changed. This discontinuous point also verifies the correctness of the derivation.

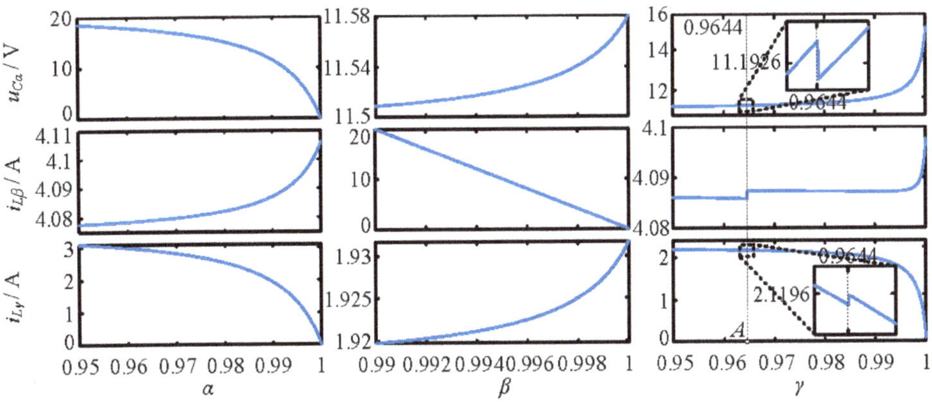

Figure 8. The effect of α, β, and γ on the ripple amplitude of the induced current, output voltage, and load current.

4.2. Verification of Small Signal Models

The simulation parameters are consistent with Set 1. To get the amplitude-frequency characteristics of the simulated circuit, frequency sweeps can be performed using MATLAB R2012a/Simulink. The scanning and calculation results are shown in Figure 9, where $G_{id}^*(s)$, $G_{ud}^*(s)$ and $G_{ird}^*(s)$ are the transfer functions from duty cycle to induced current, output voltage, and load current obtained by the **Frestimate(∗)** function, respectively. The **Frestimate(∗)** function is used for frequency response estimation of simulated models. The transfer functions can be obtained as follows:

$$\begin{cases} G_{id}(s) = \frac{5s^3+3117s^2+4.242\times10^5 s+3.992\times10^5}{s^3+334.9s^2+1381s+1278} \\ G_{ud}(s) = \frac{-7.413s^3-7135s^2+2.703\times10^5 s+2.621\times10^5}{s^3+334.9s^2+1381s+1278} \\ G_{ird}(s) = \frac{-1.477s^3-1421s^2+5.383\times10^4 s+5.242\times10^4}{s^3+334.9s^2+1381s+1278} \\ G_{id}^*(s) = \frac{4.235s^3+2717s^2+3.821\times10^5 s+4.223\times10^5}{s^3+286.7s^2+1112s+934.6} \\ G_{ud}^*(s) = \frac{-8.332s^3-8043s^2+3.123\times10^5 s+2.115\times10^5}{s^3+424.3s^2+1751s+1632} \\ G_{ird}^*(s) = \frac{-1.003s^3-1554s^2+3.768\times10^4 s+5.554\times10^4}{s^3+374.6s^2+982.8s+1697} \end{cases} . \tag{60}$$

where $G_{id}(s)$, $G_{ud}(s)$ and $G_{ird}(s)$ can be derived using Equations (54), (56) and (58). It can be seen from Equation (60) and Figure 9 that, within the tolerance of the error, the calculated results and simulation results are accordant. The experimental results verified the feasibility of applying the small signal modeling scheme to fractional-order Boost circuits with inductive loads and also verified that the derived method provides a theoretical basis for subsequent linear controller design. The experimental results show that the transfer function of the proposed model can accurately describe the amplitude-frequency and phase-frequency characteristics in the mid to low-frequency domain, verifying the feasibility of applying the small signal modeling scheme to fractional-order Boost circuits with inductive loads and also verifying the correctness of the proposed model, providing a theoretical basis for subsequent linear controller design.

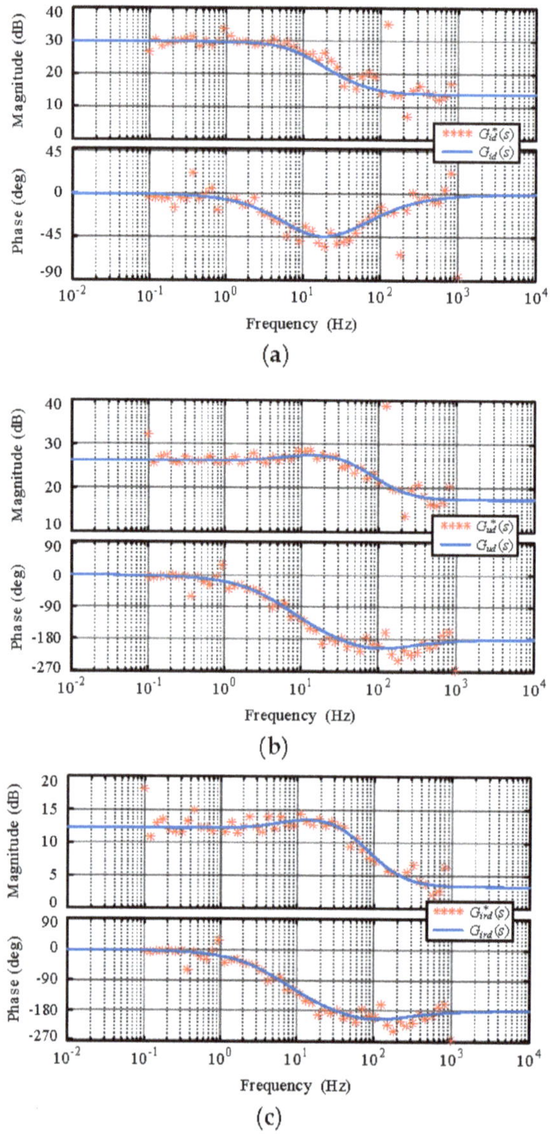

Figure 9. The amplitude-frequency characteristic. (**a**) G_{id}. (**b**) G_{ud}. (**c**) G_{ird}.

5. Conclusions

This paper presents a novel C-F definition-based modeling method for Boost converters with inductive loads using the fractional-order model, analyzes the effect of the order of fractional components on the characteristics of the converter, and verifies the validity of the C-F definition for the modeling of Boost converter circuits through simulation experiments. Firstly, a C-F definition-based mathematical model with three state variables of Boost converters with a fractional-order inductive load is constructed by using the state space averaging method. Furthermore, the quiescent operating point of the Boost converters and the ripple parameters' accurate analytical solutions of those three state variables are derived. Secondly, the transfer functions of the fractional-order Boost converters with three state variables are derived by using the small-signal linearization method. Then, circuit-oriented simulation experiments are conducted. The static operating point and ripple parameters of the circuit are obtained in the experiments. At the same time, the transfer functions of the simulated circuit are obtained through frequency sweep analysis. Those results are consistent with the numerical calculation results, verifying the correctness of the numerical derivation. Finally, the effect of the order of the capacitor, induced inductor, and load inductor on the DC component of state variable and ripple parameters is analyzed through numerical simulation. The results show that as the order of induced inductor and capacitor increases, there is a significant change in the values of voltage and current in the circuit and the ripple of the waveform is reduced. The effect of the order of the load inductance on the voltage and current in the circuit gradually increases as its value approaches 1, which is negatively correlated with the ripple amplitude of the output voltage and induced current, and positively correlated with the ripple amplitude of the load current. The order of the induced inductor mainly affects the induced current, while the order of the capacitor and load inductor mainly affects the load current and output voltage. In summary, the proposed model can comprehensively characterize the steady-state characteristics of fractional-order Boost converters with inductive loads, helping the circuit design of Boost converters. The C-F definition can be used in the modeling of Boost circuits.

The modeling method proposed in this paper is simple and easy to implement and can obtain analytical solutions of the required parameters for design. This method can be applied to other fractional-order systems with three state parameters. However, the C-F definition ignores some fractional-order characteristics to simplify derivation, which may result in some errors when describing the dynamic performance of fractional-order Boost circuits. And when considering electromagnetic induction, fatigue, or damage, the accuracy of models needs to be further improved. In the future, the mathematical model of C-F definition-based fractional-order Boost converters will be compared with other definitions, such as the Caputo definition, and Atangana–Baleanu definition, to analyze the advantages and disadvantages of different definitions in the mathematical modeling of fractional-order circuits.

Author Contributions: Conceptualization, D.Y. and X.L.; methodology, D.Y.; software, D.Y. and Y.W.; validation, D.Y., X.L. and Y.W.; formal analysis, D.Y.; investigation, D.Y. and Y.W.; resources, X.L.; data curation, D.Y.; writing—original draft preparation, D.Y.; writing—review and editing, D.Y.; visualization, D.Y.; supervision, X.L.; project administration, D.Y. and X.L.; funding acquisition, X.L. All authors have read and agreed to the published version of the manuscript.

Funding: This work is supported by the National Natural Science Foundation of China under grant 61873035.

Data Availability Statement: Data is contained within the article.

Conflicts of Interest: The authors declare no conflicts of interest. The funders had no role in the design of the study; in the collection, analyses, or interpretation of data; in the writing of the manuscript; or in the decision to publish the results.

References

1. Tarasov, V.E. On history of mathematical economics: Application of fractional calculus. *Mathematics* **2019**, *7*, 509. [CrossRef]
2. Petráš, I. Fractional calculus. In *Fractional-Order Nonlinear Systems: Modeling, Analysis and Simulation*; Springer Science & Business Media: Berlin/Heidelberg, Germany, 2011; pp. 7–42.
3. Sun, H.; Zhang, Y.; Baleanu, D.; Chen, W.; Chen, Y. A new collection of real world applications of fractional calculus in science and engineering. *Commun. Nonlinear Sci. Numer. Simul.* **2018**, *64*, 213–231. [CrossRef]
4. Chen, Y.; Petras, I.; Xue, D. Fractional order control-a tutorial. In Proceedings of the 2009 American Control Conference, St. Louis, MO, USA, 10–12 June 2009; IEEE: Piscataway, NJ, USA, 2009; pp. 1397–1411.
5. Koseoglu, M.; Deniz, F.N.; Alagoz, B.B.; Alisoy, H. An effective analog circuit design of approximate fractional-order derivative models of M-SBL fitting method. *Eng. Sci. Technol. Int. J.* **2022**, *33*, 101069. [CrossRef]

6. Suzuki, J.L.; Gulian, M.; Zayernouri, M.; D'Elia, M. Fractional modeling in action: A survey of nonlocal models for subsurface transport, turbulent flows, and anomalous materials. *J. Peridyn. Nonlocal Model.* **2023**, *5*, 392–459. [CrossRef]
7. Swaminathan, N.; Cao, Y. An overview of high-conversion high-voltage DC–DC converters for electrified aviation power distribution system. *IEEE Trans. Transp. Electrif.* **2020**, *6*, 1740–1754. [CrossRef]
8. Al-Greer, M.; Armstrong, M.; Ahmeid, M.; Giaouris, D. Advances on system identification techniques for DC–DC switch mode power converter applications. *IEEE Trans. Power Electron.* **2018**, *34*, 6973–6990. [CrossRef]
9. Song, S.; Zhang, X.; An, Y.; Ma, Y. Advanced fractional-order lithium-ion capacitor model with time-domain parameter identification method. *IEEE Trans. Ind. Electron.* **2021**, *69*, 13808–13817. [CrossRef]
10. Jiang, Y.; Zhang, B. Comparative study of Riemann–Liouville and Caputo derivative definitions in time-domain analysis of fractional-order capacitor. *IEEE Trans. Circuits Syst. II Express Briefs* **2019**, *67*, 2184–2188. [CrossRef]
11. Al-Daloo, M.; Soltan, A.; Yakovlev, A. Advance interconnect circuit modeling design using fractional-order elements. *IEEE Trans. Comput.-Aided Des. Integr. Circuits Syst.* **2019**, *39*, 2722–2734. [CrossRef]
12. Koton, J.; Dvorak, J.; Kubanek, D.; Herencsar, N. Designing series of fractional-order elements. *Analog. Integr. Circuits Signal Process.* **2021**, *106*, 553–563. [CrossRef]
13. Koton, J.; Kubanek, D.; Herencsar, N.; Dvorak, J.; Psychalinos, C. Designing constant phase elements of complement order. *Analog. Integr. Circuits Signal Process.* **2018**, *97*, 107–114. [CrossRef]
14. Nicola, M.; Nicola, C.I. Improved Performance in the Control of DC–DC Three-Phase Power Electronic Converter Using Fractional-Order SMC and Synergetic Controllers and RL-TD3 Agent. *Fractal Fract.* **2022**, *6*, 729. [CrossRef]
15. Chen, X.; Chen, Y.; Zhang, B.; Qiu, D. A modeling and analysis method for fractional-order DC–DC converters. *IEEE Trans. Power Electron.* **2016**, *32*, 7034–7044. [CrossRef]
16. Atangana, A.; Hammouch, Z. Fractional calculus with power law: The cradle of our ancestors. *Eur. Phys. J. Plus* **2019**, *134*, 429. [CrossRef]
17. Almeida, R. A Caputo fractional derivative of a function with respect to another function. *Commun. Nonlinear Sci. Numer. Simul.* **2017**, *44*, 460–481. [CrossRef]
18. Losada, J.; Nieto, J.J. Properties of a new fractional derivative without singular kernel. *Progr. Fract. Differ. Appl.* **2015**, *1*, 87–92.
19. Gabrick, E.C.; Protachevicz, P.R.; Lenzi, E.K.; Sayari, E.; Trobia, J.; Lenzi, M.K.; Borges, F.S.; Caldas, I.L.; Batista, A.M. Fractional Diffusion Equation under Singular and Non-Singular Kernel and Its Stability. *Fractal Fract.* **2023**, *7*, 792. [CrossRef]
20. Caputo, M.; Fabrizio, M. A new definition of fractional derivative without singular kernel. *Prog. Fract. Differ. Appl.* **2015**, *1*, 73–85.
21. Javed, F.; Riaz, M.B.; Iftikhar, N.; Awrejcewicz, J.; Akgül, A. Heat and mass transfer impact on differential type nanofluid with carbon nanotubes: A study of fractional order system. *Fractal Fract.* **2021**, *5*, 231. [CrossRef]
22. Sitthiwirattham, T.; Arfan, M.; Shah, K.; Zeb, A.; Djilali, S.; Chasreechai, S. Semi-analytical solutions for fuzzy Caputo–Fabrizio fractional-order two-dimensional heat equation. *Fractal Fract.* **2021**, *5*, 139. [CrossRef]
23. Idrees, M.; Alnahdi, A.S.; Jeelani, M.B. Mathematical Modeling of Breast Cancer Based on the Caputo–Fabrizio Fractal-Fractional Derivative. *Fractal Fract.* **2023**, *7*, 805. [CrossRef]
24. Cramer, E.Y.; Ray, E.L.; Lopez, V.K.; Bracher, J.; Brennen, A.; Castro Rivadeneira, A.J.; Gerding, A.; Gneiting, T.; House, K.H.; Huang, Y.; et al. Evaluation of individual and ensemble probabilistic forecasts of COVID-19 mortality in the United States. *Proc. Natl. Acad. Sci. USA* **2022**, *119*, e2113561119. [CrossRef] [PubMed]
25. Anjam, Y.N.; Shafqat, R.; Sarris, I.E.; Ur Rahman, M.; Touseef, S.; Arshad, M. A fractional order investigation of smoking model using Caputo–Fabrizio differential operator. *Fractal Fract.* **2022**, *6*, 623. [CrossRef]
26. Wang, Y.; Chen, Y.; Liao, X. State-of-art survey of fractional order modeling and estimation methods for lithium-ion batteries. *Fract. Calc. Appl. Anal.* **2019**, *22*, 1449–1479. [CrossRef]
27. Yang, N.; Xu, C.; Wu, C.; Jia, R.; Liu, C. Fractional-order cubic nonlinear flux-controlled memristor: Theoretical analysis, numerical calculation and circuit simulation. *Nonlinear Dyn.* **2019**, *97*, 33–44. [CrossRef]
28. Alilou, M.; Azami, H.; Oshnoei, A.; Mohammadi-Ivatloo, B.; Teodorescu, R. Fractional-Order Control Techniques for Renewable Energy and Energy-Storage-Integrated Power Systems: A Review. *Fractal Fract.* **2023**, *7*, 391. [CrossRef]
29. Lin, D.; Liao, X.; Dong, L.; Yang, R.; Samson, S.Y.; Iu, H.H.C.; Fernando, T.; Li, Z. Experimental study of fractional-order RC circuit model using the Caputo and Caputo–Fabrizio derivatives. *IEEE Trans. Circuits Syst. I Regul. Pap.* **2021**, *68*, 1034–1044. [CrossRef]
30. Mahdavi, J.; Emaadi, A.; Bellar, M.; Ehsani, M. Analysis of power electronic converters using the generalized state-space averaging approach. *IEEE Trans. Circuits Syst. I Fundam. Theory Appl.* **1997**, *44*, 767–770. [CrossRef]
31. Yang, C.; Xie, F.; Chen, Y.; Xiao, W.; Zhang, B. Modeling and analysis of the fractional-order flyback converter in continuous conduction mode by caputo fractional calculus. *Electronics* **2020**, *9*, 1544. [CrossRef]
32. Xie, L.; Liu, Z.; Zhang, B. A modeling and analysis method for CCM fractional order Buck-Boost converter by using R–L fractional definition. *J. Electr. Eng. Technol.* **2020**, *15*, 1651–1661. [CrossRef]
33. Wei, Z.; Zhang, B.; Jiang, Y. Analysis and modeling of fractional-order buck converter based on Riemann-Liouville derivative. *IEEE Access* **2019**, *7*, 162768–162777. [CrossRef]
34. Chen, Y.; Chen, X.; Hu, J.; Zhang, B.; Qiu, D. A symbolic analysis method for fractional-order boost converter in discontinuous conduction mode. In Proceedings of the IECON 2017-43rd Annual Conference of the IEEE Industrial Electronics Society, Beijing, China, 29 October–1 November 2017; IEEE: Piscataway, NJ, USA, 2017; pp. 8738–8743.

35. Jia, Z.; Liu, C. Fractional-order modeling and simulation of magnetic coupled boost converter in continuous conduction mode. *Int. J. Bifurc. Chaos* **2018**, *28*, 1850061. [CrossRef]
36. Fang, S.; Wang, X. Modeling and analysis method of fractional-order buck–boost converter. *Int. J. Circuit Theory Appl.* **2020**, *48*, 1493–1510. [CrossRef]
37. Sheikh, N.A.; Ching, D.L.C.; Ullah, S.; Khan, I. Mathematical and statistical analysis of RL and RC fractional-order circuits. *Fractals* **2020**, *28*, 2040030. [CrossRef]
38. Kianpoor, N.; Yousefi, M.; Bayati, N.; Hajizadeh, A.; Soltani, M. Fractional order modelling of DC–DC boost converters. In Proceedings of the 2019 IEEE 28th International Symposium on Industrial Electronics (ISIE), Vancouver, BC, Canada, 12–14 June 2019; IEEE: Piscataway, NJ, USA, 2019; pp. 864–869.
39. Sharma, M.; Rajpurohit, B.S.; Agnihotri, S.; Rathore, A.K. Development of fractional order modeling of voltage source converters. *IEEE Access* **2020**, *8*, 131750–131759. [CrossRef]
40. Leng, M.; Zhou, G.; Tian, Q.; Xu, G.; Blaabjerg, F. Small signal modeling and design analysis for boost converter with valley V 2 control. *IEEE Trans. Power Electron.* **2020**, *35*, 13475–13487. [CrossRef]
41. Siddhartha, V.; Hote, Y.V.; Saxena, S. Non-ideal modelling and IMC based PID Controller Design of PWM DC–DC Buck Converter. *IFAC-PapersOnLine* **2018**, *51*, 639–644. [CrossRef]
42. Gómez-Aguilar, J.F.; Morales-Delgado, V.F.; Taneco-Hernández, M.A.; Baleanu, D.; Escobar-Jiménez, R.F.; Mohamed Al Qurashi, M. Analytical solutions of the electrical RLC circuit via Liouville–Caputo operators with local and non-local kernels. *Entropy* **2016**, *18*, 402. [CrossRef]
43. Atangana, A.; Alkahtani, B.S.T. Extension of the resistance, inductance, capacitance electrical circuit to fractional derivative without singular kernel. *Adv. Mech. Eng.* **2015**, *7*. [CrossRef]
44. Rosales, J.; Filoteo, J.D.; González, A. A comparative analysis of the RC circuit with local and non-local fractional derivatives. *Rev. Mex. Fís.* **2018**, *64*, 647–654. [CrossRef]
45. Montesinos-García, J.J.; Barahona-Avalos, J.L.; Linares-Flores, J.; Juárez-Abad, J.A. Uncertainty Observer-Based Control for a Class of Fractional-Order Non-Linear Systems with Non-Linear Control Inputs. *Fractal Fract.* **2023**, *7*, 836. [CrossRef]
46. Liao, X.; Ran, M.; Yu, D.; Lin, D.; Yang, R. Chaos analysis of Buck converter with non-singular fractional derivative. *Chaos Solitons Fractals* **2022**, *156*, 111794. [CrossRef]
47. Liao, X.; Wang, Y.; Yu, D.; Lin, D.; Ran, M.; Ruan, P. Modeling and analysis of Buck-Boost converter with non-singular fractional derivatives. *Chaos Solitons Fractals* **2023**, *169*, 113336. [CrossRef]
48. Xie, L.; Shi, J.; Yao, J.; Wan, D. Research on the Period-Doubling Bifurcation of Fractional-Order DCM Buck–Boost Converter Based on Predictor-Corrector Algorithm. *Mathematics* **2022**, *10*, 1993. [CrossRef]
49. Abuaisha, T.; Kertzscher, J. Fractional-order modelling and parameter identification of electrical coils. *Fract. Calc. Appl. Anal.* **2019**, *22*, 193–216. [CrossRef]
50. Raorane, A.A.; Patil, M.D.; Vyawahare, V.A. Analysis of full-wave controlled rectifier with lossy inductive load using fractional-order models. In Proceedings of the 2015 International Conference on Industrial Instrumentation and Control (ICIC), Pune, India, 28–30 May 2015; IEEE: Piscataway, NJ, USA, 2015; pp. 750–755.
51. Zhu, J.; Chen, D.; Zhao, H.; Ma, R. Nonlinear dynamic analysis and modeling of fractional permanent magnet synchronous motors. *J. Vib. Control* **2016**, *22*, 1855–1875. [CrossRef]
52. Khubalkar, S.; Junghare, A.; Aware, M.; Das, S. Modeling and control of a permanent-magnet brushless DC motor drive using a fractional order proportional-integral-derivative controller. *Turk. J. Electr. Eng. Comput. Sci.* **2017**, *25*, 4223–4241. [CrossRef]
53. Tripathy, M.C.; Mondal, D.; Biswas, K.; Sen, S. Experimental studies on realization of fractional inductors and fractional-order bandpass filters. *Int. J. Circuit Theory Appl.* **2015**, *43*, 1183–1196. [CrossRef]
54. Zhang, L.; Kartci, A.; Elwakil, A.; Bagci, H.; Salama, K.N. Fractional-order inductor: Design, simulation, and implementation. *IEEE Access* **2021**, *9*, 73695–73702. [CrossRef]
55. Said, L.A.; Ismail, S.M.; Radwan, A.G.; Madian, A.H.; Abu El-Yazeed, M.F.; Soliman, A.M. On the optimization of fractional order low-pass filters. *Circuits Syst. Signal Process.* **2016**, *35*, 2017–2039. [CrossRef]
56. Yu, D.; Liao, X.; Wang, Y.; Ran, M.; Dalin; Xia, J. Modeling and Characteristic Analysis of Fractional-Order Boost Converter based on the Caputo–Fabrizio Fractional Derivatives. *Fractals* **2023**, *31*, 2350082. [CrossRef]
57. Liao, X.; Yu, D.; Lin, D.; Ran, M.; Xia, J. Characteristic Analysis of Fractional-Order RLC Circuit based on the Caputo–Fabrizio Definition. *Fractals* **2022**, *30*, 2250078. [CrossRef]

fractal and fractional

MDPI

Article

Fractional-Order Zener Model with Temperature-Order Equivalence for Viscoelastic Dampers

Kang Xu [1], Liping Chen [2], António M. Lopes [3], Mingwu Wang [1,*], Ranchao Wu [4] and Min Zhu [2]

[1] School of Civil and Hydraulic Engineering, Hefei University of Technology, Hefei 230009, China; 2019010048@mail.hfut.edu.cn

[2] School of Electrical Engineering and Automation, Hefei University of Technology, Hefei 230009, China; lip_chen@hfut.edu.cn (L.C.); zhumin@hfut.edu.cn (M.Z.)

[3] LAETA/INEGI, Faculty of Engineering, University of Porto, Rua Dr. Roberto Frias, 4200-465 Porto, Portugal; aml@fe.up.pt

[4] School of Mathematics, Anhui University, Hefei 230601, China; rcwu@ahu.edu.cn

* Correspondence: mingwu_wang@hfut.edu.cn

Abstract: Viscoelastic (VE) dampers show good performance in dissipating energy, being widely used for reducing vibration in engineering structures caused by earthquakes and winds. Experimental studies have shown that ambient temperature has great influence on the mechanical behavior of VE dampers. Therefore, it is important to accurately model VE dampers considering the effect of temperature. In this paper, a new fractional-order Zener (AEF-Zener) model of VE dampers is proposed. Firstly, the important influence of fractional orders on the energy dissipation ability of materials is analyzed. Secondly, an equivalent AEF-Zener model is developed that incorporates the ambient temperature and fractional-order equivalence principle. Finally, the chaotic fractional-order particle swarm optimization (CFOPSO) algorithm is used to determine the model's parameters. The accuracy of the AEF-Zener model is verified by comparing model simulations with experimental results. This study is helpful for designing and analyzing vibration reduction techniques for civil structures with VE dampers under the influence of temperature.

Keywords: viscoelastic damper; energy dissipation; temperature-order equivalent principle; fractional-order vibration system

1. Introduction

Earthquakes and wind are among the most catastrophic natural hazards that affect civil engineering structures. Therefore, developing new strategies for protecting building structures from damage caused by disasters has become a very important research topic [1,2]. In recent years, several control methods have been proposed to reduce structural vibrations in civil engineering structures, such as active [3,4], semi-active [5], passive [6,7], and hybrid vibration control [8]. Among them, passive control has been broadly used [9,10]. Indeed, passive vibration control devices emerged as a promising solution, and VE dampers became widely applied in building structures due to their relatively low cost and good energy dissipation performance [11].

Research on VE damping systems focuses on three main aspects, namely (i) development of VE materials with high energy dissipation, (ii) mechanical design, and (iii) analysis of the controlled structures [12,13]. In reference [14], different materials were studied under experimental dynamic loading of full-scale dampers, and a model of the dampers was developed. In references [15,16], the VE parameters of sandwich structures were identified, while a new inverse technique and an adjoint-based gradient method were developed. The dynamics of a structure with VE dampers can be well-described by differential equations of fractional order. The spline collocation method for solving systems of multi-term fractional differential equations was proposed and studied in [17]. In reference [18], several types of VE materials based on different matrix rubbers were optimized and developed, and the mechanical behavior and energy dissipation ability of VE dampers built from these materials were tested. The aforementioned research showed that VE dampers can buffer buildings efficiently against earthquakes due to their large damping capabilities. However, the properties of VE dampers are highly influenced by ambient temperature and excitation frequency, which affect their behavior. Therefore, it is crucial to accurately model VE dampers considering the effect of temperature.

Traditional VE models, such as the Kelvin and Maxwell ones, are unable to accurately capture the frequency-dependent behavior of VE materials [19]. In the past few decades, fractional calculus emerged in scientific and engineering practices [20] due to its ability to model long memory effects, enabling description of the behavior of VE dampers for a wide range of frequencies. Thus, several types of fractional-order constitutive models have been established [21]. However, the effect of ambient temperature on the performance of VE materials is still neglected in most fractional-order models, while in some previous works, it was considered through a shift factor defined by the Williams–Landel–Ferry (WLF) equation [22,23].

The fractional-order Zener model has more degrees of freedom than many other models and can better describe the dynamics of VE materials [24,25]. Indeed, the fractional-order Zener model can well-characterize the influence of frequency [26]. However, it cannot characterize the influence of temperature. In reference [27], a constitutive model was proposed to describe the self-heating effect in elastomeric materials subjected to cyclic loading. In paper [28], the frequency-temperature correspondence principle was adopted, and a method for analyzing the dynamics of structures with VE dampers was addressed. Furthermore, in references [29,30], VE damper models were developed based on molecular chain network micro structures and the temperature-frequency equivalence principle.

In the above references, the influence of temperature usually considers the frequency-temperature equivalence principle. However, temperature and frequency may influence each other, and the physical meaning of equating the influence of temperature to frequency is unclear. Therefore, the accuracy of existing models may be insufficient, and a new approach to effectively model VE dampers is required. In fact, the fractional order has certain geometric and physical significance related to the VE properties of materials [31,32]. A higher order leads to stronger viscosity and stronger energy dissipation, while a lower order causes stronger elasticity and weaker energy dissipation. Therefore, the fractional-order variation in the model can characterize the effect of ambient temperature on the dynamics of VE dampers.

Motivated by the above discussion, a new AEF-Zener model is proposed in this paper. The ability to dissipate energy from VE materials characterized by different fractional orders is analyzed, and the relationship between energy dissipation and fractional order is discussed. Furthermore, based on the temperature-order equivalence, a functional relationship between fractional-order and temperature is established to indirectly characterize the impact of ambient temperature on the performance of VE dampers. The proposed model has a clearer physical meaning and higher accuracy, especially for characterizing the loss factor parameters related to energy consumption, compared to other existing models.

The most important contributions of the paper are:

(a) The influence of fractional order on the energy dissipation capabilities of VE materials is analyzed in the time and frequency domains.
(b) A novel AEF-Zener model is proposed, and the model's parameters are determined by using a CFOPSO algorithm.
(c) The accuracy and effectiveness of the AEF-Zener model is verified by comparing model simulations with experimental results and with models that use the temperature-frequency equivalent principle.

The paper is structured into seven main parts. Section 2 recalls some elemental concepts of fractional calculus. Section 3 presents the mathematical equations of fractional-order Zener VE dampers. Section 4 analyzes the influence of fractional orders. Sections 5 and 6 describe and determine the AEF-Zener model and its parameters, respectively. Section 7 draws the conclusions.

2. Preliminary Concepts of Fractional Calculus

Fractional calculus emerged as an important tool with applications in scientific and engineering fields [33–36]. Some basic definitions concerning fractional calculus are given here for understanding later calculations and analysis.

Given a function $x(t) : R \to R$, it is referred to as C^k-class if its derivatives $x^{(1)}, x^{(2)}, \ldots,$ $x^{(k)}$ exist and are continuous (except for a finite number of points). In the following, we adopt the notation $x(t) \in C^0, C^1$, and C^∞ to denote the classes of all continuous, continuously differentiable, and smooth functions, respectively [37].

The Riemann–Liouville fractional integral of order $\alpha > 0$ of a continuous function $x(t)$ is [38]:

$$ {}_0I_t^\alpha x(t) = D^{-\alpha}x(t) = \frac{1}{\Gamma(\alpha)} \int_0^t (t-s)^{\alpha-1} x(s)ds, \quad (1) $$

where $\Gamma(\cdot)$ is the gamma function.

The Riemann–Liouville fractional derivative of order $n-1 < \alpha < n$, $n \in N$, of a continuous function $x(t) \in C^n[0,\ t]$ is [39]:

$$ {}_0^{RL}D_t^\alpha x(t) = \frac{1}{\Gamma(n-\alpha)} \frac{d^n}{dt^n} \int_0^t (t-s)^{n-\alpha-1} x(s)ds. \quad (2) $$

In discrete time, the Grünwald–Letnikov fractional derivative of order $\alpha 0$ of a function $x(t)$ can be approximated by the truncated series [40]:

$$ {}_0^{GL}D_t^\alpha x(t) \approx \frac{1}{T^\alpha} \sum_{k=0}^{r} \frac{(-1)^k \Gamma(\alpha+1) x(t-kT)}{\Gamma(k+1)\Gamma(\alpha-k+1)}, \quad (3) $$

where r is the truncation value, and T corresponds to the sampling period, respectively.

If $x(t) \in C^n[0,\ t]$, then [37]:

$$ {}_0^{RL}D_t^\alpha x(t) = {}_0^{GL}D_t^\alpha x(t). \quad (4) $$

The Riemann–Liouville fractional derivative verifies [41]:

$$ \frac{d^n}{dt^n}\left({}_0^{RL}D_t^\alpha x(t)\right) = {}_0^{RL}D_t^\alpha \left(\frac{d^n x(t)}{dt^n}\right) = {}_0^{RL}D_t^{(\alpha+n)} x(t). \quad (5) $$

For zero initial conditions in the Laplace domain, we have [42]:

$$ L(D^\alpha x(t)) = s^\alpha x(s). \quad (6) $$

3. Equation of Fractional-Order Zener VE Damper

3.1. Dynamic Equation in the Time Domain

The relationship between strain $\sigma(t)$ and stress $\gamma(t)$ is characterized by the following fractional-order Zener constitutive equation (see Figure 1) :

$$ \sigma(t) + p_1 D^\alpha \sigma(t) = q_0 \gamma(t) + q_1 D^\alpha \gamma(t), \quad (7) $$

where $\alpha \in (0,1)$ is the order of the Riemann–Liouville fractional differentiation (Equation (2)), and p_1, q_0, and q_1 are positive constant coefficients determined by the VE material's performance parameters E_1, E_2, and η.

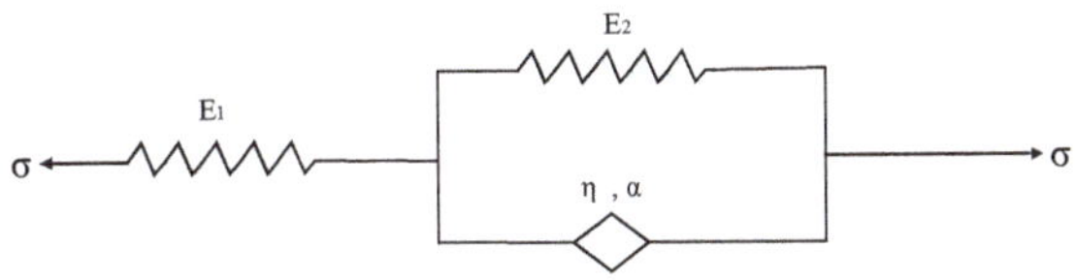

Figure 1. Fractional-order Zener model.

Figure 2 illustrates a one-degree-of-freedom fractional-order Zener damper system consisting of a mass and a damper. The strain and the stress are determined as:

$$\sigma(t) = \frac{f_d(t)}{A}, \gamma(t) = \frac{x(t)}{L}. \tag{8}$$

Combining Equations (7) and (8) results in:

$$f_d(t) + p_1 D^\alpha f_d(t) = \frac{Aq_0}{L} x(t) + \frac{Aq_1}{L} D^\alpha x(t), \tag{9}$$

where L and A stand for length and area, respectively, $f_d(t)$ denotes the damping force, and $x(t)$ represents the displacement of the damper.

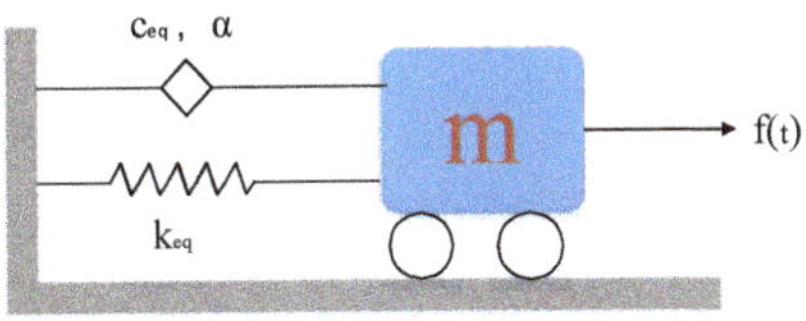

Figure 2. A single-degree-of-freedom fractional Zener VE damper system.

By Newton's second law, the dynamic equation of the damper is:

$$m\ddot{x}(t) + f_d(t) = f(t). \tag{10}$$

From Equations (10) and (5), one has:

$$p_1 m D^{2+\alpha} x(t) + p_1 D^\alpha f_d(t) = p_1 D^\alpha f(t). \tag{11}$$

Equations (10) and (11) give:

$$p_1 m D^{2+\alpha} x(t) + m\ddot{x}(t) + f_d(t) + p_1 D^\alpha f_d(t) = p_1 D^\alpha f(t) + f(t). \tag{12}$$

Substituting Equation (9) into (12) and letting $k = Aq_0/L$ and $c = Aq_1/L$ leads to:

$$p_1 m D^{2+\alpha} x(t) + m\ddot{x}(t) + cD^\alpha x(t) + kx(t) = p_1 D^\alpha f(t) + f(t), \tag{13}$$

where $f(t)$ is the disturbance force, and p_1 falls into either Case 1 or Case 2:

Case 1. If $p_1 = 0$ or $p_1 \to 0$, then Equation (13) can be rewritten as:

$$m\ddot{x}(t) + cD^\alpha x(t) + kx(t) = f(t); \tag{14}$$

Case 2. If $p_1 > 0$, with the following state transformation, then:

$$x(t) = p_1 D^\alpha y(t) + y(t). \tag{15}$$

Substituting Equation (15) into Equation (13) leads to:

$$mp_1 D^{2+\alpha} y(t) + m\ddot{y}(t) + cD^{\alpha} y(t) + ky(t) = f(t). \quad (16)$$

With $mp_1 D^{2+\alpha} y(t) + m\ddot{y}(t) = m\ddot{x}(t)$, let $cD^{\alpha} y(t) = c' D^{\alpha} x(t)$, $ky(t) = k' x(t)$, Equation (16) can be equivalently transformed into:

$$m\ddot{x}(t) + c' D^{\alpha} x(t) + k' x(t) = f(t). \quad (17)$$

From the above, we establish the equivalent dynamic equation of the fractional-order Zener VE damper with a single degree of freedom:

$$\begin{cases} m\ddot{x}(t) + c_{eq} D^{\alpha} x(t) + k_{eq} x(t) = f(t), \\ f_d(t) = k_{eq} x(t) + c_{eq} D^{\alpha} x(t), \end{cases} \quad (18)$$

where c_{eq} is the damping, and k_{eq} is the equivalent stiffness, which are related to the values of α, p_1, q_0, q_1, frequency ω, and temperature T. We usually analyze them in the frequency domain.

3.2. Dynamic Equation in the Frequency Domain

The Laplace transform (Equation (6)) on Equation (7) results in:

$$\sigma(s) + p_1 s^{\alpha} \sigma(s) = q_0 \gamma(s) + q_1 s^{\alpha} \gamma(s). \quad (19)$$

Therefore, the transfer function of Equation (19) is:

$$G(s) = \frac{\sigma(s)}{\gamma(s)} = \frac{q_0 + q_1 s^{\alpha}}{1 + p_1 s^{\alpha}}. \quad (20)$$

By replacing s with $i\omega$, with $i^{\alpha} = \cos(\alpha\pi/2) + i \cdot \sin(\alpha\pi/2)$, we obtain the complex modulus:

$$G^*(\omega) = G_1(\omega) + iG_2(\omega), \quad (21)$$

where $i = \sqrt{-1}$, and the storage and loss modulus, $G_1(\omega)$ and $G_2(\omega)$, are the real and imaginary components of the complex modulus, respectively. Hence, we have:

$$\begin{cases} G_1(\omega) = \dfrac{\left[q_0 + p_1 q_1 \omega^{2\alpha} + (q_1 + p_1 q_0)\omega^{\alpha} \cos\frac{\alpha\pi}{2}\right]}{\left[1 + p_1^2 \omega^{2\alpha} + 2p_1 \omega^{\alpha} \cos\frac{\alpha\pi}{2}\right]}, \\ G_2(\omega) = \dfrac{(q_1 - p_1 q_0)\omega^{\alpha} \sin\frac{\alpha\pi}{2}}{\left[1 + p_1^2 \omega^{2\alpha} + 2p_1 \omega^{\alpha} \cos\frac{\alpha\pi}{2}\right]}, \\ \eta = \dfrac{(q_1 - p_1 q_0)\omega^{\alpha} \sin\frac{\alpha\pi}{2}}{\left[q_0 + p_1 q_1 \omega^{2\alpha} + (q_1 + p_1 q_0)\omega^{\alpha} \cos\frac{\alpha\pi}{2}\right]}, \end{cases} \quad (22)$$

where $\eta = G_2(\omega)/G_1(\omega)$ is the loss factor.

Then, the mechanical properties of the VE damper, namely the equivalent stiffness and damping, k_{eq} and c_{eq}, respectively, can be calculated and analyzed with the following equations:

$$k'_{eq} = \frac{n_v \cdot G_1 \cdot A_v}{h_v}, \quad (23)$$

$$c'_{eq} = \frac{n_v \cdot G_2 \cdot A_v}{\omega \cdot h_v}, \quad (24)$$

where n_v is the number of layers of VE material between the steel plates that compose the VE damper, and A_v and h_v are the shear area and thickness of each VE layer, respectively.

4. The Influence of Fractional-Order α

Numerical simulations are carried out to demonstrate the influence of the fractional order α on the VE damper energy dissipation capacity. From Section 3, one can observe that the fractional order α is related to the dynamic properties of the VE material in the time and frequency domains.

4.1. Analysis in the Time Domain

The coefficients in the fractional-order model of the Zener VE damper (Equation (18)) are taken as $m = 1, c_{eq} = 0.5, k_{eq} = 1$, and $\alpha \in (0, 1)$, and the disturbance is assumed to be a step signal:

$$f(t) = \begin{cases} 0, & 0 < t < 1, \\ 10, & 1 \leq t. \end{cases} \tag{25}$$

It follows from Equation (18) that:

$$x(t) = \frac{1}{k_{eq}}(f(t) - m\ddot{x}(t) - c_{eq} \cdot {}_{RL}D^{\alpha}x(t)). \tag{26}$$

Figure 3 illustrates the Simulink block diagram programming adopted for the fractional-order equation with zero initial values. The fractional-order operator D^{α} can be approximated using MATLAB2019a programming based on Equations (3) and (4). Vibration responses of the fractional-order Zener VE damper with different fractional orders are shown in Figure 4. One can see that the energy dissipation capacity of the VE damper is stronger with the increase in the fractional order α.

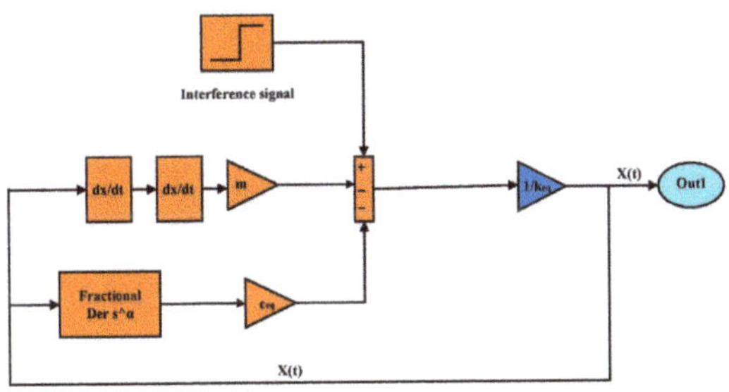

Figure 3. Simulink block diagram for the fractional equation with zero initial values.

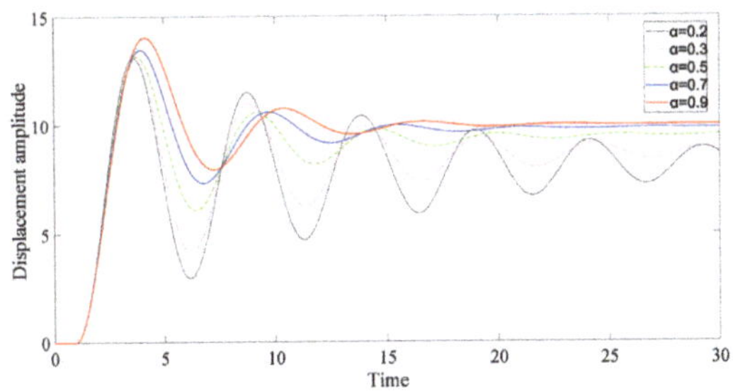

Figure 4. Vibration responses of the fractional Zener VE damper with different fractional order α.

4.2. Analysis in the Frequency Domain

In this simulation, the coefficients of the fractional-order Zener VE damper (Equation (22)) are taken as $p_1 = 0.0015, q_0 = 0.5, q_1 = 1.25, \omega \in (0.1, 2]$, and $\alpha \in (0, 1)$.

The responses of the storage modulus and loss factor, G_1 and η, respectively, of the fractional-order Zener VE damper with different fractional orders are shown in Figures 5 and 6, respectively. Figures 7 and 8 show two responses with different fractional orders and frequencies. From Figures 5 and 6, we verify that the fractional order α has a positive correlation with the change in G_1 and a negative correlation with the change in η. Figures 7 and 8 indicate that frequency also has a great influence on the dynamic performance of the damper.

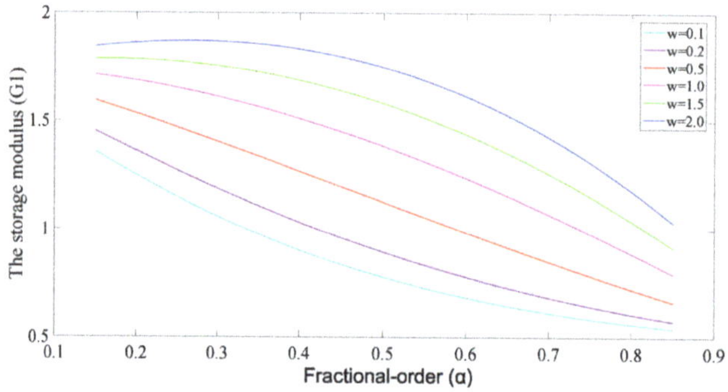

Figure 5. The storage modulus G_1 of the VE damper at different frequencies and fractional orders.

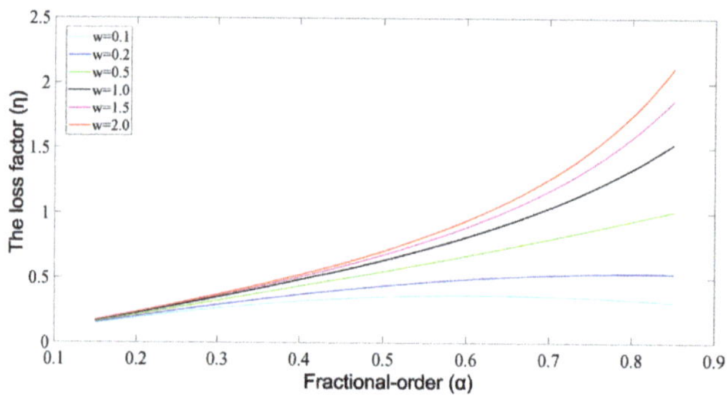

Figure 6. The loss factor η of the VE damper at different frequencies and fractional orders.

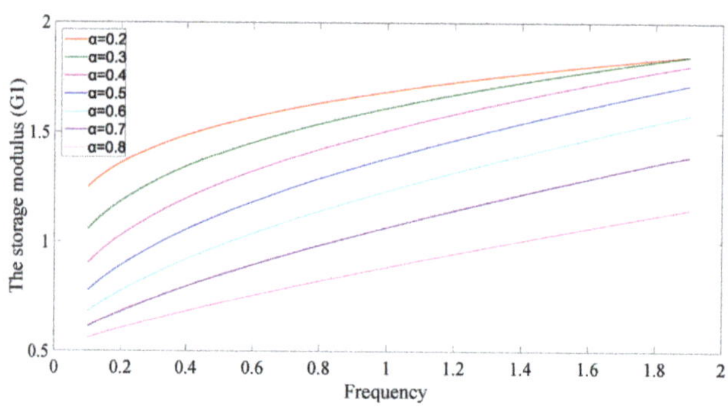

Figure 7. The storage modulus G_1 of the VE damper at different fractional orders and frequencies.

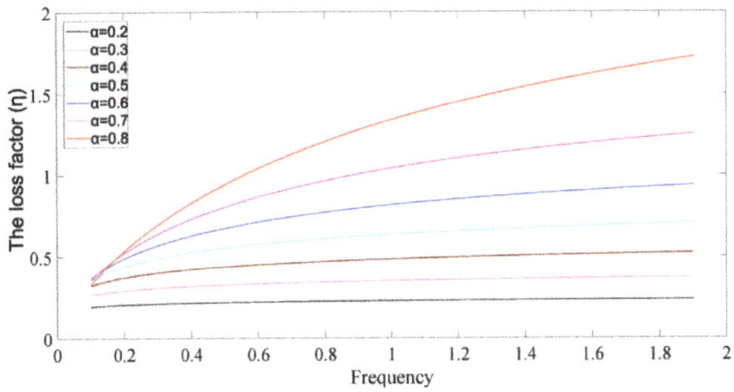

Figure 8. The loss factor η of the VE damper at different fractional orders and frequencies.

The above simulations confirm that the fractional order α is related to the energy dissipation capacity and dynamic performance of the damper. The higher the order is, the stronger the viscosity and the energy dissipation are.

5. Temperature-Order Equivalent Mathematical Model

5.1. Temperature-Order Equivalent Principle

Experimental results show that temperature and frequency affect the dynamics of VE dampers and that temperature has a more prominent effect, as illustrated in Figures 9 and 10 [29]. From Equation (22), it can be seen that the influence of frequency is described well. However, the fractional-order Zener model can not characterize the effect of temperature. Therefore, we establish the necessary relationship by introducing a new mathematical model that considers the temperature change and fractional-order equivalence, given by:

$$\begin{cases} G_1(\omega, T) = G_1(\omega, \alpha_1(T)), \\ \eta(\omega, T) = \eta(\omega, \alpha_2(T)), \end{cases} \tag{27}$$

where α_1 and α_2 are:

$$\begin{cases} \alpha_1(T) = \sum_{i=1}^{5} a_i T^i + b_1, \\ \alpha_2(T) = 1 - (\sum_{i=1}^{5} c_i T^i + b_2). \end{cases} \tag{28}$$

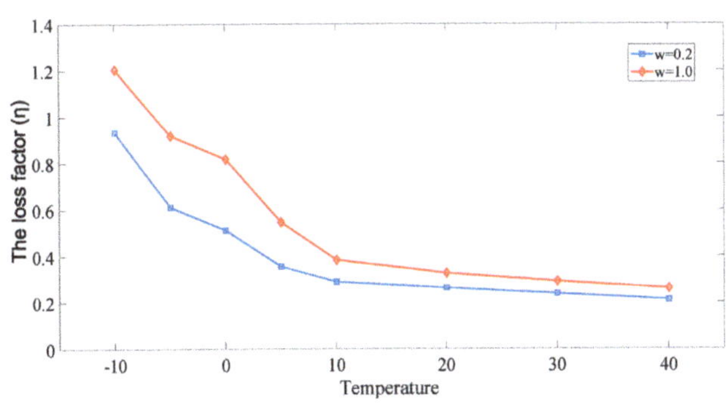

Figure 9. The loss factor η of the VE damper at different temperatures.

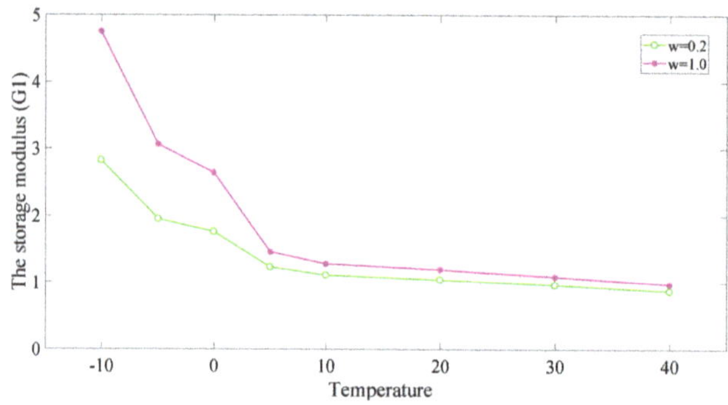

Figure 10. The storage modulus G_1 of the VE damper at different temperatures.

Thus, Equation (22) can be rewritten as:

$$\begin{cases} G_1 = \dfrac{\left[q_0 + p_1 q_1 \omega^{2\alpha_1} + (q_1 + p_1 q_0)\omega^{\alpha_1}\cos\frac{\alpha_1 \pi}{2}\right]}{\left[1 + p_1^2 \omega^{2\alpha_1} + 2p_1\omega^{\alpha_1}\cos\frac{\alpha_1 \pi}{2}\right]}, \\ \eta = G_2/G_1 = \dfrac{(q_1 - p_1 q_0)\omega^{\alpha_2}\sin\frac{\alpha_2 \pi}{2}}{\left[q_0 + p_1 q_1 \omega^{2\alpha_2} + (q_1 + p_1 q_0)\omega^{\alpha_2}\cos\frac{\alpha_2 \pi}{2}\right]}. \end{cases} \tag{29}$$

5.2. Model Modification

As the influence of temperature on the properties of VE dampers is related to frequency, the temperature and fractional-order equivalent relationship with frequency correction can be obtained as:

$$\begin{cases} G_1(\omega, T) = G_1(\omega, \alpha_1^*(T, \omega)), \\ \eta(\omega, T) = \eta(\omega, \alpha_2^*(T, \omega)). \end{cases} \tag{30}$$

For simplifying the analysis, we first fix $\omega = 0.5$. Then, α_1^* and α_2^* are calculated as:

$$\begin{cases} \alpha_1^*(T, \omega) = \alpha_1(T, 0.5) + k_1(\omega - 0.5), \\ \alpha_2^*(T, \omega) = \alpha_2(T, 0.5) - k_2(\omega - 0.5), \end{cases} \tag{31}$$

where k_1 and k_2 are determined by:

$$\begin{cases} k_1 = \sum_{i=1}^{5} a_i^* T^i + b_1^*, \\ k_2 = \sum_{i=1}^{5} c_i^* T^i + b_2^*. \end{cases} \tag{32}$$

Therefore, by considering the temperature effect and the frequency modified model, the new AEF-Zener model is given by:

$$\begin{cases} G_1 = \dfrac{\left[q_0 + p_1 q_1 \omega^{2\alpha_1^*} + (q_1 + p_1 q_0)\omega^{\alpha_1^*}\cos\frac{\alpha_1^* \pi}{2}\right]}{\left[1 + p_1^2 \omega^{2\alpha_1^*} + 2p_1\omega^{\alpha_1^*}\cos\frac{\alpha_1^* \pi}{2}\right]}, \\ \eta = G_2/G_1 = \dfrac{(q_1 - p_1 q_0)\omega^{\alpha_2^*}\sin\frac{\alpha_2^* \pi}{2}}{\left[q_0 + p_1 q_1 \omega^{2\alpha_2^*} + (q_1 + p_1 q_0)\omega^{\alpha_2^*}\cos\frac{\alpha_2^* \pi}{2}\right]}. \end{cases} \tag{33}$$

Further, we have:

$$k_{eq}' = \frac{n_v \cdot G_1(\omega, \alpha^*) \cdot A_v}{h_v}, \tag{34}$$

$$c'_{eq} = \frac{n_v \cdot G_2(\omega, \alpha^*) \cdot A_v}{\omega \cdot h_v}, \tag{35}$$

where the values of parameters p_1, q_0, q_1, α_1^*, and α_2^* in Equation (33) are used to define the material properties. It should be noted that this model reflects the impact of ambient temperature on the dynamic behaviors of the VE dampers through the fractional order.

6. Parameter Identification and Experimental Comparison

In this section, the storage modulus and loss factor, G_1 and η, respectively, that represent the mechanical properties of the VE damper are used to determine the parameters of the equivalent model. The experimental data from the dynamic tests in reference [29] were used. Herein, we propose a new chaotic fractional-order particle swarm optimization (CFOPSO) algorithm to accurately determine the model's parameters.

6.1. Parameter Identification with the CFOPSO

The PSO is a simple and easy-to-implement algorithm. The PSO can be generalized using fractional-order tools to yield the fractional-order PSO algorithm, which can better balance global and local searching capabilities [43]. Chaotic mapping can be used to generate evenly chaotic numbers between 0 and 1, as shown in Figure 11. The population initialization is carried out by using chaotic sequences contributing to an increase in the performance of the algorithm [44]. The values are mapped to initialization particle individuals according to the following formula:

$$\begin{cases} y_{i+1} = \mu y_i(1 - y_i), \\ \chi = \chi_{Lb} + (\chi_{Ub} - \chi_{Lb}) y_{i+1}, \end{cases} \tag{36}$$

where i is the number of iterations, and μ is the bifurcation parameter. The symbols χ_{Ub} and χ_{Lb} are the upper and lower limits of each individual in each dimension, and y_{i+1} is the mapped individual.

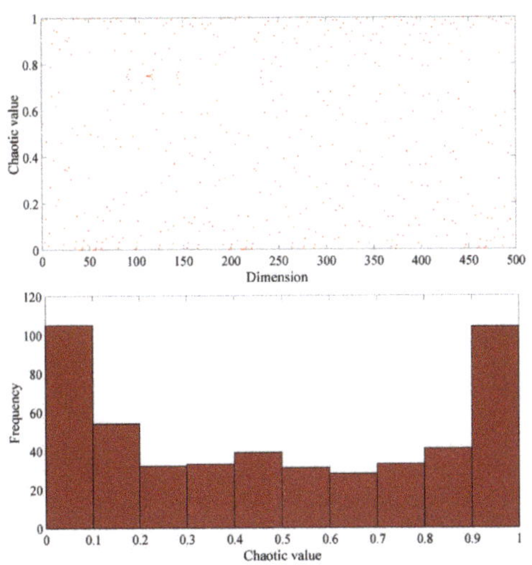

Figure 11. Chaotic mapping generating chaotic numbers.

The velocity and position of the particles are updated using:

$$\begin{cases} D^{\alpha} v_{ij}(t+1) = c_1\phi_1[Pb_{ij}(t) - \chi_{ij}(t)] + c_2\phi_2[Gb_{gj}(t) - \chi_{ij}(t)], \\ \chi_{ij}(t+1) = \chi_{ij}(t) + v_{ij}(t+1), \end{cases} \tag{37}$$

where $Pb_{ij}(t)$ is its best position for each particle found so far, $Gb_{gj}(t)$ is the best position of the swarm, c_1 and c_2 denote the coefficients of the particle acceleration, and ϕ_1 and ϕ_2 are random numbers in the interval $[0, 1]$.

Considering the first four terms of the differential derivative given by Equation (3), one has:

$$\begin{aligned} v_{ij}(t+1) &= \alpha v_{ij}(t) + \frac{1}{2}\alpha(1-\alpha)v_{ij}(t-1) \\ &+ \frac{1}{6}\alpha(1-\alpha)(2-\alpha)v_{ij}(t-2) \\ &+ \frac{1}{24}\alpha(1-\alpha)(2-\alpha)(3-\alpha)v_{ij}(t-3) \\ &+ c_1\phi_1[Pb_{ij}(t) - \chi_{ij}(t)] + c_2\phi_2[Gb_{gj}(t) - \chi_{ij}(t)], \end{aligned} \tag{38}$$

where α at the i-th iteration is:

$$\alpha_i = \alpha_{max} - \frac{\alpha_{max} - \alpha_{min}}{i_{max}} i, \quad \alpha_i \in [0.4, 0.9], \tag{39}$$

with i_{max} denoting the maximum number of iterations.

The parameter values are found by minimizing the fitness function, $f(.)$, which represents the error between the calculated $(G_1(i), \eta(i))$ and experimental $(\widehat{G}_1(i), \widehat{\eta}(i))$ values, as defined in:

$$\min f(\cdot) = \min \sum_{i=1}^{M} \left[|G_1(i) - \widehat{G}_1(i)| + |\eta(i) - \widehat{\eta}(i)| \right], \tag{40}$$

where the symbol M is the number of sampling points. Figure 12 schematically illustrates the CFOPSO algorithm. Table 1 lists the parameter values of the CFOPSO algorithm.

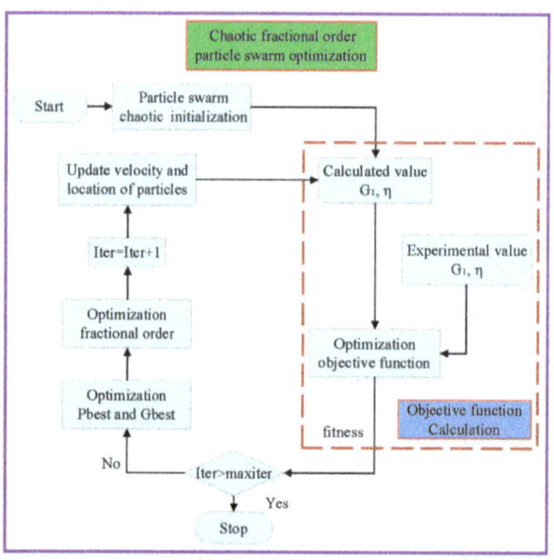

Figure 12. Flowchart of the CFOPSO algorithm.

Table 1. Parameters of the CFOPSO algorithm.

CFOPSO Parameter	Value
Number of particles	$N = 50$
Number of iterations/Repeated experiments	$i = 200/E = 40$
Scaling factors	$c_1 = c_2 = 1.5$
Chaotic bifurcation parameter	$\mu = 4.0$

The experimental data with a displacement of 1.0 mm are adopted for parameter determination and fitting. With reference to the parameter values in previous fractional models, the range of current parameter values is set as $p_1 \in (0, 2.5 \times 10^{-6}]$, $q_0 \in (0, 2]$, $q_1 \in (0, 5]$, $\alpha_1 \in (0, 1)$, and $\alpha_2 \in (0, 1)$. The process of model parameter determination and fitting is:

Step 1: Determine the parameters p_1, q_0, q_1, α_1, and α_2 in Equation (29) with $T = 10$ °C and $\omega = 0.5$ rad/s using the CFOPSO algorithm;

Step 2: With fixed parameters p_1, q_0, and q_1, determine the values of α_1 and α_2 with $T = -10$ °C, -5 °C, 0 °C, 5 °C, 20 °C, 30 °C, 40 °C, and $\omega = 0.5$ rad/s;

Step 3: Use curve-fitting to find the parameters in the functions that relate α_1 and α_2 to temperature T;

Step 4: Repeat Steps 1 to 3 with $\omega = 0.1$ rad/s, 0.2 rad/s, and 1.0 rad/s, with the fixed parameters p_1, q_0, and q_1;

Step 5: Set the model at $\omega = 0.5$ rad/s as the reference model. Fit the effects of other frequencies into the fractional orders α_1^* and α_2^* through two slope functions. Use curve-fitting to determine the parameters in the functions that relate k_1 and k_2 to temperature T.

Finally, the new AEF-Zener model's parameters in Equation (33) have been determined.

Table 2 lists the parameter values of the AEF-Zener model ($\omega = 0.5$ rad/s) obtained with the CFOPSO algorithm. The values of k_1 and k_2 determined by slope curve-fitting are shown in Table 3.

Table 2. Parameters of the AEF-Zener model ($\omega = 0.5$ rad/s).

Parameters	P_1	q_0	q_1	a_1
Values	1.02×10^{-6}	0.651	3.849	-6.82×10^{-9}
Parameters	a_2	a_3	a_4	a_5
Values	4.076×10^{-7}	1.369×10^{-5}	−0.0013	0.0301
Parameters	b_1	c_1	c_2	c_3
Values	0.6526	-7.37×10^{-9}	7.039×10^{-7}	-1.449×10^{-5}
Parameters	c_4	c_5	b_2	
Values	-0.454×10^{-3}	0.0213	0.574	

Table 3. Parameters of the modified AEF-Zener model (k_1, k_2).

Parameters	a_1^*	a_2^*	a_3^*	a_4^*
Values	4.911×10^{-8}	-4.656×10^{-6}	1.537×10^{-4}	−0.00212
Parameters	a_5^*	b_1^*	c_1^*	c_2^*
Values	0.00995	0.2227	-4.314×10^{-8}	4.291×10^{-6}
Parameters	c_3^*	c_4^*	c_5^*	b_2^*
Values	0.2227	0.001589	0.004628	−0.1724

6.2. Comparison between Numerical and Experimental Results

To assess the accuracy of the proposed AEF-Zener model, the parameters G_1 and η with varying loading frequencies and ambient temperatures were computed based on Equation (33). The numerical calculations and experimental data are compared in Figures 13–16 and Table 4. It can be seen that the model has high precision.

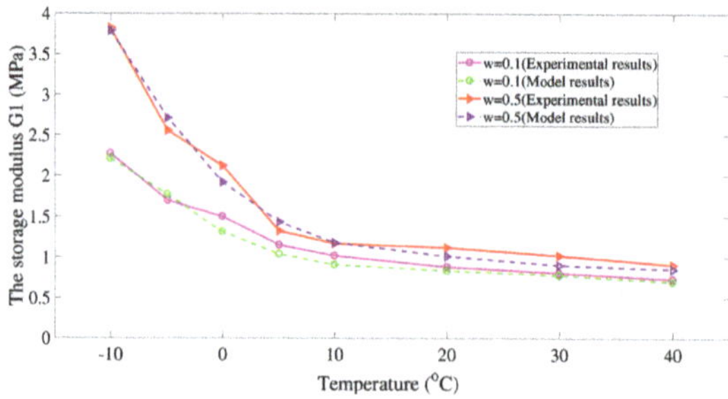

Figure 13. Comparison between numerical and experimental results of G_1 ($\omega = 0.1, 0.5$).

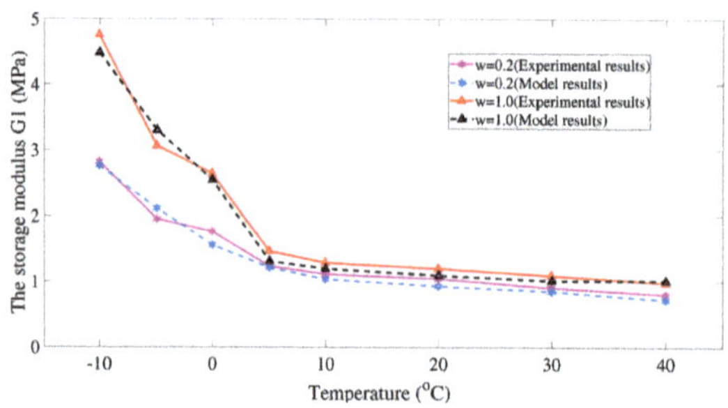

Figure 14. Comparison between numerical and experimental results of G_1 ($\omega = 0.2, 1.0$).

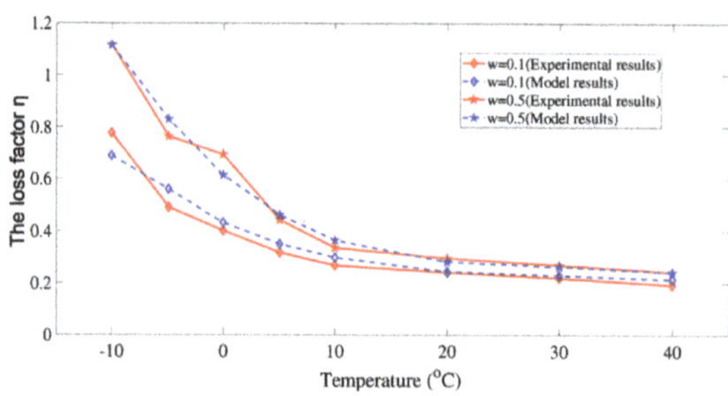

Figure 15. Comparison between numerical and experimental results of η ($\omega = 0.1, 0.5$).

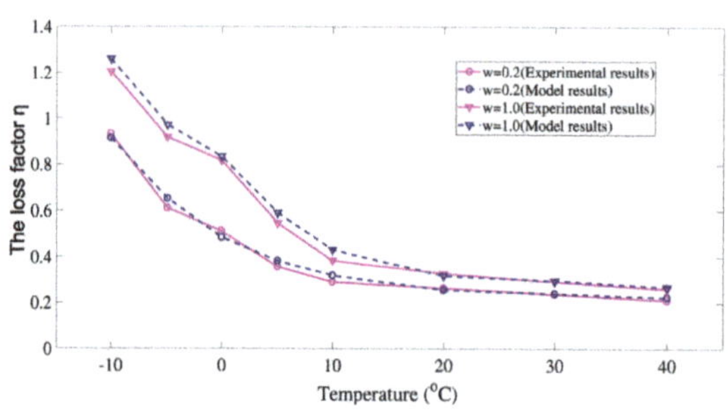

Figure 16. Comparison between numerical and experimental results of η ($\omega = 0.2, 1.0$).

Table 4. Comparison between experimental data and numerical results for the AEF-Zener model.

		Storage Modulus, G_1 (MPa)		Loss Factor, η	
ω (rad/s)	T (°C)	Experimental	Numerical	Experimental	Numerical
	−10	2.2740	2.2129	0.7765	0.6886
	−5	1.6951	1.7699	0.4904	0.5591
	0	1.5043	1.3159	0.4012	0.4321
0.1	5	1.1530	1.0412	0.3170	0.3498
	10	1.0232	0.9092	0.2681	0.2985
	20	1.0037	0.9068	0.2413	0.2447
	30	0.8111	0.7819	0.2201	0.2306
	40	0.7360	0.7014	0.1940	0.2157
	−10	2.8233	2.7623	0.9332	0.9156
	−5	1.9408	2.1160	0.6119	0.6533
	0	1.7612	1.5584	0.5132	0.4863
0.2	5	1.2341	1.2118	0.3573	0.3831
	10	1.1123	1.0350	0.2905	0.3190
	20	1.0481	0.9313	0.2612	0.2566
	30	0.9068	0.8531	0.2380	0.2412
	40	0.8034	0.7221	0.2121	0.2245
	−10	3.8227	3.7887	1.1168	1.1153
	−5	2.5560	2.7139	0.7635	0.8305
	0	2.1240	1.9211	0.6923	0.6135
0.5	5	1.3250	1.4382	0.4423	0.4618
	10	1.1710	1.1824	0.3353	0.3641
	20	1.1262	1.0158	0.2940	0.2817
	30	1.0231	0.9062	0.2693	0.2640
	40	0.9114	0.8565	0.2433	0.2429
	−10	4.7551	4.4795	1.2049	1.2601
	5	3.0626	3.2987	0.9186	0.9722
	0	2.6408	2.5450	0.8185	0.8356
1.0	5	1.4614	1.3090	0.5468	0.5912
	10	1.2840	1.1941	0.3848	0.4322
	20	1.1967	1.0929	0.3274	0.3176
	30	1.0897	1.0123	0.2920	0.2968
	40	0.9786	1.0116	0.2605	0.2690

The root-mean-square errors between numerical and experimental results are given in Table 5. When the frequencies are chosen as 0.1, 0.2, 0.5, and 1.0 rad/s, the errors for the values of G_1 are 9.65%, 11.16%, 11.63%, and 15.41%, respectively. The errors for η are 4.47%, 2.23%, 3.89%, and 3.64%, respectively. As the frequency increases, its impact on the parameters may increase, which may lead to an increase in errors for high frequencies. In addition, the relative errors of the storage modulus and loss factor, G_1 and η, at various frequencies are less than 20%, which are within the requirements usually adopted in engineering applications.

Table 5. Root-mean-square error of G_1 and η.

	Storage Modulus, G_1	Loss Factor, η
Frequency (rad/s)	Root-Mean-Square Error (%)	Root-Mean-Square Error (%)
0.1	9.65	4.47
0.2	11.16	2.23
0.5	11.63	3.89
1.0	15.41	3.64

To further verify the effectiveness of the AEF-Zener model, taking the frequency of 1.0 rad/s, we compare its results with those of the EFMCS model (that considers the temperature–frequency equivalent principle) [45] and the experimental data. The storage modulus and the loss factor for the displacement of 1.0 mm and temperatures of −10 °C to 40 °C are illustrated in Figures 17 and 18, respectively, and summarized in Tables 6 and 7.

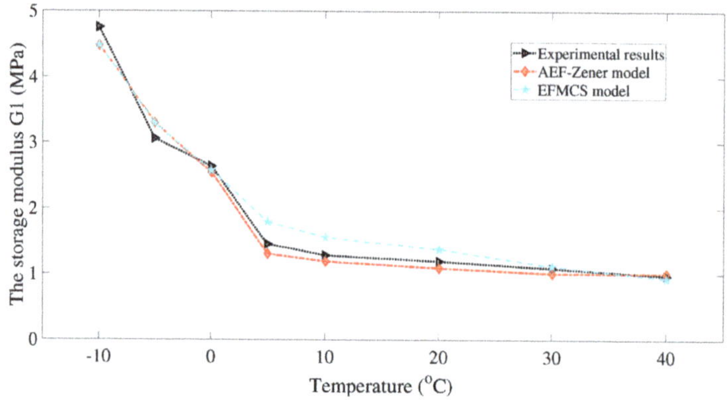

Figure 17. Comparison between numerical and experimental results of G_1 with $T(°C) = -10, -5, 0, 5, 10, 20, 30, 40$ when $d = 1.0$ mm and $\omega = 1.0$ rad/s.

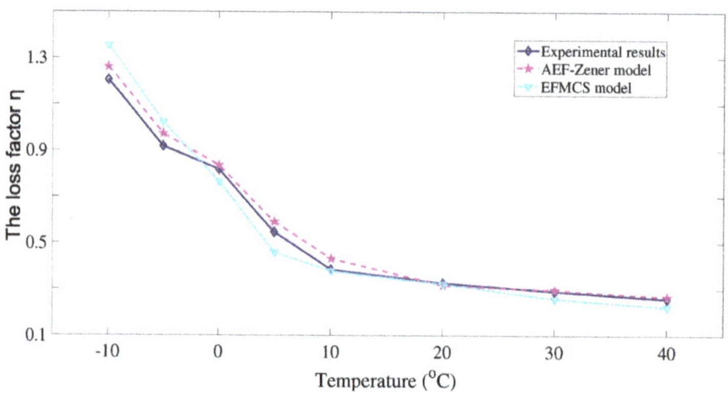

Figure 18. Comparison between numerical and experimental results of η with $T(°C) = -10, -5, 0, 5, 10, 20, 30, 40$ when $d = 1.0$ mm and $\omega = 1.0$ rad/s.

Table 6. The experimental and numerical results comparison of G_1 for different frequencies when $d = 1.0$ mm and $\omega = 1.0$ rad/s.

	Storage Modulus, G_1 (MPa)			Error	
T(°C)	**Experimental**	**AEF Model**	**EFMCS Model**	**AEF Model**	**EFMCS Model**
−10	4.7551	4.4795	4.4803	5.80%	5.78%
−5	3.0626	3.2987	3.2900	7.71%	7.41%
0	2.6408	2.5450	2.5777	3.63%	2.39%
5	1.4614	1.3090	1.7995	9.28%	23.14%
10	1.2840	1.1941	1.5653	7.00%	21.73%
20	1.1967	1.0929	1.3847	8.67%	15.71%
30	1.0897	1.0123	1.1218	7.10%	2.95%
40	0.9786	1.0116	0.9389	3.37%	4.06%

Table 7. The experimental and numerical results comparison of η for different frequencies when $d = 1.0$ mm and $\omega = 1.0$ rad/s.

	Loss Factor, η			Error	
T(° C)	Experimental	AEF Model	EFMCS Model	AEF Model	EFMCS Model
−10	1.2049	1.2601	1.3549	4.58%	7.52%
−5	0.9186	0.9722	1.0225	5.83%	11.31%
0	0.8185	0.8356	0.7666	2.09%	6.34%
5	0.5468	0.5912	0.4608	8.12%	15.73%
10	0.3848	0.4322	0.3784	12.32%	1.66%
20	0.3274	0.3176	0.3234	3.00%	1.22%
30	0.2920	0.2968	0.2597	1.64%	11.06%
40	0.2605	0.2690	0.2253	3.26%	13.51%

For the storage modulus, at different temperatures, the average and the maximum errors between experimental data and simulation results for the AEF-Zener and the EFMCS models are 6.57% and 10.40%, and 9.28% and 23.14%, respectively. For the loss factor, the average and the maximum errors are 5.11% and 8.54%, and 12.32% and 15.73%, respectively. This shows that both errors for the AEF-Zener model are smaller than those for the EFMCS.

Additionally, at the temperature of 20 °C, the AEF-Zener model simulation results are compared with those obtained with Xu's model [29] and with experimental data. Figures 19 and 20 depict the storage modulus and the loss factor when the displacement is 1.0 mm and the frequencies vary between 0.1 rad/s and 1.0 rad/s, respectively. Tables 8 and 9 summarize the results.

For the storage modulus, the average and the maximum errors for the AEF-Zener and the Xu models are 7.23% and 9.34%, and 11.14% and 11.80%, respectively. For the loss factor, the errors are 2.59% and 3.90%, and 4.18% and 9.07%, respectively. This confirms that the AEF-Zener model is better than the Xu model.

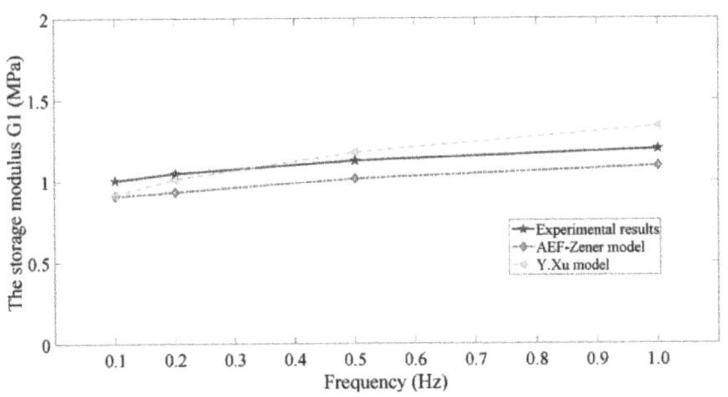

Figure 19. Comparison of numerical and experimental results of G_1 with $\omega = 0.1, 0.2, 0.5, 1.0$ when $d = 1.0$ mm and $T = 20$ °C.

Table 8. The experimental and numerical results comparison of G_1 for different frequencies when $d = 1.0$ mm and $T = 20$ °C.

	Storage Modulus, G_1 (MPa)			Error	
ω (rad/s)	Experimental	AEF Model	Xu's Model	AEF Model	Xu's Model
0.1	1.0037	0.9068	0.9128	9.65%	9.05%
0.2	1.0481	0.9313	1.0119	11.14%	3.45%
0.5	1.1262	1.0158	1.1784	9.80%	4.63%
1.0	1.1967	1.0929	1.3379	8.67%	11.80%

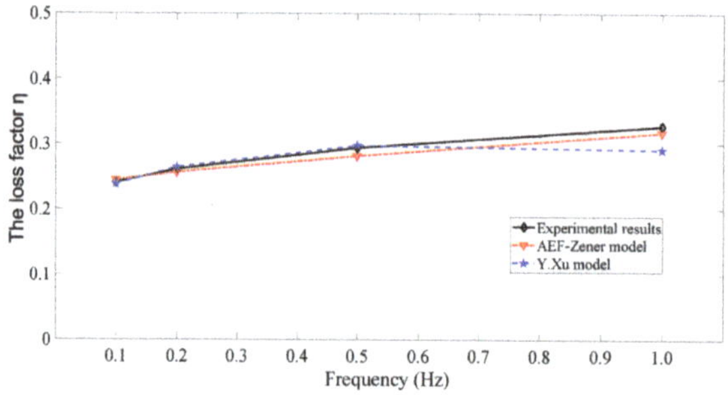

Figure 20. Comparison of numerical and experimental results of η with $\omega = 0.1, 0.2, 0.5, 1.0$ when $d = 1.0$ mm and $T = 20$ °C.

Table 9. The experimental and numerical results comparison of η for different frequencies when $d = 1.0$ mm and $T = 20$ °C.

	Loss Factor, η			Error	
ω (rad/s)	Experimental	AEF Model	Xu's Model	AEF Model	Xu's Model
0.1	0.2413	0.2447	0.2390	1.41%	0.95%
0.2	0.2612	0.2566	0.2646	1.76%	1.30%
0.5	0.2940	0.2817	0.2977	4.18%	4.28%
1.0	0.3274	0.3176	0.2917	2.99%	9.07%

From the above analysis, we verify that the numerical results obtained with the proposed AEF-Zener model are close to the experimental ones, which means that the temperature-order equivalence principle can well characterize the effect of temperature for VE dampers. In addition, by comparing the new model with the EFMCS and the Xu models, we confirmed that the AEF-Zener model has superior accuracy and availability. In general, the AEF-Zener model is accurate enough to reflect the mechanical behavior and energy dissipation ability of VE dampers at a low frequency. The model can be conveniently applied to the dynamic analysis of structures with VE dampers.

7. Simulation Analysis of Structures with VE Dampers

In this section, simulations of structures with and without VE dampers under earthquake action are carried out. The equation of motion of the structure with VE dampers can be written as:

$$M\ddot{x}(t) + C\dot{x}(t) + Kx(t) + c_d\dot{x}(t) + k_d x(t) = -Ml\ddot{x_g}, \tag{41}$$

where x, $\dot{x}$, and $\ddot{x} \in R^{n\times 1}$ stand for displacement, velocity, and acceleration vectors of the building, respectively; M, C, and $K \in R^{n\times n}$ are the mass, stiffness, and damping matrices, respectively; l is a vector with all elements equal to 1; and $k_d = \mathrm{diag}(k_{di}, \ldots, k_{dn})$ and $c_d = \mathrm{diag}(c_{di}, \ldots, c_{dn})$, with k_{di} and c_{di} standing for the sum of equivalent stiffness and damping of all VE dampers in the i-th floor for $i = 1, \ldots, n$, are parameters.

The ground acceleration $\ddot{x_g}$ is modulated with amplitude 0.24 g and 0.12 g to adopt the El Centro and Taft earthquake seismic waves for 25 s and 30 s, as shown in Figure 21. In addition, the Rayleigh damping is given by $C = \alpha_1 M + \beta_1 K$, where $\alpha_1, \beta_1 \in R$ are calculated from the damping ratio of the modes of vibration. Matrices M and K can be represented by:

$$M = \begin{bmatrix} m_1 & 0 & \cdots & 0 & 0 \\ 0 & m_2 & \cdots & 0 & 0 \\ \vdots & \vdots & \vdots & \ddots & \vdots \\ 0 & 0 & \cdots & m_{n-1} & 0 \\ 0 & 0 & \cdots & 0 & m_n \end{bmatrix}_{n\times n},$$

$$K = \begin{bmatrix} k_1+k_2 & -k_2 & \cdots & 0 & 0 \\ -k_2 & k_2+k_3 & \cdots & 0 & 0 \\ \vdots & \vdots & \ddots & \vdots & \vdots \\ 0 & 0 & \cdots & k_{n-1}+k_n & -k_n \\ 0 & 0 & \cdots & -k_n & k_n \end{bmatrix}_{n\times n}.$$

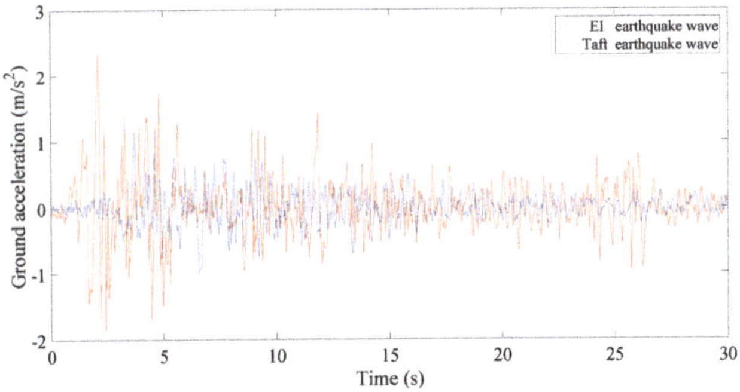

Figure 21. El-Centro and Taft earthquake seismic waves.

Example : The application of the AEF-Zener model for a three-story building structure with 10 VE dampers on each story is illustrated in Figure 22. The parameters of the structure are summarized in Table 10. The sizes of the VE dampers are $n_v = 2$, $A_v = 0.36\ \mathrm{m}^2$, and $h_v = 10$ mm, respectively. The VE dampers can be placed in any location where shear deformation of the VE layers is allowed to occur. The ambient temperature is set as $T = 7.3\ °\mathrm{C}$. The first natural frequency of the vibration mode is $\omega = 0.881$ rad/s. Equations (33)–(35) can be used to calculate the equivalent stiffness and damping.

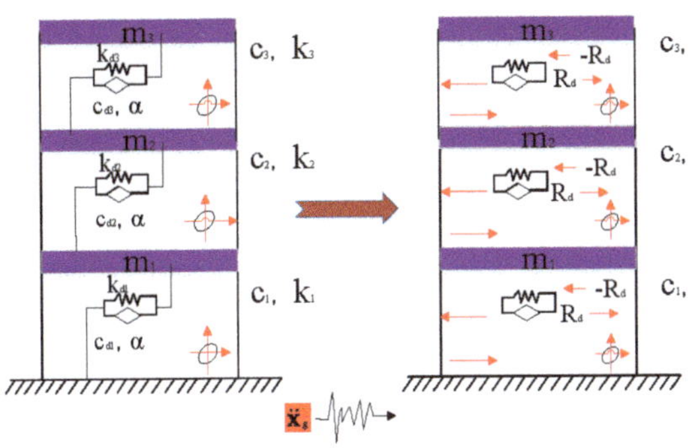

Figure 22. A three-story building with VE dampers.

Table 10. Building parameters for the example.

Floor	1	2	3
Quality (kg)	2.40×10^5	1.20×10^5	1.20×10^5
Rigidity (N/m)	1.08×10^6	3.60×10^5	2.16×10^5

Figures 23–25 show the displacements of the first to third floors, without and with VE dampers, respectively, in the El Centro earthquake. Figure 26 show the maximum displacements in the El-Centro earthquake. The corresponding floor displacements in the Taft earthquake are shown in Figures 27–29, respectively. Figure 30 show the maximum displacements in the Taft earthquake.

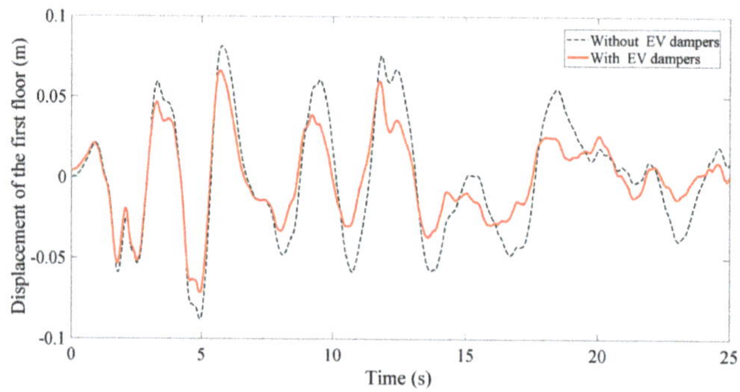

Figure 23. First floor displacement of the building in the example in the El Centro earthquake.

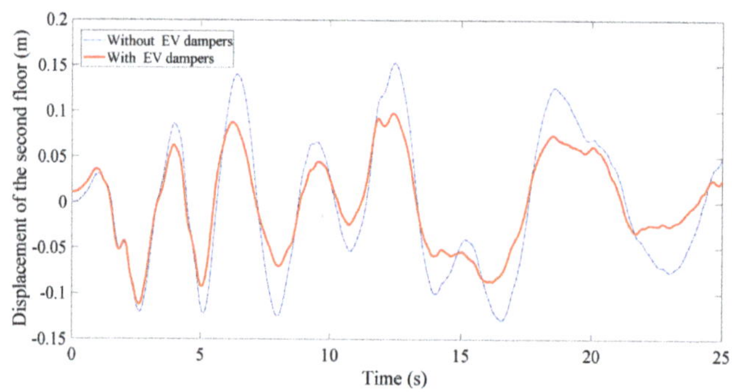

Figure 24. Second floor displacement of the building in the example in the El Centro earthquake.

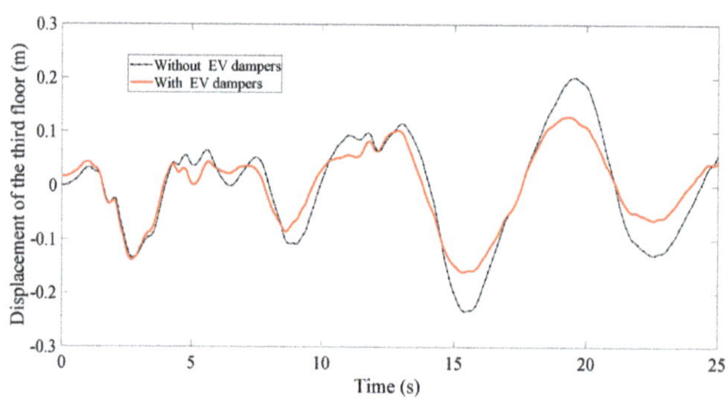

Figure 25. Third floor displacement of the building in the example in the El Centro earthquake.

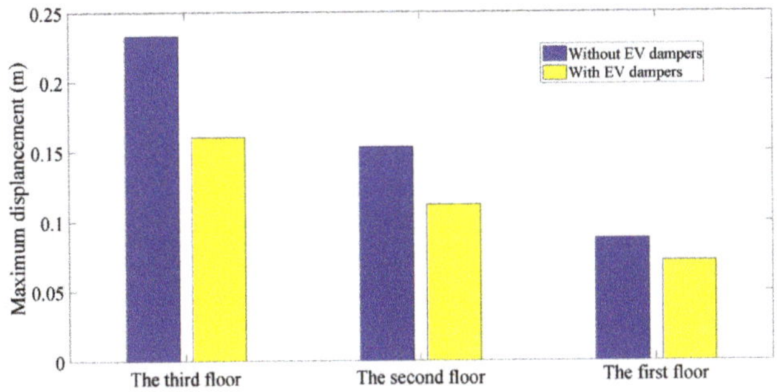

Figure 26. The maximum displacement of each floor in the El Centro earthquake.

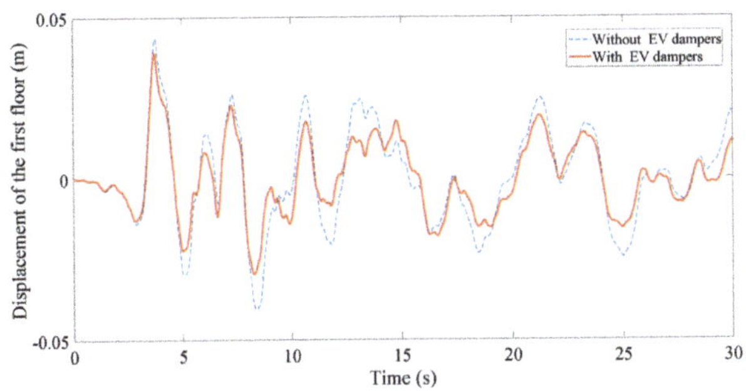

Figure 27. First floor displacement of the building in the example in the Taft earthquake.

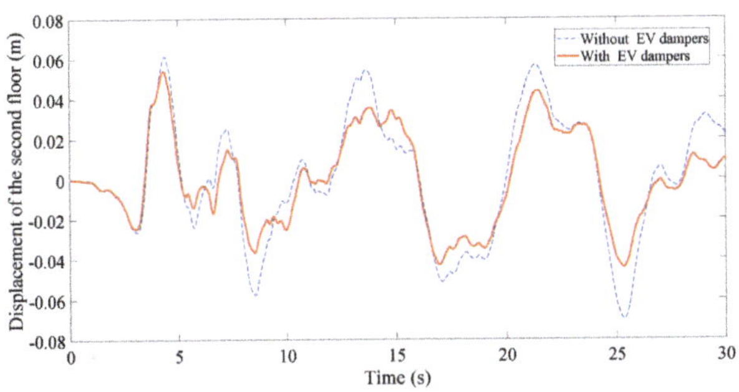

Figure 28. Second floor displacement of the building in the example in the Taft earthquake.

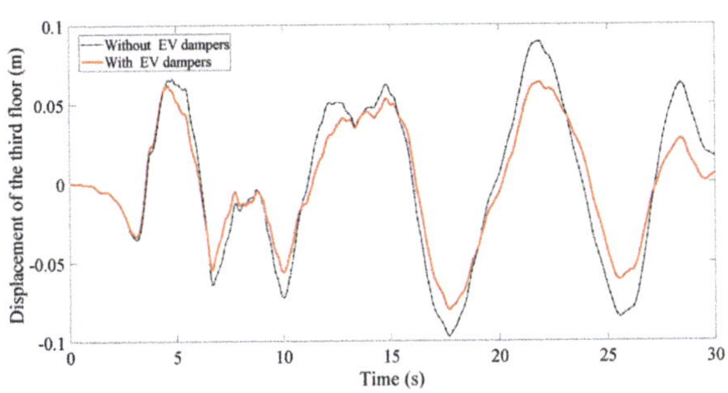

Figure 29. Third floor displacement of the building in the example in the Taft earthquake.

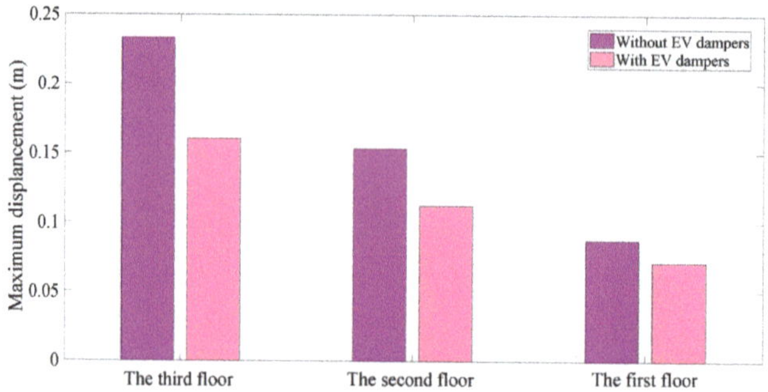

Figure 30. The maximum displacement of each floor in the Taft earthquake.

It can be seen that the structure with VE dampers has good seismic performance at the ambient temperature $T = 7.3$ °C. Indeed, compared with the case without VE dampers, VE dampers reduce the maximum displacement of each floor by more than 45.4%, 36.67%, and 22.97%, respectively, in the El Centro earthquake. Moreover, the maximum displacement decreases by more than 20.5%, 29.84%, and 11.53% under Taft wave excitation, respectively.

It is obvious that VE dampers are effective for seismic reduction, and the proposed AEF-Zener model can be applied to the analysis of the seismic performance and the design of structures with VE dampers in consideration of ambient temperature.

8. Conclusions

A new AEF-Zener model of VE dampers that takes into account temperature and the fractional-order equivalence principle was proposed. Firstly, the relationship between fractional order and energy dissipation of VE materials was analyzed in the time and frequency domains. Secondly, based on experimental data, the relationship between ambient temperature and energy dissipation of VE materials was analyzed. Finally, with the equivalence principle of temperature and fractional order, a new model able to describe the influence of temperature was established, and the model parameters were determined using a CFOPSO algorithm. Comparing the numerical results of the new AEF-Zener model with those of other models and with experimental data, it was shown that the proposed AEF-Zener model has good accuracy and availability, particularly in characterizing the loss factor for energy consumption. The proposed AEF-Zener model can be applied to design VE dampers in consideration of ambient temperature.

Author Contributions: Methodology, L.C.; software, M.Z.; validation and data curation, R.W.; writing—original draft preparation, K.X.; writing—review and editing, A.M.L.; supervision and project administration, M.W. All authors have read and agreed to the published version of the manuscript.

Funding: This work was supported by the National Natural Science Foundation of China (No. 62073114; 11971032).

Data Availability Statement: Data available on request due to restrictions eg privacy or ethical.

Conflicts of Interest: The authors declare no conflict of interest.

References

1. Huang, J.; Rao, Y.; Qiu, H.; Lei, Y. Generalized algorithms for the identification of seismic ground excitations to building structures based on generalized Kalman filtering under unknown input. *Adv. Struct. Eng.* **2020**, *23*, 2163–2173. [CrossRef]
2. He, Q.; Yin, A.; Fan, Z.; He, L. Seismic responses analysis of multi-story suspended floors system. *J. Vibroeng.* **2021**, *23*, 167–182. [CrossRef]
3. Gómez, F.; Yu, W. Discrete-time tri-directional active control of building structures. *Eng. Struct.* **2021**, *243*, 112689. [CrossRef]
4. Xu, K.; Chen, L.; Wang, M.; Lopes, A.M.; Tenreiro Machado, J.; Zhai, H. Improved decentralized fractional PD control of structure vibrations. *Mathematics* **2020**, *8*, 326. [CrossRef]

5. Hu, W.; Gao, Y.; Yang, B. Semi-active vibration control of two flexible plates using an innovative joint mechanism. *Mech. Syst. Signal Process.* **2019**, *130*, 565–584. [CrossRef]
6. Nasab, M.S.E.; Kim, J. Fuzzy analysis of a viscoelastic damper in seismic retrofit of structures. *Eng. Struct.* **2022**, *250*, 113473. [CrossRef]
7. Ocak, A.; Nigdeli, S.M.; Bekdaş, G. Passive control via mass dampers: A review of state-of-the-art developments. *Optimization of Tuned Mass Dampers*; Springer: Cham, Switzerland, 2022; pp. 15–40.
8. Stanikzai, M.H.; Elias, S.; Chae, Y. Recent advances in hybrid vibration-control systems. *Pract. Period. Struct. Des. Constr.* **2022**, *27*, 03122003. [CrossRef]
9. Feudo, S.L.; Touzé, C.; Boisson, J.; Cumunel, G. Nonlinear magnetic vibration absorber for passive control of a multi–storey structure. *J. Sound Vib.* **2019**, *438*, 33–53. [CrossRef]
10. Xu, Z.D.; Dong, Y.R.; Chen, S.; Guo, Y.Q.; Li, Q.Q.; Xu, Y.S. Development of hybrid test system for three-dimensional viscoelastic damping frame structures based on Matlab-OpenSees combined programming. *Soil Dyn. Earthq. Eng.* **2021**, *144*, 106681. [CrossRef]
11. Mokhtari, M.; Permoon, M.; Haddadpour, H. Dynamic analysis of isotropic sandwich cylindrical shell with fractional viscoelastic core using Rayleigh–Ritz method. *Compos. Struct.* **2018**, *186*, 165–174. [CrossRef]
12. Xu, Y.; Xu, Z.D.; Guo, Y.Q.; Dong, Y.; Ge, T.; Xu, C. Tests and modeling of viscoelastic damper considering microstructures and displacement amplitude influence. *J. Eng. Mech.* **2019**, *145*, 04019108. [CrossRef]
13. Dadkhah Khiabani, E.; Ghaffarzadeh, H.; Shiri, B.; Katebi, J. Spline collocation methods for seismic analysis of multiple degree of freedom systems with visco-elastic dampers using fractional models. *J. Vib. Control* **2020**, *26*, 1445–1462. [CrossRef]
14. Asano, M.; Masahiko, H.; Yamamoto, M. The experimental study on viscoelastic material dampers and the formulation of analytical model. In Proceedings of the 12th World Conference on Earthquake Engineering, Nagoya, Japan, 30 January–4 February 2000.
15. Barkanov, E.; Skukis, E.; Petitjean, B. Characterisation of viscoelastic layers in sandwich panels via an inverse technique. *J. Sound Vib.* **2009**, *327*, 402–412. [CrossRef]
16. Hamdaoui, M.; Ledi, K.; Robin, G.; Daya, E.M. Identification of frequency-dependent viscoelastic damped structures using an adjoint method. *J. Sound Vib.* **2019**, *453*, 237–252. [CrossRef]
17. Dadkhah, E.; Shiri, B.; Ghaffarzadeh, H.; Baleanu, D. Visco-elastic dampers in structural buildings and numerical solution with spline collocation methods. *J. Appl. Math. Comput.* **2020**, *63*, 29–57. [CrossRef]
18. Xu, Z.D.; Liao, Y.X.; Ge, T.; Xu, C. Experimental and theoretical study of viscoelastic dampers with different matrix rubbers. *J. Eng. Mech.* **2016**, *142*, 04016051. [CrossRef]
19. Shu, Z.; You, R.; Zhou, Y. Viscoelastic Materials for Structural Dampers: A Review. *Constr. Build. Mater.* **2022**, *342*, 127955. [CrossRef]
20. Zhang, X.; Wu, R.C. Modified projective synchronization of fractional-order chaotic systems with different dimensions. *Acta Math. Appl. Sin. Engl. Ser.* **2020**, *36*, 527–538. [CrossRef]
21. Xu, Z.D.; Ge, T.; Liu, J. Experimental and theoretical study of high-energy dissipation-viscoelastic dampers based on acrylate-rubber matrix. *J. Eng. Mech.* **2020**, *146*, 04020057. [CrossRef]
22. Arikoglu, A. A new fractional derivative model for linearly viscoelastic materials and parameter identification via genetic algorithms. *Rheol. Acta* **2014**, *53*, 219–233. [CrossRef]
23. Xu, Y.; Xu, Z.D.; Guo, Y.Q.; Sarwar, W.; She, W.; Geng, Z.F. Study on viscoelastic materials at micro scale pondering supramolecular interaction impacts with DMA tests and fractional derivative modeling. *J. Appl. Polym. Sci.* **2023**, *140*, e53660. [CrossRef]
24. Sun, H.; Zhang, Y.; Baleanu, D.; Chen, W.; Chen, Y. A new collection of real world applications of fractional calculus in science and engineering. *Commun. Nonlinear Sci. Numer. Simul.* **2018**, *64*, 213–231. [CrossRef]
25. Bonfanti, A.; Kaplan, J.L.; Charras, G.; Kabla, A. Fractional viscoelastic models for power-law materials. *Soft Matter* **2020**, *16*, 6002–6020. [CrossRef] [PubMed]
26. Markou, A.A.; Manolis, G.D. A fractional derivative Zener model for the numerical simulation of base isolated structures. *Bull. Earthq. Eng.* **2016**, *14*, 283–295. [CrossRef]
27. Rodas, C.O.; Zaïri, F.; Naït-Abdelaziz, M. A finite strain thermo-viscoelastic constitutive model to describe the self-heating in elastomeric materials during low-cycle fatigue. *J. Mech. Phys. Solids* **2014**, *64*, 396–410. [CrossRef]
28. Lewandowski, R. Influence of temperature on the dynamic characteristics of structures with viscoelastic dampers. *J. Struct. Eng.* **2019**, *145*, 04018245. [CrossRef]
29. Xu, Y.; Xu, Z.D.; Guo, Y.Q.; Ge, T.; Xu, C.; Huang, X. Theoretical and experimental study of viscoelastic damper based on fractional derivative approach and micromolecular structures. *J. Vib. Acoust.* **2019**, *141*, 031010. [CrossRef]
30. Ge, T.; Xu, Z.D.; Guo, Y.Q.; Huang, X.H.; He, Z.F. Experimental investigation and multiscale modeling of ve damper considering chain network and ambient temperature influence. *J. Eng. Mech.* **2022**, *148*, 04021124. [CrossRef]
31. Cao, J.; Chen, Y.; Wang, Y.; Zhang, H. Numerical analysis of nonlinear variable fractional viscoelastic arch based on shifted Legendre polynomials. *Math. Methods Appl. Sci.* **2021**, *44*, 8798–8813. [CrossRef]
32. Sun, L.; Chen, Y. Numerical analysis of variable fractional viscoelastic column based on two-dimensional Legendre wavelets algorithm. *Chaos Solitons Fractals* **2021**, *152*, 111372. [CrossRef]

33. Moghaddam, B.; Mendes Lopes, A.; Tenreiro Machado, J.; Mostaghim, Z. Computational scheme for solving nonlinear fractional stochastic differential equations with delay. *Stoch. Anal. Appl.* **2019**, *37*, 893–908. [CrossRef]
34. Ortigueira, M.D.; Machado, J.T. The 21st century systems: An updated vision of continuous-time fractional models. *IEEE Circuits Syst. Mag.* **2022**, *22*, 36–56. [CrossRef]
35. Ortigueira, M.D.; Valério, D. *Fractional Signals and Systems*; Walter de Gruyter GmbH & Co KG: Berlin, Germany, 2020; Volume 7.
36. Ortigueira, M.D. *Fractional Calculus for Scientists and Engineers*; Springer Science & Business Media: Berlin/Heidelberg, Germany, 2011; Volume 84
37. Majidabad, S.S.; Shandiz, H.T.; Hajizadeh, A. Decentralized sliding mode control of fractional-order large-scale nonlinear systems. *Nonlinear Dyn.* **2014**, *77*, 119–134. [CrossRef]
38. Xiao, M.; Tao, B.; Zheng, W.X.; Jiang, G. Fractional-order PID controller synthesis for bifurcation of fractional-order small-world networks. *IEEE Trans. Syst. Man Cybern. Syst.* **2019**, *51*, 4334–4346. [CrossRef]
39. Yuan, J.; Gao, S.; Xiu, G.; Wang, L. Mechanical energy and equivalent viscous damping for fractional Zener oscillator. *J. Vib. Acoust.* **2020**, *142*, 041004. [CrossRef]
40. Shahri, E.S.A.; Alfi, A.; Machado, J.T. Fractional fixed-structure H_∞ controller design using augmented Lagrangian particle swarm optimization with fractional order velocity. *Appl. Soft Comput.* **2019**, *77*, 688–695. [CrossRef]
41. Wang, C.; Zhou, X.; Jin, Y.; Shi, X. Variable fractional order sliding mode control for seismic vibration suppression of building structure. *J. Vib. Control.* **2022**, *28*, 3794–3807. [CrossRef]
42. Li, H.; Gomez, D.; Dyke, S.J.; Xu, Z. Fractional differential equation bearing models for base-isolated buildings: Framework development. *J. Struct. Eng.* **2020**, *146*, 04019197. [CrossRef]
43. Xu, K.; Cheng, T.; Lopes, A.M.; Chen, L.; Zhu, X.; Wang, M. Fuzzy Fractional-Order PD Vibration Control of Uncertain Building Structures. *Fractal Fract.* **2022**, *6*, 473. [CrossRef]
44. Zheng, Y.; Huang, Z.; Tao, J.; Sun, H.; Sun, Q.; Sun, M.; Dehmer, M.; Chen, Z. A novel chaotic fractional-order beetle swarm optimization algorithm and its application for load-frequency active disturbance rejection control. *IEEE Trans. Circuits Syst. II Express Briefs* **2021**, *69*, 1267–1271. [CrossRef]
45. Xu, Y.; Xu, Z.D.; Guo, Y.Q.; Jia, H.; Huang, X.; Wen, Y. Mathematical modeling and test verification of viscoelastic materials considering microstructures and ambient temperature influence. *Mech. Adv. Mater. Struct.* **2021**, *29*, 7063–7074. [CrossRef]

fractal and fractional

MDPI

Article

Fractional Photoconduction and Nonlinear Optical Behavior in ZnO Micro and Nanostructures

Victor Manuel Garcia-de-los-Rios [1], Jose Alberto Arano-Martínez [1], Martin Trejo-Valdez [2], Martha Leticia Hernández-Pichardo [2], Mónica Araceli Vidales-Hurtado [3] and Carlos Torres-Torres [1,*]

1 Sección de Estudios de Posgrado e Investigación, Escuela Superior de Ingeniería Mecánica y Eléctrica Unidad Zacatenco, Instituto Politécnico Nacional, Mexico City 07738, Mexico
2 Escuela Superior de Ingeniería Química e Industrias Extractivas, Instituto Politécnico Nacional, Mexico City 07738, Mexico
3 Centro de Investigación en Ciencia Aplicada y Tecnología Avanzada Unidad Querétaro, Instituto Politécnico Nacional, Santiago de Querétaro, Querétaro 76090, Mexico
* Correspondence: ctorrest@ipn.mx

Abstract: A fractional description for the optically induced mechanisms responsible for conductivity and multiphotonic effects in ZnO nanomaterials is studied here. Photoconductive, electrical, and nonlinear optical phenomena exhibited by pure micro and nanostructured ZnO samples were analyzed. A hydrothermal approach was used to synthetize ZnO micro-sized crystals, while a spray pyrolysis technique was employed to prepare ZnO nanostructures. A contrast in the fractional electrical behavior and photoconductivity was identified for the samples studied. A positive nonlinear refractive index was measured on the nanoscale sample using the z-scan technique, which endows it with a dominant real part for the third-order optical nonlinearity. The absence of nonlinear optical absorption, along with a strong optical Kerr effect in the ZnO nanostructures, shows favorable perspectives for their potential use in the development of all-optical switching devices. Fractional models for predicting electronic and nonlinear interactions in nanosystems could pave the way for the development of optoelectronic circuits and ultrafast functions controlled by ZnO photo technology.

Keywords: fractional calculus; nonlinear optics; photoconductivity; Kerr effect; ZnO nanomaterials

1. Introduction

Zinc oxide (ZnO) is a fascinating semiconductor material which has gained particular interest in recent years due to its characteristic wide bandgap energy (E_g) that promotes an easy electron interchange between its conduction and valence band [1]. Also, due to its unique physical properties [2], and versatility in being designed by different processing routes [3], this material is suitable for applications in highly sensitive gas sensors, transparent electrodes, and a variety of optoelectronic and piezoelectric devices like solar cells [4]. Moreover, ZnO is a low-cost material that can be synthesized by hydrothermal effects, sol-gel methods, chemical vapor deposition (CVD), spray pyrolysis, and other techniques [5]. It is worth mentioning that the physico-chemical properties exhibited by the ZnO depend on their structure size, shape, and morphology, which are crucial for their successful application in various fields [6,7]. The high surface/volume ratio of ZnO nanomaterials has a significant impact on electrical features, compared to the bulk phase case. Defect structures present at grain boundaries of nanostructures, such as dangling bonds, vacancies, and micropores, significantly affect energy transport phenomena. A decrease in nanoscale size increases the defect ion concentration, which tends to segregate at grain boundaries and leads to grain boundary defect barrier formation [8,9]. On the other hand, considering that the morphology of ZnO nanostructures affects the amount of surface oxygen, it has been reported that oxygen vacancies in ZnO nanostructures can be responsible for an increase in electrical conductivity [10].

Diverse potential applications of ZnO nanostructures for optoelectronic, electronic, and biomedical functions have been pointed out [11]. High electron mobility and strong luminescence exhibited by ZnO nanostructures make them useful in light-emitting diodes (LEDs), while high biocompatibility makes them useful for drug delivery and tissue engineering [12].

Moreover, the ZnO exhibits UV-protection properties attractive for UV-blocking coatings with different low-cost nanofabrication processes, and in this direction, their photoconductive and nonlinear optical properties have been investigated for a wide range of applications. The design of opto-piezo-electronic materials like highly sensitive sensors [13] and energy collectors for both piezotronic logic nanodevices [14] and piezotronic transistors [15] has been demonstrated in ZnO. The photon absorption of ZnO for valence band excitations [16] and a decreased transmittance at shorter wavelengths [17] can be employed for developing ultrafast functions and nonlinear materials. A large nonlinear optical (NLO) response has the ability to manipulate light, which is the base for modern data transmission [18] and harmonic generation [19].

Regarding the vectorial nature of light and the physical mechanisms responsible for the optically induced electronic effects, NLO properties in ZnO nanosystems are dependent on wavelength, incident polarization, and pulse duration able to tune a variety of electronic excitations [20–30]. In this work, we report the modification of photoconductive, electrical, and NLO effects exhibited by ZnO-based materials prepared by two different processing routes. A fractional description allowed us to analyze electronic characteristics and photoinduced properties using nanosecond pulses that proved to be of interest as a base for the design and development of optoelectronic and all-optical devices.

2. Materials and Methods

2.1. Synthesis of the ZnO Samples and Morphology Characterization

For the preparation of the ZnO microstructures in film form, a combination of hydrothermal synthesis and intermittent spray was employed, similar to the procedure of Wang et al. [31]. For the synthesis, a mixture of 1.53 g of zinc acetate ($Zn(O_2CCH_3)_2$) and 12.47 g of sodium citrate ($Na_3C_6H_5O_7$) was dissolved in 70 mL of deionized water and stirred for 20 min to form a clear solution. Subsequently, a sodium hydroxide solution (1 mol/L) was added to the product and stirred for 30 min to adjust the pH to 14. Then, the solution was transferred to an autoclave and placed in an oven at 150 °C for 24 h. Subsequently, it was allowed to cool at room temperature and filtered using a vacuum pump. The resulting product was washed with deionized water and anhydrous ethanol twice and diluted in 10 mL of deionized water. The obtained product was ultrasonically cleaned for 20 min. Finally, the solution was sprayed intermittently every 10 s on a SiO_2 substrate, previously ultrasonically cleaned with ethanol, and then preheated to 320 °C, following the method of Ravichandran and Philominathan [32]. Also, the spray pyrolysis technique was used for the generation of nanostructures by depositing a total of 15 layers on preheated $10 \times 25 \times 1$ mm^3 SiO_2 substrates ultrasonically cleaned with ethanol for 20 min and then after with deionized water at 430 °C on a graphite surface over a tin bath.

For the fabrication of the ZnO nanostructures, a precursor solution of 2.65 g of zinc acetylacetone ($Zn(C_5H_7O_2)_2$), 12.54 mL of deionized water, 83.88 mL of methanol (CH_3OH), and 3.58 mL of acetic acid ($C_2H_4O_2$) was made and stirred for about 10 min. The deposition was performed by nebulizing the precursor solution on the substrates with a vapor exposition of 105 s, at an input pressure of 7 L/min and output of 3 L/min, with a stabilizing time of 10 min between each deposit. With this, multiple ZnO nanostructured thin films were obtained.

The ZnO samples were characterized using a Nova200 Nanolab, Dual Beam Microscope, Field Emission Scanning Electron Beam, Scanning Electron Microscope (SEM), which has 1.1 nm of resolution, and a Focused Ion Beam with 1.7 nm for obtaining high-resolution images for the analysis of a large portion of the surface and the characterization of its morphology. From SEM analysis, it was possible to achieve the visualization of the sample porosity and the orientation of the crystallization phase on the surface. Experimental data for the material thickness over the substrate were obtained by spectroscopic ellipsometry (Uvisel HORIBA Jobin Yvon ellipsometer model LT M200AGMS) with an incident angle of 70°, a 1200 μm spot, and a spectral range of 1.5 to 5.5 eV with increments of 0.0500 eV, and a high-pressure Xenon lamp of 75 W was used for both samples.

2.2. Optical and Electrical Properties Characterization

For the characterization of the optical properties, a UV spectrophotometer (Perkin Elmer XLS) was used to obtain the absorbance of the micro and nanostructured ZnO samples. Moreover, the electrical conductivity was evaluated using a two-probe ohmmeter model MUT-202 (Truper, Mexico); the measurement was carried out by applying copper electrodes over the samples with a separation distance of 1.5 cm. The electrical impedance (Z) as a function of electrical frequency was obtained with an Autolab potentiostat (Autolab/PGSTAT302N high-power potentiostat/galvanostat) connected to the same electrodes of the analyzed samples.

Photoconductivity under optical irradiation from a Nd:YVO_4 laser system (Spectra-Physics Explorer® One™ XP) at 532 nm wavelength, linear polarization, and 50 KHz was also studied. In order to describe the buildup persistent photoconductivity (σ) for semiconductors, we consider [33]:

$$\sigma(I) = \sigma_D + (\sigma_{\max} - \sigma_D)\,(1 - \exp(-\alpha_1 I)), \tag{1}$$

where σ_D is the initial material electrical current in darkness, and σ_{max} is the maximum data value of photoconduction, which was assumed to be the value at maximum irradiance (100%) of the laser system employed. Also, α_1 is described as a decay constant of the buildup process system.

In order to describe the fractional order photoconductivity, different values of the optical irradiance were systematically evaluated with fractional calculus. The implementation of this derivation was carried out to analyze the gradual fractional order contribution of the intensity and its relationship with the experimental photoconduction buildup process. For this, we found the best fitting for the study of the photoconduction effect with the Caputo fractional derivative. The following expression was employed [34]:

$$\frac{d^n}{dx^n}[{}^{RL}_{a}I^{\phi}_{x}(f(t))] = \frac{d^n}{dx^n}\left[\frac{1}{\Gamma(\phi)}\int_a^x (x-t)^{\phi-1} f(t)dt\right], \tag{2}$$

where ϕ is the fractional order exponent that takes different fractional values ($0 < \phi < 1$), x and a are derivative limits, $\Gamma(\phi)$ is the gamma function. The understanding of this formula requires the obtention of the Riemann–Liouville fractional integral (${}^{RL}_{a}I^{\phi}_{x}$) of the analyzed function.

2.3. Experimental Setups for NLO Effects

The z-scan technique setup was used to characterize the NLO properties of the analyzed samples. With this technique, it is possible to determine the possible Kerr nonlinearity and nonlinear absorption effects by analyzing the closed and open aperture configurations, respectively. In this research, the experimental setup was designed for a range between −4 and 4 mm for the manifestation of the nonlinear optical transmittance. For both samples, an incident irradiance of 10.3 and 14.58 GW/cm^2 was used for open and closed configurations, under the same laboratory conditions provided by a 532 nm wavelength with 4 nanosecond pulses emitted by a Continuum SL II-10 Nd:YAG Laser system. The z-scan setup used for this work can be seen in Figure 1a. An approximation of the optical transmittance T_o in the nonlinear media for the open aperture configuration of the z-scan can be obtained by considering the following equations [35]:

$$T_o(z, \Delta\Phi_o) = 1 - \frac{(\beta I_o L_e f f)}{(2\sqrt{2}(1 + z^2/z_o^2))}, \tag{3}$$

$$L_{eff} = \frac{(1 - e^{(-\alpha_o L)})}{\alpha_o}, \tag{4}$$

where z is the position, $z_0 = kw_0^2/2$, $k = 2\pi/\lambda$, with λ being the probe laser wavelength, β represents the two-photon absorption coefficient, L_{eff} is the effective length, L is the sample length, I_o is the peak irradiance at focus on the propagation axis, and α_o is the linear absorption coefficient. In a similar way, for the closed aperture configuration using a Gaussian beam with waist radius w_o travelling in the propagation direction, the normalized transmittance T_c, as a function of the position (z), is given by [36]:

$$T_c(z, \Delta\Phi_o) = 1 - \frac{(4\Delta\Phi_o(z/z_o))}{(z^2/(z_o^2) + 9)(z^2/(z_o^2) + 1)}, \tag{5}$$

$$\Delta\Phi_o = k\Delta n_o L_{eff}, \tag{6}$$

where $\Delta\Phi_o$ is the optical phase change when the laser passes through the sample, and Δn_o is the refractive index change equal to the product of the nonlinear refractive index n_2 and I_o.

To further investigate the NLO effects, a two-wave-mixing (TWM) setup, shown in Figure 1b, was used to explore the vectorial nature of the nonlinear response. Irradiation at 532 nm wavelength with 4 nanosecond pulses was provided by a Continuum SL II-10 Nd:YAG Laser system, focused by a 50 mm optical lens. The results of the high optical irradiation of the sample were captured by a pair of photodetectors connected to an ADS1102CAL ATTEN, 100 MHz capacity digital oscilloscope. In order to numerically estimate the transmitted irradiance of the TWM interaction, an approximation of the wave equation [37] can be described as:

$$\nabla^2 E_\pm = -\frac{n_\pm^2 \omega^2}{c^2} E_\pm \tag{7}$$

where $E_\pm$ represents the electric fields that propagate through the samples in their circular components as E_+ and E_-, while ω represents the optical frequency of the light. The refraction index is denoted by n, and c is the speed of light.

The nonlinear refractive index for circular polarized light, being right-handed (n_+) or left-handed (n_-) can be considered:

$$n_\pm^2 = n_o^2 + 4\pi(\chi_{1122}^{(3)}\left|E_\pm\right|2 + (\chi_{1122}^{(3)} + \chi_{1212}^{(3)})\left|E_\pm\right|2), \tag{8}$$

where n_o is the refractive index at low irradiance, and $\chi_{1122}^{(3)}$ and $\chi_{1212}^{(3)}$ are the independent components of the third-order optical susceptibility tensor of the system.

Furthermore, to numerically estimate the contribution of different micro and nanostructures on the sample as a function of the volume fraction ρ, the nonlinear third-order susceptibility can be approximated as follows:

$$\chi_{(n+m)}^{(3)} = (1 - \rho)\chi_n^{(3)} + \rho\chi_m^{(3)}, \tag{9}$$

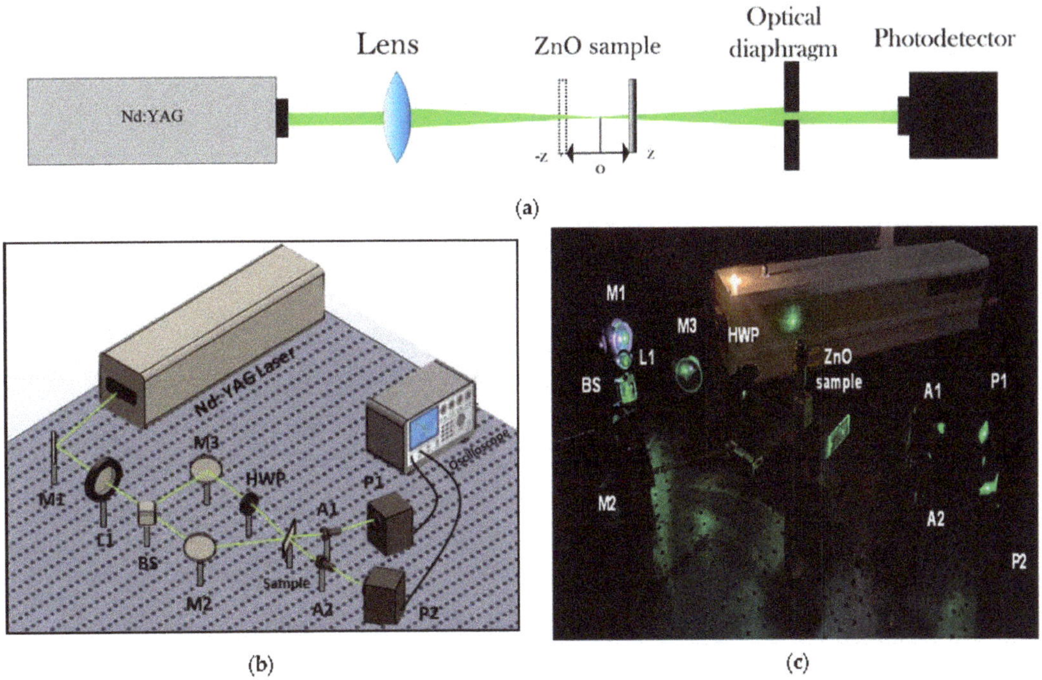

Figure 1. (**a**) Z-scan experimental setup for the open and closed configuration by focusing the high-intensity irradiation with a biconvex lens and with the help of an optical diaphragm before the detector. (**b**,**c**) TWM experimental setup to observe the NLO response as a function of different angles of polarization; for this setup, L1 is an optical lent, BS corresponds to a beam splitter, M1 to M3 are mirrors, HWP represents a half wave polarizer, A1 and A2 are polarizers, and P1 and P2 are photodetectors.

The sum of the nonlinear third-order susceptibility of the integrated nanocrystals $\chi_n^{(3)}$ with microcrystals $\chi_m^{(3)}$ on the sample is represented as $\chi_{n+m}^{(3)}$. For further analysis, the mathematical expression used to obtain the transmitted irradiance I, as a function of the propagation distance L, the absorption coefficient α_o, and the incident irradiance I_0 from a coherent optical source analyzed through a nonlinear optical absorptive medium is:

$$I(L) = \frac{I_0 \exp(-\alpha_o L)}{1 + \beta I_o L_{eff}}, \tag{10}$$

3. Results and Discussion

3.1. Morphology Characterization

The results in Figure 2 show representative images of the surface of the ZnO thin films. It was possible to observe the morphology of the micro and nanostructures, obtaining micro-structured desert rose-like ZnO (RD-ZnO) crystals of about 6 μm in diameter which compose the thin film. In a similar way, from the images of the nanostructures, we observe nanoflake-like crystals which form the nanomaterial. The estimated flake thickness ranged from 30 to 150 nm. Furthermore, an ellipsometry test was carried out to determine the nanoscale thickness of the thin film, obtaining an approximate value of 688 nm. The material thickness was attributed to the spray pyrolysis technique utilized for both samples.

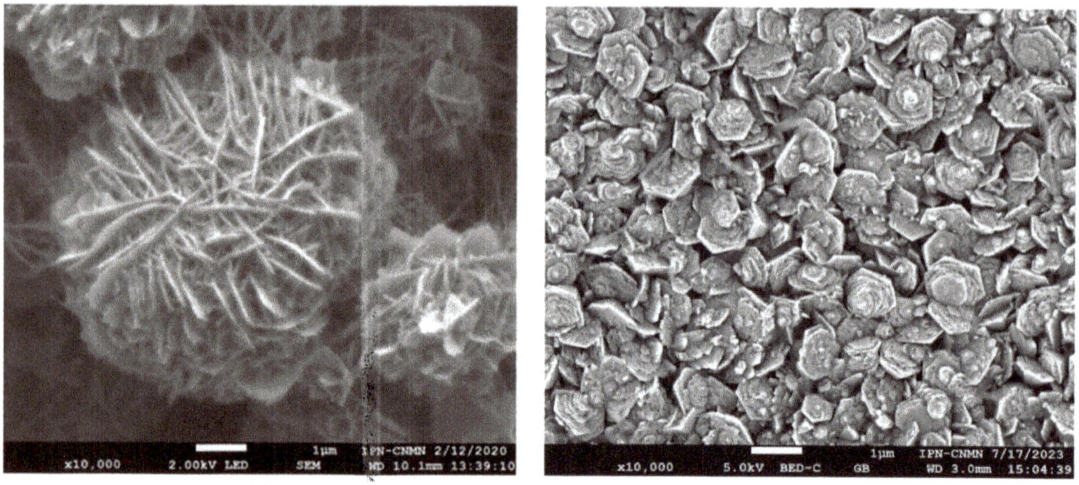

(**a**) (**b**)

Figure 2. SEM images: (**a**) ZnO microstructures and (**b**) ZnO nanostructures.

3.2. UV-VIS Observations

The absorbance of the analyzed ZnO is shown in Figure 3a. It was found that the absorbance spectra of the samples have a special preference for the UV low frequencies at wavelength regions from about 260 to 400 nm. The obtained Tauc plots for the absorbance spectra are shown in Figure 3b. It was determined that the binding energy was about 3.15 eV and 3.76 eV for the nano and microstructures, respectively. The nanoscale contribution of the petals in the microstructures seems to be responsible for a higher bandgap than the correspondent magnitude in the flake-like nanostructures studied.

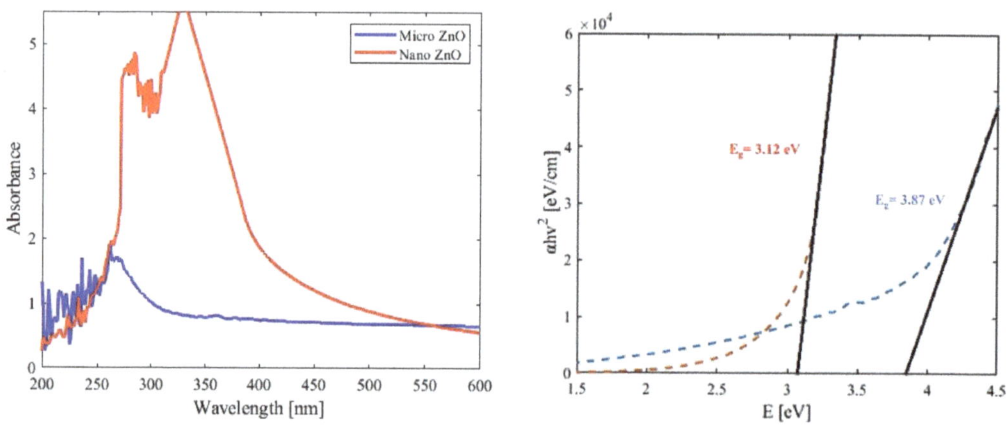

(**a**) (**b**)

Figure 3. (**a**) UV-Vis data obtained for the ZnO samples showing the absorbance as a function of the wavelength. (**b**) Graphical Tauc plots for obtaining the energy bandgap.

3.3. Photoconductivity Response

The electrical response under laser irradiation measured by an Autolab potentiostat indicated an impedance decrease as a function of the frequency, denoting an n-type semiconductor behavior in the ZnO nanostructured material when analyzing with Nova 1.1

software. The micro-structured sample presented high electrical resistivity, which cannot be measured when analyzing with the potentiostat; this behavior is in good agreement with similar works for other synthetized ZnO microstructures which reported low electrical conductivity values in a range of 1–100 S/cm. The best numerical simulation was obtained by considering a Resistor-Capacitor (RC) system that induced the impedance drop for the photoconductivity data results and their equivalent RC circuit showing capacitive behavior, presented in Figure 4a for the overall results.

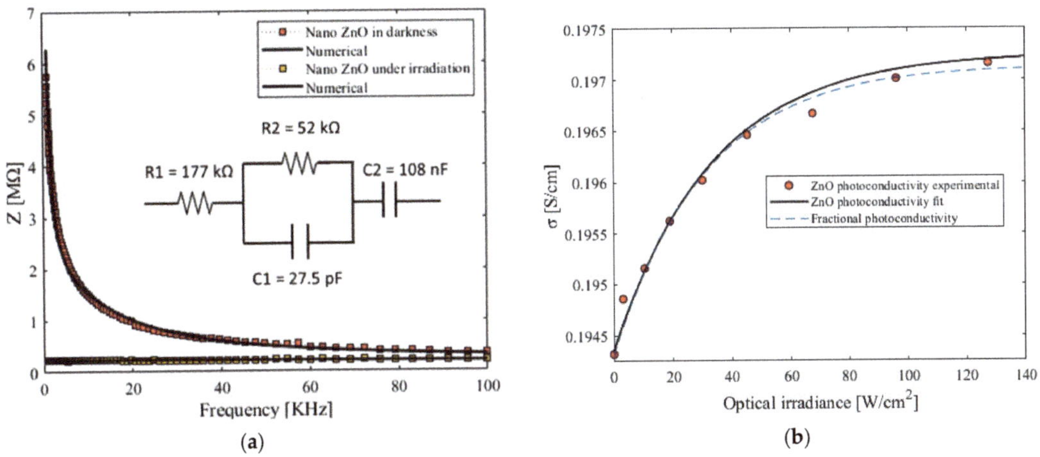

Figure 4. (**a**) Graphical representation of the impedance data in darkness and under irradiation obtained from the Autolab potentiostat for the ZnO nanostructures and their respective best fitting electrical RC circuit. (**b**) Experimental and numerical photoconductivity data obtained under 532 nm wavelength excitation at different optical irradiances for the ZnO nanostructures. The parameters of this experiment correspond to $\sigma_D = 0.194$ S/cm; $\sigma_{max} = 0.19716$ S/cm. Also shown are the numerical simulations of the best fractional order exponent for the irradiance-dependent photoconductivity of the nano ZnO sample using Caputo fractional derivative.

Furthermore, experimentation to evaluate the photoconduction influenced by the light intensity on thin films was undertaken as shown in Figure 4b. The results indicated an exponential growth from the initial steady state (or current in darkness) to the irradiation state. The change from the initial darkness current on the semiconductors could be attributed to the excited charge carriers that change with the irradiation of the light, which makes them photoconductive. Also, it was assumed that the interface heating the mechanism behind the conduction phenomena modifies the velocity of the carriers. Such an amount of heat could be obtained from the high-intensity irradiation of the light beams, which produces multiphotonic effects. From these results, an exponential growth in photoconduction can be seen as a function of higher irradiances for both samples. An important aspect of the conductivity behavior in semiconductors is the temperature dependence; in this type of material, a large amount of temperature differential is required to induce a notable change in the charge carrier's mobility. Thus, the numerical interpretation of some fractional values of the dependent variable was obtained by putting Equations (1) in (2) with different fractional order values of I.

A comparison was made between different fractional derivative theories to probe the effectiveness on these equations, like Grünwald–Letnikov and Riemann–Liouville, determining that the Caputo fractional derivative was the best for the fitting. The results of the Caputo fractional derivative can be observed in detail in Figure 4b, showing the relation of the conductivity as a function of the light intensity. Comparative results in ZnO nanostructures have been previously reported [38,39]. These are explained as the oxygen vacancies that directly affect the electron–hole interactions of the charge carriers, which permit the electrical conduction. The implications of this effect are investigated for uses in photodetectors, gas sensors, and other optoelectronic systems. It should be mentioned that optical absorbance effects are interesting for applications in a handful of solar cells systems, electronics, and optoelectronics [40]. In addition, ZnO micro and nanostructures have been compared in their photoconductive potential, which showed results that indicated an enhancement in photo response in nano ZnO materials [41], which also leads to an increase in NLO response.

3.4. Results of the z-Scan Analysis

The z-scan traces for the open and closed apertures and the best numerical fitting for the ZnO nanostructured thin film are presented in Figure 5. A significant Kerr effect on the sample inducing a change in the refractive index at high irradiances was clearly observed. On the other side, the micro-structured ZnO was irradiated under the same conditions but showed a Kerr response with at least a decrease of one order of magnitude not far from the error bar ±15%. Also, a positive change in the nonlinear absorption index was found for the open aperture, which reveals the existence of a significant multiphonic effect in the nanostructures at high irradiances. In addition, the numerical interpretation of the overall results allows us to calculate the nonlinear refractive index and absorption coefficient of the samples. The approximated nonlinear refractive index value obtained was $n_2 = 1.36 \times 10^{-11}$ cm^2/W for the ZnO nanostructured sample.

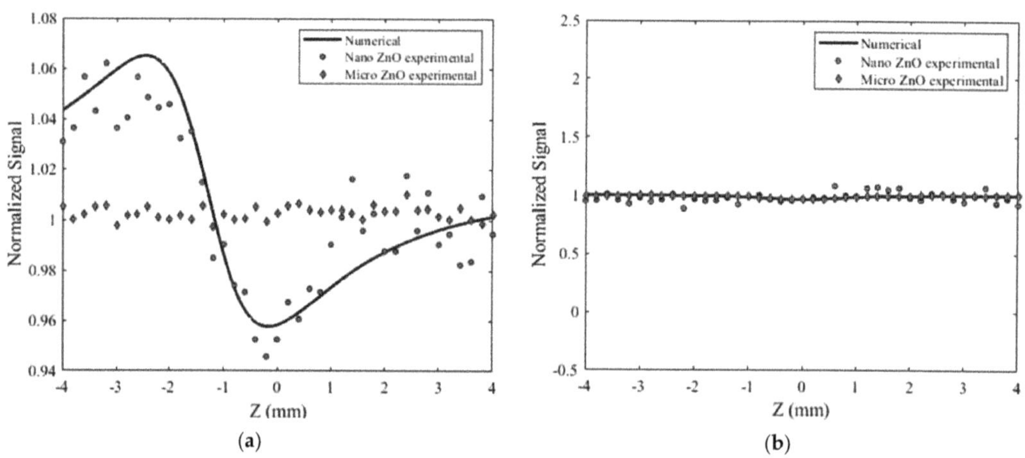

Figure 5. Results for the z-scan for the ZnO micro and nanostructures (**a**) closed aperture, (**b**) open aperture.

The z-scan results indicate a positive nonlinear refractive index in the nanosecond regime. The sign in the nonlinear refractive index might vary depending on many factors responsible for the physical mechanisms of nonlinearity [42], material thickness, incident irradiance, and different preparation techniques, like RF magnetron sputtering [43] or chemical vapor deposition [44]. Also, previous works have reported that the crystallization form of the ZnO could have influenced its optical and NLO response.

3.5. Nanosecond TWM Studies

Figure 6a depicts the transmitted optical irradiance obtained as a function angle of polarization for both ZnO samples in the TWM mixing experiments. The obtained curves show a clear relation between the optical properties and the crystal size that forms the ZnO structures, one of the principal factors that influence different physical properties of ZnO thin films. Thus, the overall results indicate a direct correlation between the two-sized structures and the optical response at a maximum angle of polarization. Complementarily, the nanosized crystals presented the stronger enhancement on transmittance at least three times larger than the microcrystals (at data $\times 100$). In view of these considerations, it is possible to speculate a particle size dependence responsible for the variations in the Kerr transmittance that increased from the polarization of the light. The possibility of obtaining different optical signals with hybrid materials is rather attractive in optoelectronics in order to generate different nonlinearities and all-optical functions. The modulation of a normalized nonlinear refractive index in the ZnO nanostructures as a function of their volume fraction in respect to microstructures and the angle of polarization is illustrated in Figure 6b. The numerical data plotted in Figure 6b were estimated using Equations (7)–(10) and the finite difference method.

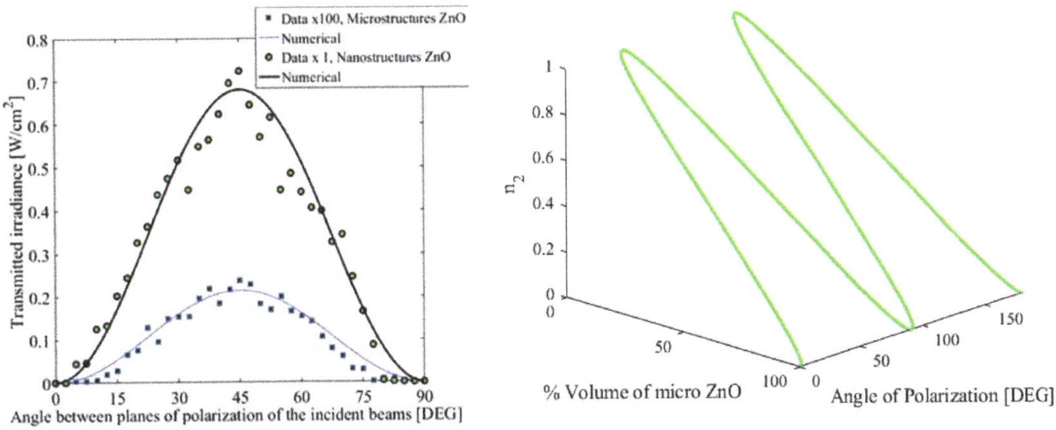

Figure 6. (**a**) Graphical representation of the NLO response comparison between micro and nanocrystals as a function of the angle of polarization. (**b**) Numerical simulation for describing the modulation of the nonlinear refraction in ZnO nanostructures and its relation between the angle of polarization considering a variation in the volume fraction of incorporated micro ZnO structures.

Third-order optical nonlinearities can be controlled by irradiance, polarization, and concentration of different sizes and morphologies of crystals in ZnO nanostructures [45]. In addition, it has been reported that ZnO nanocrystals, nanofilms, nanowires [46], and bulk structures can be used as nonlinear media to obtain higher-frequency conversion efficiencies from nonlinear effects [47,48]. Also, various ZnO-based nanohybrids have been examined for the enhancement of their nonlinear optical interactions [49–56]. In this work, we highlight the importance of describing a fractional model and optically induced electronic behavior with influence on photoconductivity and electronic mechanisms responsible for Kerr nonlinearity. We propose the tuning of ZnO systems via the combination of micro and nanostructures that can be assisted by a fractional description for predicting electronic and optically induced functions with potential applications for optoelectronics and all-optical devices.

4. Conclusions

Fractional electrical studies for describing conductivity effects in low-dimensional systems are reported. Photoconductive and capacitive behavior was identified in the nanostructured ZnO thin film studied, while inhibition of conductivity was obtained when the samples were in a micro-structured form. An enhancement in NLO effects and electrical conductivity was obtained via the preparation of ZnO in a nanostructured form.

A red shift in the optical resonance of nanostructured ZnO was observed in respect to micro-structured ZnO. TWM experiments and z-scan explorations were conducted for the characterization of NLO response of the studied ZnO samples. The NLO effects revealed the existence of a nanosecond Kerr effect at 532 nm, which was attributed to an electronic physical mechanism responsible for the third-order optical nonlinearities. The results of the NLO nature demonstrate the potential to combine nano and microstructures to modulate electrical, electromagnetic, and NLO effects in ZnO circuits and optoelectronic platforms.

Author Contributions: Investigation, V.M.G.-d.-l.-R., J.A.A.-M., M.T.-V., M.L.H.-P., M.A.V.-H. and C.T.-T.; writing—original draft, V.M.G.-d.-l.-R., J.A.A.-M., M.T.-V., M.L.H.-P., M.A.V.-H. and C.T.-T.; writing—review and editing, V.M.G.-d.-l.-R., J.A.A.-M., M.T.-V., M.L.H.-P., M.A.V.-H. and C.T.-T.; conceptualization, C.T.-T. All the authors contributed equally to the proposal and development of this research. The manuscript was written with the contribution of all the authors. All authors have read and agreed to the published version of the manuscript.

Funding: This research was funded by Instituto Politécnico Nacional (SIP-2023) and Consejo Nacional de Humanidades, Ciencias y Tecnologías (CF-2023-I-2042).

Data Availability Statement: Data and materials are available upon reasonable request to C. Torres-Torres (ctorrest@ipn.mx).

Acknowledgments: The authors kindly acknowledge the financial support from the Instituto Politécnico Nacional, COFAA-IPN, and Consejo Nacional de Humanidades, Ciencias y Tecnologías (CONAHCyT). The authors are also thankful to the Central Microscopy facilities at the Centro de Nanociencias y Micro y Nanotecnologías del Instituto Politécnico Nacional.

Conflicts of Interest: The authors declare no conflict of interest.

References

1. Vyas, S. A short review on properties and applications of zinc oxide based thin films and devices: ZnO as a promising material for applications in electronics, optoelectronics, biomedical and sensors. *Johns. Matthey Technol. Rev.* **2020**, *64*, 202–218. [CrossRef]
2. Sharma, D.K.; Shukla, S.; Sharma, K.K.; Kumar, V. A review on ZnO: Fundamental properties and applications. *Mater. Today Proc.* **2022**, *49*, 3028–3035. [CrossRef]
3. Borysiewicz, M.A. ZnO as a functional material, a review. *Crystals* **2019**, *9*, 505. [CrossRef]
4. Abed, S.; Aida, M.S.; Bouchouit, K.; Arbaoui, A.; Iliopoulos, K.; Sahraoui, B. Non-linear optical and electrical properties of ZnO doped Ni Thin Films obtained using spray ultrasonic technique. *Opt. Mater.* **2011**, *33*, 968–972. [CrossRef]
5. Shahzad, S.; Javed, S.; Usman, M. A review on synthesis and optoelectronic applications of nanostructured ZnO. *Front. Mater.* **2021**, *8*, 613825. [CrossRef]
6. Sharma, S.; Kumar, K.; Thakur, N.; Chauhan, S.; Chauhan, M.S. The effect of shape and size of ZnO nanoparticles on their antimicrobial and photocatalytic activities: A green approach. *Bull. Mater. Sci.* **2020**, *43*, 1–10. [CrossRef]
7. Rahman, A.; Harunsani, M.H.; Tan, A.L.; Khan, M.M. Zinc oxide and zinc oxide-based nanostructures: Biogenic and phytogenic synthesis, properties and applications. *Bioprocess Biosyst. Eng.* **2021**, *44*, 1333–1372. [CrossRef]
8. Parvez Ahmad, M.D.; Venkateswara Rao, A.; Suresh Babu, K.; Narsinga Rao, G. Particle size effect on the dielectric properties of ZnO nanoparticles. *Mater. Chem. Phys.* **2019**, *224*, 79–84. [CrossRef]
9. Aljawfi Rezq, R.N.; Rahman, F.; Batoo Khalid, M. Effect of grain size and grain boundary defects on electrical and magnetic properties of Cr doped ZnO nanoparticles. *J. Mol. Struct.* **2014**, *1065–1066*, 199–204. [CrossRef]
10. Hwang, S.-H.; Kim, Y.K.; Hong, S.H.; Lim, S.K. Effect of the Morphology and Electrical Property of Metal-Deposited ZnO Nanostructures on CO Gas Sensitivity. *Nanomaterials* **2020**, *10*, 2124. [CrossRef]
11. Yathisha, R.O.; Arthoba Nayaka, Y. Structural, Optical and Electrical Properties of ZnO Nanostructures Synthesized under Different Microwave Power. *Russ. J. Electrochem.* **2021**, *57*, 784–794. [CrossRef]
12. Long, P.; Peng, H.; Sun, B.; Lan, J.; Wan, J.; Fei, Y.; Ye, X.; Qu, S.; Ye, G.; He, Y.; et al. Modulation of ZnO Nanostructure for Efficient Photocatalytic Performance. *Nanoscale Res. Lett.* **2022**, *17*, 118. [CrossRef]
13. Qiao, S.; Liu, J.; Fu, G.; Ren, K.; Li, Z.; Wang, S.; Pan, C. ZnO nanowire based CIGS solar cell and its efficiency enhancement by the piezo-phototronic effect. *Nano Energy* **2018**, *49*, 508–514. [CrossRef]
14. Dan, M.; Hu, G.; Li, L.; Zhang, Y. High performance piezotronic logic nanodevices based on GaN/InN/GaN topological insulator. *Nano Energy* **2018**, *50*, 544–551. [CrossRef]
15. Hu, G.; Zhang, Y.; Li, L.; Wang, Z.L. Piezotronic transistor based on topological insulators. *ACS Nano* **2017**, *12*, 779–785. [CrossRef] [PubMed]
16. Khalid, N.R.; Hammad, A.; Tahir, M.B.; Rafique, M.; Iqbal, T.; Nabi, G.; Hussain, M.K. Enhanced photocatalytic activity of Al and Fe co-doped ZnO nanorods for methylene blue degradation. *Ceram. Int.* **2019**, *45*, 21430–21435. [CrossRef]

17. Kurtaran, S. Al doped ZnO thin films obtained by spray pyrolysis technique: Influence of different annealing time. *Opt. Mater.* **2021**, *114*, 110908. [CrossRef]
18. Lou, A.J.T.; Marks, T.J. A twist on nonlinear optics: Understanding the unique response of π-twisted chromophores. *Acc. Chem. Res.* **2019**, *52*, 1428–1438. [CrossRef] [PubMed]
19. Waszkowska, K.; Krupka, O.; Kharchenko, O.; Figà, V.; Smokal, V.; Kutsevol, N.; Sahraoui, B. Influence of ZnO nanoparticles on nonlinear optical properties. *Appl. Nanosci.* **2020**, *10*, 4977–4982. [CrossRef]
20. Paul, S.; Balasubramanian, K. Charge transfer induced excitons and nonlinear optical properties of ZnO/PEDOT: PSS nanocomposite films. *Spectrochim. Acta Part A Mol. Biomol. Spectrosc.* **2021**, *245*, 118901. [CrossRef]
21. Kepceoğlu, A.; Gezgin, S.Y.; Gündoğdu, Y.; Küçükçelebi, H.; Kılıç, H.Ş. Nonlinear optical properties of zinc oxide thin films produced by pulsed laser deposition. *Mater. Today Proc.* **2019**, *18*, 1819–1825. [CrossRef]
22. Sindhu, H.S.; Maidur, S.R.; Patil, P.S.; Choudhary, R.J.; Rajendra, B.V. Nonlinear optical and optical power limiting studies of Zn1-xMnxO thin films prepared by spray pyrolysis. *Optik* **2019**, *182*, 671–681. [CrossRef]
23. Haghighatzadeh, A.; Mazinani, B.; Ostad, M.; Shokouhimehr, M.; Dutta, J. Hollow ZnO microspheres self-assembled from rod-like nanostructures: Morphology-dependent linear and Kerr-type nonlinear optical properties. *J. Mater. Sci. Mater. Electron.* **2021**, *32*, 23385–23398. [CrossRef]
24. Shehata, A.; Tawfik, W.Z.; Mohamed, T. Cobalt enhanced nonlinear optical properties and optical limiting of zinc oxide irradiated by femtosecond laser pulses. *JOSA B* **2020**, *37*, A1–A8. [CrossRef]
25. Ciprian, R.; Baratto, C.; Giglia, A.; Koshmak, K.; Vinai, G.; Donarelli, M.; Ferroni, M.; Campanini, M.; Comini, E.; Ponzoni, A.; et al. Magnetic gas sensing exploiting the magneto-optical Kerr effect on ZnO nanorods/Co layer system. *RSC Adv.* **2016**, *6*, 42517–42521. [CrossRef]
26. Hua, S.; Zhang, W. Anisotropy of 2PA, 3PA, and Kerr effect in nonpolar ZnO. *Opt. Lett.* **2021**, *46*, 4065–4068. [CrossRef] [PubMed]
27. Zhang, S.; Lu, H.; Rui, G.; Lv, C.; He, J.; Cui, Y.; Gu, B. Preparation of Ag@ ZnO core–shell nanostructures by liquid-phase laser ablation and investigation of their femtosecond nonlinear optical properties. *Appl. Phys. B* **2020**, *126*, 1–9. [CrossRef]
28. Moreira, L.; Falci, R.F.; Darabian, H.; Anjos, V.; Bell, M.J.V.; Kassab, L.R.P.; Bordon, C.D.S.; Doualan, J.L.; Camy, P.; Moncorgé, R. The effect of excitation intensity variation and silver nanoparticle codoping on nonlinear optical properties of mixed tellurite and zinc oxide glass doped with Nd_2O_3 studied through ultrafast z-scan spectroscopy. *Opt. Mater.* **2018**, *79*, 397–402. [CrossRef]
29. Ortíz-Trejo, F.; Trejo-Valdez, M.; Campos-López, J.P.; Castro-Chacón, J.H.; Torres-Torres, C. Multipath data storage by third-order nonlinear optical properties in zinc oxide nanostructures. *Appl. Sci.* **2020**, *10*, 5688. [CrossRef]
30. Wen, X.; Han, Y.; Yao, C.; Zhang, K.; Li, J.; Sun, W.; Li, Q.; Zhang, M.; Wu, J.D. The photoluminescence, ultrafast nonlinear optical properties, and carrier dynamics of 1D In-doped ZnO nanostructures: Experiment and mechanism. *Opt. Mater.* **2018**, *77*, 67–76. [CrossRef]
31. Wang, H.; Wang, C.; Chen, Q.; Ren, B.; Guan, R.; Cao, X.; Yang, X.; Duan, R. Interface-defect-mediated photocatalysis of mesocrystalline ZnO assembly synthesized in-situ via a template-free hydrothermal approach. *Appl. Surf. Sci.* **2017**, *412*, 517–528. [CrossRef]
32. Ravichandran, K.; Philominathan, P. Fabrication of antimony doped tin oxide (ATO) films by an inexpensive, simplified spray technique using perfume atomizer. *Mater. Lett.* **2008**, *62*, 2980–2983. [CrossRef]
33. Jiang, H.X.; Lin, J.Y. Chapter 6: Persistent photoconductivity in III-nitrides. In *III-Nitride Semiconductors: Electrical, Structural and Defects Properties*; Elsevier Science: Amsterdam, The Netherlands, 2000; pp. 151–191.
34. Matar, M.M.; Abbas, M.I.; Alzabut, J.; Kaabar, M.K.A.; Etemad, S.; Rezapour, S. Investigation of the p-Laplacian nonperiodic nonlinear boundary value problem via generalized Caputo fractional derivatives. *Adv. Differ. Equ.* **2021**, *2021*, 1–18. [CrossRef]
35. Sandeep, K.M.; Bhat, S.; Dharmaprakash, S.M. Nonlinear absorption properties of ZnO and Al doped ZnO thin films under continuous and pulsed modes of operations. *Opt. Laser Technol.* **2018**, *102*, 147–152. [CrossRef]
36. Walden, S.L.; Fernando, J.F.; Shortell, M.P.; Jaatinen, E.A. Accurate determination of nonlinear refraction in ZnO and Au composite nanostructures. *Opt. Mater. Express* **2020**, *10*, 653–661. [CrossRef]
37. Boyd, R.W. *Nonlinear Optics*, 3rd ed.; Elsevier Academic Press: San Diego, CA, USA, 2009.
38. Nair, V.G.; Jayakrishnan, R.; John, J.; Salam, J.A.; Anand, A.M.; Raj, A. Anomalous photoconductivity in chemical spray pyrolysis deposited nano-crystalline ZnO thin films. *Mater. Chem. Phys.* **2020**, *247*, 122849. [CrossRef]
39. Worasawat, S.; Tasaki, K.; Hatanaka, Y.; Neo, Y.; Mimura, H.; Pecharapa, W. Growth of ZnO nano-rods and its photoconductive characteristics on the photo-catalytic properties. *Mater. Today Proc.* **2019**, *17*, 1379–1385. [CrossRef]
40. Kokate, S.K.; Jagtap, C.V.; Baviskar, P.K.; Jadkar, S.R.; Pathan, H.M.; Mohite, K.C. CdS sensitized cadmium doped ZnO solar cell: Fabrication and characterizations. *Optik* **2018**, *157*, 628–634. [CrossRef]
41. Acharya, S.; Biswal, S.K.; Sarangi, S.N. Effect of structure and morphology on the UV photo detection of ZnO nanostructures and microstructures. *Chem. Phys.* **2021**, *523*, 99–105. [CrossRef]
42. Trejo-Valdez, M.; Torres-Torres, C.; Castro-Chacón, J.H.; Graciano-Armenta, G.A.; García-Gil, C.I.; Khomenko, A.V. Modification of the picosecond optical absorptive nonlinearity by a nanosecond irradiation in a nanostructured ZnO thin film. *Opt. Laser Tech.* **2013**, *49*, 75–80. [CrossRef]
43. Abdallah, B.; Zidan, M.D.; Allahham, A. Syntheses, structural and nonlinear optical characteristics of ZnO films using Z-scan technique. *Silicon* **2021**, *13*, 4139–4146. [CrossRef]

44. Sony, T.; Zaker, T.A.; Zakar, A.T.; Mohammed, H.N. Nonlinear Optical Properties of ZnO Thin Film at Low Laser Intensity Using Z-scan Technique. *Rafidain J. Sci.* **2021**, *30*, 32–38. [CrossRef]
45. Chamundeeswari, A.; Das, S.J.; Mageshwari, P.S.; Vijayakumar, G.; Deepapriya, S.; Rodney, J.D.; Infantiya, S.G.; Jensipriya, A.; Reena, R.S.; Rathikha, R. Structural, non-linear optical analysis of ZnO-CdO nanocomposite. *AIP Conf. Proc.* **2020**, *2244*, 060001. [CrossRef]
46. Tran, D.; Valdes, C.; Sadoqi, M.; Kityk, I.; Long, G. Second Harmonic Generation On Hydrothermal Grown Zno Nanowires And Colloidal Nanostructures Films. *APS March Meet. Abstr.* **2019**, *2019*, T70–T303.
47. Ma, Q.; Pan, C.; Xue, Y.; Fang, Z.; Zhang, S.; Wu, B.; Wu, E. Plasmon Enhanced Second Harmonic Generation from ZnO Nanofilms on Vertical Au Nanorod Arrays. *Nanomaterials* **2021**, *11*, 2597. [CrossRef] [PubMed]
48. Volmert, R.; Weber, N.; Meier, C. Nanoantennas embedded in zinc oxide for second harmonic generation enhancement. *J. Appl. Phys.* **2020**, *128*, 043107. [CrossRef]
49. Rout, A.; Boltaev, G.S.; Ganeev, R.A.; Rao, K.S.; Fu, D.; Rakhimov, R.Y.; Kurbanov, S.S.; Urolov, S.Z.; Shaymardanov, Z.S.; Guo, C. Low-and high-order nonlinear optical studies of ZnO nanocrystals, nanoparticles, and nanorods. *Eur. Phys. J. D* **2019**, *73*, 1–8. [CrossRef]
50. Waszkowska, K.; Chtouki, T.; Krupka, O.; Smokal, V.; Figà, V.; Sahraoui, B. Effect of UV-Irradiation and ZnO nanoparticles on nonlinear optical response of specific photochromic polymers. *Nanomaterials* **2021**, *11*, 492. [CrossRef]
51. Upadhya, K.; Deekshitha, U.G.; Antony, A.; Ani, A.; Kityk, I.V.; Jedryka, J.; Wojciechowski, A.; Ozga, K.; Poornesh, P.; Kulkarni, S.D.; et al. Second and third harmonic nonlinear optical process in spray pyrolysed Mg: ZnO thin films. *Opt. Mater.* **2020**, *102*, 109814. [CrossRef]
52. Haider, A.J.; Sultan, F.I.; Haider, M.J.; Taha, B.A.; Al-Musawi, S.; Edan, M.S.; Jassim, C.S.; Arsad, N. Characterization of laser dye concentrations in ZnO nanostructures for optimization of random laser emission performance. *Int. J. Mod. Phys. B* **2023**, 2450111. [CrossRef]
53. Radičić, R.; Maletić, D.; Blažeka, D.; Car, J.; Krstulović, N. Synthesis of silver, gold, and platinum doped zinc oxide nanoparticles by pulsed laser ablation in water. *Nanomaterials* **2022**, *12*, 3484. [CrossRef] [PubMed]
54. Nikov, R.; Dikovska, A.; Nedyalkov, N.; Nikova, T.; Karashanova, D. Nanosecond laser ablation of composite thin films in liquid. *J. Phys. Conf. Ser.* **2021**, *1859*, 012012. [CrossRef]
55. Perez-Lopez, C.A.; Perez-Taborda, J.A.; Riascos, H.; Avila, A. The influence of pulsed laser ablation in liquids parameters on the synthesis of ZnO nanoparticles. *J. Phys. Conf. Ser.* **2020**, *1541*, 012019. [CrossRef]
56. Zandalazini, C.; Oliva, M.; Ferrero, J.C. Highly c-axis oriented ZnO thin films on glass substrate by pulsed laser deposition: Fluence-dependent effects. *J. Nanoelectron. Optoelectron.* **2019**, *14*, 1461–1467. [CrossRef]

fractal and fractional

MDPI

Article

Fractional Partial Differential Equation Modeling for Solar Cell Charge Dynamics

Waleed Mohammed Abdelfattah [1,*], Ola Ragb [2], Mohamed Salah [2], Mohamed S. Matbuly [2] and Mokhtar Mohamed [3,*]

[1] College of Engineering, University of Business and Technology, Jeddah 23435, Saudi Arabia
[2] Department of Engineering Mathematics and Physics, Faculty of Engineering, Zagazig University, Zagazig P.O. Box 44519, Egypt; ormohamed@eng.zu.edu.eg (O.R.); msalaheldin@zu.edu.eg (M.S.); msabdelkreem@eng.zu.edu.eg (M.S.M.)
[3] Basic Science Department, Faculty of Engineering, Delta University for Science and Technology, Gamasa 11152, Egypt
* Correspondence: w.abdelfattah@ubt.edu.sa (W.M.A.); mokhtar.alsaidi@deltauniv.edu.eg (M.M.)

Abstract: This paper presents a groundbreaking numerical approach, the fractional differential quadrature method (FDQM), to simulate the complex dynamics of organic polymer solar cells. The method, which leverages polynomial-based differential quadrature and Cardinal sine functions coupled with the Caputo-type fractional derivative, offers a significant improvement in accuracy and efficiency over traditional methods. By employing a block-marching technique, we effectively address the time-dependent nature of the governing equations. The efficacy of the proposed method is validated through rigorous numerical simulations and comparisons with existing analytical and numerical solutions. Each scheme's computational characteristics are tailored to achieve high accuracy, ensuring an error margin on the order of 10^{-8} or less. Additionally, a comprehensive parametric study is conducted to investigate the impact of key parameters on device performance. These parameters include supporting conditions, time evolution, carrier mobilities, charge carrier densities, geminate pair distances, recombination rate constants, and generation efficiency. The findings of this research offer valuable insights for optimizing and enhancing the performance of organic polymer solar cell devices.

Keywords: fractional derivative; block marching; differential quadrature; renewable energy; organic solar cells; Caputo

1. Introduction

Organic solar cells (OSCs) have emerged as a promising renewable energy technology due to their low cost, flexibility, and potential for large-scale deployment [1]. However, their performance is significantly influenced by complex factors such as charge carrier transport, recombination, and energy loss mechanisms. To accurately model and optimize these devices, it is crucial to develop robust numerical methods that can capture the intricate dynamics of charge carrier transport [2–4]. Fractional calculus provides a powerful mathematical tool for modeling non-local and memory effects, which are prevalent in many physical systems, including organic solar cells. By incorporating fractional derivatives into the governing equations, we can more accurately describe the complex behavior of charge carriers and their interactions within the device.

The latest generation of photovoltaic technologies [5] are classified into two types: organic polymer cells [6,7] and electrochemical cells [8,9]. The focus of this paper will be on organic polymer cells. This kind is a renewable source of electrical energy with several advantages, including cheap production costs [10,11] and facile processing on flexible substrates [12,13]. The bulk heterojunction (BHJ) architecture significantly improves the efficiency of organic polymer cells. This approach involves blending electron donor and acceptor materials in solution and casting the resulting mixture into a thin film. The film is then sandwiched between two electrodes [6,7], as depicted in Figure 1. After excitons dissociate in bulk heterojunction OSCs, electrons move to the acceptor's lowest unoccupied molecular orbital (LUMO), which is similar to the conduction band in conventional semiconductors, and holes move to the donor's highest occupied molecular orbital (HOMO), which is similar to the valence band in conventional semiconductors. In this situation, the mix of donor and acceptor materials functions as a new organic material with a narrower band gap, consisting of the acceptor's LUMO and the donor's HOMO [14,15].

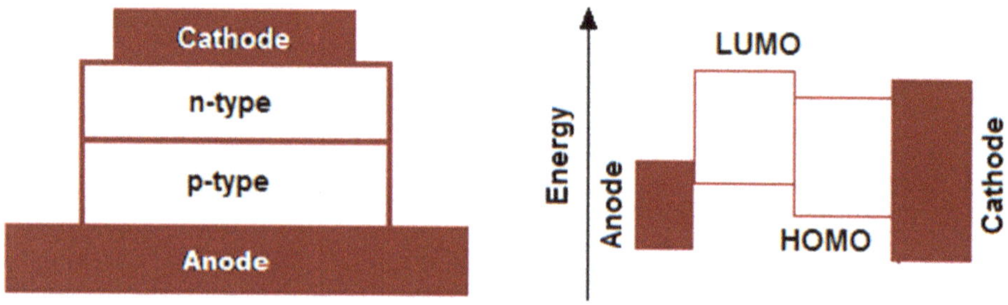

Figure 1. Energy band diagram of a heterojunction organic solar cell.

While extensive experimental research has been conducted on solar cell design [13], analytical and numerical studies remain relatively limited [16]. Falco et al. [17] employed a combination of finite element and Newton–Raphson methods to investigate photocurrent transients in organic polymer solar cells. Buxton et al. [18] utilized finite difference methods to simulate the behavior of polymer solar cells. Hwang et al. [19] explored the transient photocurrent response of organic photovoltaic devices using numerical modeling of drift-diffusion equations. Van Mensfoort et al. [20] characterized iterative approaches for solving drift-diffusion equations and investigated the impact of disorder on device performance. Blom et al. [21] employed Braun's theory to analyze the influence of electric field and temperature on photocurrent in PPV:PCBM blends. However, these numerical approaches can be computationally challenging and may suffer from issues such as ill-conditioning [22,23].

While significant progress has been made in the field of organic solar cell modeling, several challenges remain. Existing numerical methods often struggle to accurately capture the complex, non-linear behavior of charge carrier transport, especially in the presence of fractional-order dynamics. Additionally, many models rely on simplifying assumptions that may not fully capture the intricate processes occurring within organic solar cells. Fractional-order differential equations offer a powerful framework for modeling complex systems with memory effects and non-local behavior. These equations, which generalize classical differential equations by incorporating fractional derivatives, have found applications in a wide range of fields [24,25], including viscoelasticity, biology, fluid mechanics [26], and physics [27]. Depending on the specific application, fractional derivatives can be applied to time, space, or both [28]. Researchers have developed various techniques to solve fractional differential equations, including transform methods (Laplace, Mellin, Fourier) and numerical methods. Recent studies have explored the use of the Atangana–Baleanu fractional derivative operator [29], the modified Adomian decomposition method [30], the Akbari–Ganji technique [31], and the natural transform decomposition method [32] to solve fractional diffusion equations.

Nonlinear dynamics in organic solar cells require solving fractional drift-diffusion equations, which pose significant numerical challenges, particularly in higher dimensions. Various numerical methods, such as finite difference [33], Galerkin [34], collocation [35], homotopy analysis transform [36], and finite volume element methods [37], have been proposed to approximate one-dimensional fractional drift-diffusion equations. Recent advancements include the use of matrix transform techniques [38], shifted Grünwald–Letnikov difference operators [39], radial basis function finite difference methods [40], and finite-volume/finite-difference approaches [41].

In this paper, we propose a novel numerical approach, the fractional differential quadrature method (FDQM), to simulate the nonlinear dynamics of organic polymer solar cells and address the previous limitations. This method offers several advantages, including high accuracy, computational efficiency, and flexibility. The FDQM can accurately capture the non-local and memory effects inherent in fractional-order systems. The method is computationally efficient, especially for high-dimensional problems. The FDQM can be applied to a wide range of fractional differential equations, including those with complex boundary conditions. By addressing these challenges and leveraging the power of fractional calculus, our proposed approach offers a significant advancement in the field of organic solar cell modeling. This approach leverages the strengths of polynomial-based differential quadrature [42] and Cardinal sine functions [43], coupled with the Caputo fractional derivative, to accurately solve the governing system of fractional partial differential equations (FPDEs) and ordinary differential equations (ODEs). By addressing the limitations of traditional integer-order models, our approach enables a more comprehensive understanding of the underlying physics and provides valuable insights for optimizing device performance. When compared to previous analytical [19,44] and numerical (finite element and finite difference techniques) [17,45] approaches, the resultant numerical findings are very efficient and accurate. Furthermore, we present several parametric studies to demonstrate the reliability of the proposed methods by investigating the effects of fractional-order derivatives, supporting conditions, different times, different mobilities, different densities, different geminate pair distances, and the influence of varying geminate recombination rate constants and generation efficiencies on the resulting photocurrent.

The paper is organized as follows: Section 2 presents the mathematical formulation of the problem. Section 3 details the numerical methods employed. Sections 4 and 5 present the numerical results and a discussion of the findings. Finally, Section 6 summarizes the main conclusions of the study.

2. Formulation of the Problem

Organic solar cells (OSCs) are a promising renewable energy technology that converts sunlight directly into electricity. A typical OSC device consists of a photoactive layer sandwiched between two electrodes. The photoactive layer is composed of a blend of donor and acceptor materials, which absorb sunlight and generate excitons. These excitons then dissociate into free charge carriers (electrons and holes) at the donor–acceptor interface. The generated charge carriers are transported to the electrodes, where they are collected to produce electrical current.

When modeling bulk heterojunction (BHJ) solar cells using one-dimensional fractional drift-diffusion equations, the governing equations are modified to account for the fractional derivative terms. Fractional derivatives allow for the inclusion of non-local and memory effects in the charge transport processes. The modified equations for BHJ solar cells can be expressed as follows [8,13,16,33]:

2.1. Fractional Continuity Equation for Electrons

The fractional continuity equation for electrons incorporates the fractional derivative term to describe the non-local transport behavior. In one dimension, it can be written as [33]:

$$\frac{\partial^{\alpha} n(x,t)}{\partial t^{\alpha}} = \frac{\mu_n k_B T}{q}\frac{\partial^{\beta} n(x,t)}{\partial x^{\beta}} - \mu_n \frac{\partial^{\alpha}}{\partial x^{\alpha}}\left(n\frac{\partial \varnothing(x,t)}{\partial x}\right) + k_{diss}X - \gamma np \tag{1}$$

$$\text{where} \begin{cases} \alpha \in]0,1[\text{ and } \beta \in]1,2[\text{ are the fractional order derivative} \\ \text{n is the number of electrons } (\text{cm}^{-3}) \\ \text{p is the number of holes } (\text{cm}^{-3}) \\ \text{X is the charge pair densities } (\text{cm}^{-3}) \\ \varnothing \text{ is the electrostatic potential } (\text{V}) \\ \text{T is the absolute temperature } (\text{K}) \\ \text{t is the time } (\text{s}) \\ \gamma \text{ is the The bimolecular recombination rate } (\text{cm}^3/\text{s}) \\ \text{k}_{\text{diss}} \text{ is The dissociation of charge pairs rate } (\text{s}^{-1}) \\ \mu_{\text{n}} \text{ is The carrier mobilities for electron } (\text{cm}^2/\text{Vs}) \\ \text{x is the x–axis direction } (\text{cm}) \\ \text{q is the elementary charge} > 0 \ (\text{C}) \\ \text{k}_{\text{B}} \text{ is Boltzmann's constant } (\text{eV/K}) \end{cases}.$$

2.2. Fractional Continuity Equation for Holes

Similar to electrons, the fractional continuity equation for holes incorporates the fractional derivative term to describe non-local transport. In one dimension, it can be written as [33]:

$$\frac{\partial^\alpha p(x,t)}{\partial t^\alpha} = \frac{\mu_p k_B T}{q}\frac{\partial^\beta p(x,t)}{\partial x^\beta} + \mu_p \frac{\partial^\alpha}{\partial x^\alpha}\left(p\frac{\partial \varnothing(x,t)}{\partial x}\right) + k_{diss}X - \gamma np \tag{2}$$

where μ_p is The carrier mobilities for hole (cm^2/Vs).

2.3. Poisson's Equation

Poisson's equation remains the same as in the classical model, relating the electric field to the charge densities in the device. It can be written as [28]:

$$\frac{\partial^2 \varnothing(x,t)}{\partial x^2} = \frac{q}{\varepsilon}(p - n + n_d - n_a) \tag{3}$$

where ε is the dielectric permittivity of the blend. n_d and n_a are the densities of ionized donor and acceptor impurities, respectively.

2.4. Charge Pair Density Equation

The volume density of geminate charge pairs (X) is described by the following equation [28]:

$$\frac{\partial X}{\partial t} = G(x,t) + \gamma np - (k_{diss} + k_{rec})X \tag{4}$$

where $G(x,t)$ is the charge pairs generation rate. k_{rec} is The monomolecular recombination rate.

2.5. Current Density Equations

The current density equations describe the flow of charge carriers in the device. They are modified to include the fractional drift terms as follows [8,9]:

$$J_n = q\mu_n nE - \mu_n k_B T\frac{\partial^\alpha n}{\partial x^\alpha} \tag{5}$$

$$J_p = q\mu_p pE + \mu_p k_B T\frac{\partial^\alpha p}{\partial x^\alpha} \tag{6}$$

$$J = q(J_p - J_n), \qquad q > 0 \tag{7}$$

where $\begin{cases} J_n \text{ and } J_p \text{ are the electron and hole current densities, respectively } (A/cm^2) \\ E = -\frac{\partial \varnothing}{\partial x} \text{ is the electric field magnitude} \\ J \text{ is the total current density } (A/cm^2) \end{cases}$.

To establish the initial conditions, we solve the system of Equations (1)–(4) at steady state. This entails setting the α-order time derivatives of the electron density, hole density, and charge pair density to zero:

$$\frac{\mu_n k_B T}{q}\frac{d^\beta n}{dx^\beta} - \mu_n \frac{d^\alpha}{dx^\alpha}\left(n\frac{d\varnothing}{dx}\right) + k_{diss}X - \gamma np = 0 \tag{8}$$

$$\frac{\mu_p k_B T}{q}\frac{d^\beta p}{dx^\beta} + \mu_p \frac{d^\alpha}{dx^\alpha}\left(p\frac{d\varnothing}{dx}\right) + k_{diss}X - \gamma np = 0 \tag{9}$$

$$\frac{d^2\varnothing}{dx^2} = \frac{q}{\varepsilon}(p - n + n_d - n_a) \tag{10}$$

$$G + \gamma np - (k_{diss} + k_{rec})X = 0 \tag{11}$$

The boundary conditions can be described as [8,13,16,33,42]:

$$\begin{bmatrix} n(0) \\ p(0) \\ n(L) \\ p(L) \end{bmatrix} = \begin{bmatrix} N_c\, e^{(-B_n/k_B T)} \\ N_v\, e^{-(E_{gap}-B_n/k_B T)} \\ N_c\, e^{-(E_{gap}-B_p/k_B T)} \\ N_v\, e^{(-B_p/k_B T)} \end{bmatrix} \tag{12}$$

where n(0), p(0), n(L), p(L) represent the concentrations (or densities) of electrons (n) and holes (p) at the boundaries x = 0 and x = L. Units: particles/cm^3 or cm^{-3}. If the contact for electron (hole) is ohmic, there is no energy barrier for electron (hole). The boundary condition for the potential is

$$\varnothing(L) - (0) = \frac{E_{gap} - B_n - B_p}{q} - V_a \tag{13}$$

where B_n and B_p are the electron and hole energy barrier, respectively. N_c and N_v (cm^{-3}) are the effective density of states of conduction band and valence band. E_{gap} is band gap energy. V_a is the applied voltage [46,47].

3. Method of Solution

We try to develop a mathematical solution for organic polymer solar cells. These cells are complex and involve several factors, including the movement of charged particles (diffusion reaction), imbalances in electrical charge (electrostatic convection), and chemical reactions (kinetic ordinary differential equation). To solve this problem, we apply a special mathematical technique (differential quadrature) that uses different types of shape functions (polynomial and cardinal sine) alongside a step-by-step approach (block marching technique).

This work dives into fractional derivatives, a mathematical concept with various definitions. We will be focusing on the most widely accepted one, developed by Caputo.

3.1. Caputo's Fractional Derivative

Leveraging the established framework of the Riemann–Liouville fractional derivative [48], Caputo introduced a new way to define fractional derivatives. This definition, known as Caputo's fractional derivative, is expressed in the following equation, as shown by Weilbeer [49]:

If $\lambda \in R^+$, "κ" is a positive integer, and $\kappa - 1 < \lambda < \kappa$. Thus, the Riemann–Liouville fractional derivative, a generalization of the classical derivative, is defined for a function $u(t)$ of order $\lambda,(\alpha,\beta)$, is defined as:

$$D_a^{\lambda} u(t) = \frac{1}{\Gamma(\kappa-\lambda)} \frac{d^{\kappa}}{dt^{\kappa}} \int_a^t (t-x)^{\kappa-\lambda-1} u^{\kappa}(x) dx\,, \tag{14}$$

There is a specific way to calculate the fractional derivative of a function, introduced by Caputo. This method involves taking a regular integer-order derivative a certain number of times (based on the order λ) and then applying a mathematical integral over a specific interval.

$$D_a^{\lambda} u(t) = \begin{cases} \frac{1}{\Gamma(\kappa-\lambda)} \frac{d^{\kappa}}{dt^{\kappa}} \int_a^t (t-x)^{\kappa-\lambda-1} u^{\kappa}(x) dx, & \kappa - 1 < \lambda < \kappa \\ \frac{d^{\kappa} u}{dt^{\kappa}}, & \kappa = \lambda \end{cases} \tag{15}$$

where the integration begins at the value represented by "a". The notation $D_a^{\lambda} u(t)$ represents how the function $u(t)$ changes over time, but in a more general way than regular derivatives. It is a fractional derivative of $u(t)$.

For $\lambda = \kappa$, the equation recovers the standard integer-order derivative.

Moving on, we will define the differential quadrature method. This approach relies on different functionalities (represented by "shape functions") to tackle problems:

3.2. Using Lagrange Polynomials Within the Differential Quadrature Method (PDQM)

Within the framework of this shape function, the functional evaluations of an arbitrary unknown function $u(t)$ at a predetermined set of N grid points can be represented as the vector [50].

$$u(t_i) = \sum_{j=1}^{N} \frac{\prod_{k=1}^{N} [t_i - t_k]}{(t_i - t_j) \prod_{k \neq 1,\; j=1}^{N} [t_j - t_k]} u(t_j), \qquad (i = 1:N) \tag{16}$$

Consequently, the expressions for the various derivatives of the unknown function $u(t)$ can be derived as follows:

$$\left.\frac{\partial^n u}{\partial t^n}\right|_{t=t_i} = \sum_{j=1}^{N} \mathcal{R}_{ij}^{(n)} u(t_j), \qquad (i = 1:N) \tag{17}$$

where $\mathcal{R}_{ij}^{(n)}$ represents the weighting coefficient associated with the nth derivative. However, the accuracy of the DQM hinges critically upon the determination of these weighting coefficients. Consequently, the specific values of $\mathcal{R}_{ij}^{(n)}$ depend on the chosen shape function.

Therefore, the weighting coefficients $\mathcal{R}_{ij}^{(1)}$ associated with the first derivative and $\mathcal{R}_{ij}^{(2)}$ associated with the second derivative can be obtained by differentiating Equation (16).

$$\mathcal{R}_{ij}^{(1)} = \begin{cases} \frac{1}{(t_i - t_j)} \prod_{k=1,\; k \neq i,j}^{N} \frac{(t_i - t_k)}{(t_j - t_k)} & i \neq j \\ -\sum_{j=1,\; j \neq i}^{N} \mathcal{R}_{ij}^{(1)} & i = j \end{cases}, \qquad \mathcal{R}_{ij}^{(2)} = \left[\mathcal{R}_{ij}^{(1)}\right]\left[\mathcal{R}_{ij}^{(1)}\right], \tag{18}$$

3.3. Using Cardinal Sine Within the Differential Quadrature Method (SDQM)

Within this methodology, the Cardinal sine function is adopted as the shape function. This enables the approximation of the unknown function $u(t)$ and its nth derivatives via a weighted linear summation of nodal values, u_i, for i ranging from $-N$ to N, as expressed in the following equation [51]:

$$S_j(t_i,\Delta)=\frac{sin\left(\frac{\pi}{\Delta}(t_i-t_j)\right)}{\frac{\pi}{\Delta}(t_i-t_j)} \tag{19}$$

$$u(t_i)=\sum_{j=-N}^{N}\frac{sin\left(\frac{\pi}{\Delta}(t_i-t_j)\right)}{\frac{\pi}{\Delta}(t_i-t_j)}u(t_j), \qquad (i=-N:N) \tag{20}$$

where Δ is the positive step size, and N represents the number of grid points employed in the discretization.

Consequently, the expressions for the various derivatives of the unknown function $u(t)$ can be derived as follows [52]:

$$\left.\frac{\partial u}{\partial t}\right|_{t=t_i}=\sum_{j=-N}^{N}\mathcal{R}_{ij}^{(1)}u(t_j), \qquad \left.\frac{\partial^2 u}{\partial t^2}\right|_{t=t_i}=\sum_{j=-N}^{N}\mathcal{R}_{ij}^{(2)}u(t_j) \qquad (i=-N:N) \tag{21}$$

Therefore, the weighting coefficients $\mathcal{R}_{ij}^{(1)}$ associated with the first derivative and $\mathcal{R}_{ij}^{(2)}$ associated with the second derivative can be obtained by differentiating Equation (20).

$$\mathcal{R}_{ij}^{(1)}=\begin{cases}\frac{(-1)^{i-j}}{\Delta(i-j)} & i\neq j\\ 0 & i=j\end{cases}, \quad \mathcal{R}_{ij}^{(2)}=\begin{cases}\frac{2(-1)^{1+i-j}}{(\Delta(i-j))^2} & i\neq j\\ \frac{-\pi^2}{3\Delta^2} & i=j\end{cases} \tag{22}$$

Within the Caputo framework, the weighting coefficients utilized in the fractional derivative formulations of PDQM and SDQM can be acquired by applying Equations (14) and (15) to Equations (17) and (21), respectively. This procedure results in the following expressions:

a. The Caputo fractional derivative of order α, where α is a real number within the open interval (0, 1), is defined as:

$$D^{\alpha}u(t)=\begin{cases}\frac{1}{\Gamma(1-\alpha)}\int_a^t(t-x)^{-\alpha}\,\grave{u}(x)dx=\sum_{j=1}^{N}\mathcal{R}_{ij}^{\alpha}\,u(t_j,x) & 0<\alpha<1\\ \sum_{j=1}^{N}\mathcal{R}_{ij}^{(1)}u(t_j,x) & \alpha=1\end{cases} \tag{23}$$

b. The Caputo fractional derivative of order β, where β is a real number within the open interval (1, 2), is defined as [27]:

$$D^{\beta}u(t)=\begin{cases}\frac{1}{\Gamma(2-\beta)}\int_a^t(t-x)^{1-\beta}\,\grave{u}(x)dx=\sum_{j=1}^{N}\mathcal{R}_{ij}^{\beta}\,u(t_j,x) & 1<\beta<2\\ \sum_{j=1}^{N}\mathcal{R}_{ij}^{(2)}u(t_j,x) & \beta=2\end{cases} \tag{24}$$

Subsequently, the weighting coefficients are determined through the following expression:

$$\mathcal{R}_{ij}^{\alpha}=A^{1-\alpha}\mathcal{R}_{ij}^{(1)}-\frac{\mathcal{R}_{1.j}^{(1)}}{\Gamma(2-\alpha)}(t-a)^{1-\alpha} \tag{25}$$

$$\mathcal{R}_{ij}^{\beta}=B^{2-\beta}\mathcal{R}_{ij}^{(2)}-\frac{\mathcal{R}_{1.j}^{(2)}}{\Gamma(3-\beta)}(t-a)^{2-\beta} \tag{26}$$

where A_{ij} and B_{ij} represent the fractional weighting coefficients for the Caputo derivatives of order $\alpha \in (0,1)$ and $\beta \in (1,2)$, respectively. These coefficients are calculated as follows: $A_{ij} = \mathcal{R}_{ij}^{(1)} - \mathcal{R}_{1j}^{(1)}$ and $B_{ij} = \mathcal{R}_{ij}^{(2)} - \mathcal{R}_{1j}^{(2)}$.

The validity of Equations (25) and (26) can be established through the following demonstration:

For $\alpha \in (0,1)$ let,

$$J^{\alpha}u(t) = \frac{1}{\Gamma(\alpha)}\int_{a}^{t} (t-x)^{\alpha-1}u(x)dx$$

Then,

$$\begin{gathered} \dot{u}(a) = d\,u(a) \to d = \mathcal{R}_{1,j}^{(1)} \\ J^{\alpha}\dot{u}(a) = d\,J^{\alpha}u(a) = d\frac{u(a)}{\Gamma(\alpha)}\int_{a}^{t} (t-x)^{\alpha-1}\,dx = \frac{u(a)}{\Gamma(\alpha+1)}d\,(t-a)^{\alpha} \end{gathered} \tag{27}$$

Therefore,

$$J_a^{1-\alpha}\dot{u}(a) = \frac{u(a)}{\Gamma(2-\alpha)}d\,(t-a)^{1-\alpha} \tag{28}$$

Furthermore,

$$\int_{a}^{t} u(t)dt = \sum_{j=1}^{N}\left(\mathcal{R}_{ij}^{(1)} - \mathcal{R}_{1j}^{(1)}\right)u(t_j,x) \to A_{ij} = \mathcal{R}_{ij}^{(1)} - \mathcal{R}_{1j}^{(1)} \tag{29}$$

Then,

$$\begin{gathered} J^{1}u(t) = \int_{a}^{t} u(x)dx = Au(t) \\ \text{and} \\ J^{2}u(t) = \int_{a}^{t}\int_{a}^{t} u(x)dx = \int_{a}^{t} (t-x)u(x)dx = A^{2}u(t) \end{gathered} \tag{30}$$

So,

$$J^{\alpha}u(t) = A^{\alpha}u(t) \to J^{1-\alpha}\dot{u}(t) = A^{1-\alpha}\mathcal{R}_{ij}^{(1)}u(t) \tag{31}$$

Within the same framework, the weighting coefficients associated with the Caputo fractional derivative of order $\beta \in (1,2)$ can be ascertained by employing an analogous procedure.

Building upon the prior analysis of governing Equations (8)–(11) under steady-state conditions, a more concise representation can be derived using DQM. This simplified form is presented below:

$$\begin{gathered} \frac{\mu_n k_B T}{q}\sum_{j=1}^{N} \mathcal{R}_{ij}^{\beta}n_j - \mu_n n_i \sum_{j=1}^{N} \mathcal{R}_{ij}^{\beta}\varnothing_j - \mu_n \sum_{k=1}^{N} \mathcal{R}_{ik}^{(1)}\varnothing_k \sum_{j=1}^{N} \mathcal{R}_{ij}^{\alpha}n_j + k_{diss}\sum_{j=1}^{N} \delta_{ij}X_j \\ -\gamma \sum_{k=1}^{N} \delta_{ik}n \sum_{kj=1}^{N} \delta_{ij}p_j = 0, \end{gathered} \tag{32}$$

$$\begin{gathered} \frac{\mu_p k_B T}{q}\sum_{j=1}^{N} \mathcal{R}_{ij}^{\beta}p_j + \mu_p p_i \sum_{j=1}^{N} \mathcal{R}_{ij}^{\beta}\varnothing_j + \mu_p \sum_{k=1}^{N} \mathcal{R}_{ik}^{(1)}\varnothing_k \sum_{j=1}^{N} \mathcal{R}_{ij}^{\alpha}p_j + k_{diss}\sum_{j=1}^{N} \delta_{ij}X_j \\ -\gamma \sum_{k=1}^{N} \delta_{ik}n_k \sum_{j=1}^{N} \delta_{ij}p_j = 0, \end{gathered} \tag{33}$$

$$\sum_{j=1}^{N} \mathcal{R}_{ij}^{(2)}\varnothing_j = \frac{q}{\varepsilon}\left(\sum_{j=1}^{N} \delta_{ij}p_j - \sum_{j=1}^{N} \delta_{ij}n_j + n_d - n_a\right) \tag{34}$$

$$\gamma \sum_{k=1}^{N} \delta_{ik} n \sum_{kj=1}^{N} \delta_{ij} p_j - (k_{diss} + k_{rec}) \sum_{j=1}^{N} \delta_{ij} X_j = -G \tag{35}$$

Consequently, this analysis enables the determination of the initial conditions for $n,\ p,\ X,$ and $\varnothing$ at time $t = 0$.

In order to address time-dependent partial differential equations (PDEs) and convert them into a system of algebraic equations, the block-marching method is employed. This technique offers enhanced accuracy for the DQM regardless of the chosen shape function. A detailed explanation of this method is provided subsequently:

3.4. Differential Quadrature Discretization via the Block-Marching Method

The governing Equations (1)–(4) represent one-dimensional phenomena that evolve over time. To solve such time-dependent models, the block-marching method [53] is implemented. This technique discretizes the semi-infinite domain in the time direction (t) by segmenting it into a series of finite time intervals denoted by $\delta t^1, \delta t^2, \delta t^3, \ldots,$etc. Each individual block encompasses a single time interval (δt) and the entire spatial domain in the x-direction, ranging from x = 0 to x = L_x.

To maintain consistency within the block-marching scheme, all blocks employ a uniform grid distribution. This is achieved by ensuring equal time increments across all blocks, denoted by $\delta t^1 = \delta t^2 = \delta t^3 = \ldots,\ ect.$ The reference [54] provides details regarding the specific mesh sizes adopted in both the x-direction (spatial) and t-direction (temporal) for each nth block:

$$x_i = \frac{1}{2} L_x \left(1 - cos\left(\frac{\pi(i-1)}{N-1}\right)\right), \qquad (i = 1:N) \tag{36}$$

$$t_i = \delta t\left((\mathcal{H} - 1) + \frac{1}{2}\left(1 - cos\left(\frac{\pi(k-1)}{L-1}\right)\right)\right), \qquad (k = 1:L) \tag{37}$$

Within this framework, $\mathcal{H}$ represents the total number of blocks employed in the discretization process. N signifies the number of grid points used to discretize the spatial domain (x-direction), and L indicates the specific time level associated with each block.

Following the analysis of the governing Equations (1)–(4) presented earlier, a simplified form can be expressed as:

$$\begin{aligned} \frac{\mu_n k_B T}{q} \sum_{j=1}^{N} \mathcal{R}_{ij}^{\beta} n_j - \mu_n n_i \sum_{j=1}^{N} \mathcal{R}_{ij}^{\beta} \varnothing_j - \mu_n \sum_{k=1}^{N} \mathcal{R}_{ik}^{(1)} \varnothing_k \sum_{j=1}^{N} \mathcal{R}_{ij}^{\alpha} n_j + k_{diss} \sum_{j=1}^{N} \delta_{ij} X_j \\ -\gamma \sum_{k=1}^{N} \delta_{ik} n_k \sum_{j=1}^{N} \delta_{ij} p_j = \sum_{j=1}^{N} \overline{\mathcal{R}}_{ij}^{\alpha} n_j, \end{aligned} \tag{38}$$

$$\begin{aligned} \frac{\mu_p k_B T}{q} \sum_{j=1}^{N} \mathcal{R}_{ij}^{\beta} p_j + \mu_p p_i \sum_{j=1}^{N} \mathcal{R}_{ij}^{\beta} \varnothing_j + \mu_p \sum_{k=1}^{N} \mathcal{R}_{ik}^{(1)} \varnothing_k \sum_{j=1}^{N} \mathcal{R}_{ij}^{\alpha} p_j + k_{diss} \sum_{j=1}^{N} \delta_{ij} X_j \\ -\gamma \sum_{k=1}^{N} \delta_{ik} n_k \sum_{j=1}^{N} \delta_{ij} p_j = \sum_{j=1}^{N} \overline{\mathcal{R}}_{ij}^{\alpha} p_j, \end{aligned} \tag{39}$$

$$\sum_{j=1}^{N} \mathcal{R}_{ij}^{(2)} \varnothing_j = \frac{q}{\varepsilon}\left(\sum_{j=1}^{N} \delta_{ij} p_j - \sum_{j=1}^{N} \delta_{ij} n_j + n_d - n_a\right) \tag{40}$$

$$G + \gamma \sum_{k=1}^{N} \delta_{ik} n_k \sum_{j=1}^{N} \delta_{ij} p_j - (k_{diss} + k_{rec}) \sum_{j=1}^{N} \delta_{ij} X_j = \sum_{j=1}^{N} \overline{\mathcal{R}}_{ij}^{(1)} X_j \tag{41}$$

Within this framework, $\overline{\mathcal{R}}_{ij}^{\alpha}$ denotes the weighting coefficient associated with the fractional derivative of order α in the time domain (t). Here, $\overline{\mathcal{R}}_{ij}^{(1)}$ specifically represents the weighting coefficient for the first-order time derivative.

To incorporate the influence of boundary conditions on the overall system behavior, the governing Equations (38)–(41) are augmented with the boundary conditions (12) and (13) applicable to all cases. Subsequently, the iterative quadrature technique, as detailed in references [16,17,32], is employed to transform this system into a linear algebraic problem:

1- The initial step involves solving Equations (38)–(41) as a linear system:

$$\frac{\mu_n k_B T}{q}\sum_{j=1}^{N}\mathcal{R}_{ij}^{\beta} n_j + k_{diss}\sum_{j=1}^{N}\delta_{ij}X_j = \sum_{j=1}^{N}\overline{\mathcal{R}}_{ij}^{\alpha} n_j, \quad (42)$$

$$\frac{\mu_p k_B T}{q}\sum_{j=1}^{N}\mathcal{R}_{ij}^{\beta} p_j + k_{diss}\sum_{j=1}^{N}\delta_{ij}X_j = \sum_{j=1}^{N}\overline{\mathcal{R}}_{ij}^{\alpha} p_j, \quad (43)$$

$$\sum_{j=1}^{N}\mathcal{R}_{ij}^{(2)}\varnothing_j = \frac{q}{\varepsilon}\left(\sum_{j=1}^{N}\delta_{ij}p_j - \sum_{j=1}^{N}\delta_{ij}n_j + n_d - n_a\right) \quad (44)$$

$$G - (k_{diss} + k_{rec})\sum_{j=1}^{N}\delta_{ij}X_j = \sum_{j=1}^{N}\overline{\mathcal{R}}_{ij}^{(1)} X_j \quad (45)$$

2- Subsequently, an iterative solution procedure is implemented to solve the system of equations. This iterative process continues until a pre-defined convergence criterion is satisfied.

$$\left|\frac{n_{r+1}}{n_r}\right| < 1 \left|\frac{p_{r+1}}{p_r}\right| < 1$$

where $r = 0, 1, 2, \ldots$

$$\begin{aligned}\frac{\mu_n k_B T}{q}\sum_{j=1}^{N}\mathcal{R}_{ij}^{\beta} n_{r+1,\,j} - \mu_n n_{r,i}\sum_{j=1}^{N}\mathcal{R}_{ij}^{\beta}\varnothing_j - \mu_n\sum_{k=1}^{N}\mathcal{R}_{ik}^{(1)}\varnothing_k\sum_{j=1}^{N}\mathcal{R}_{ij}^{\alpha} n_{r,\,j} + k_{diss}\sum_{j=1}^{N}\delta_{ij}X_j \\ -\gamma\sum_{k=1}^{N}\delta_{ik}n_{r,\,k}\sum_{j=1}^{N}\delta_{ij}p_{r+1,\,j} = \sum_{j=1}^{N}\overline{\mathcal{R}}_{ij}^{\alpha} n_{r+1,\,j},\end{aligned} \quad (46)$$

$$\begin{aligned}\frac{\mu_p k_B T}{q}\sum_{j=1}^{N}\mathcal{R}_{ij}^{\beta} p_{r+1,\,j} + \mu_p p_{r,\,i}\sum_{j=1}^{N}\mathcal{R}_{ij}^{\beta}\varnothing_j + \mu_p\sum_{k=1}^{N}\mathcal{R}_{ik}^{(1)}\varnothing_k\sum_{j=1}^{N}\mathcal{R}_{ij}^{\alpha} p_{r,\,j} + k_{diss}\sum_{j=1}^{N}\delta_{ij}X_j \\ -\gamma\sum_{k=1}^{N}\delta_{ik}n_{r+1,\,k}\sum_{j=1}^{N}\delta_{ij}p_{r,\,j} = \sum_{j=1}^{N}\overline{\mathcal{R}}_{ij}^{\alpha} p_{r+1,\,j},\end{aligned} \quad (47)$$

$$\sum_{j=1}^{N}\mathcal{R}_{ij}^{(2)}\varnothing_j = \frac{q}{\varepsilon}\left(\sum_{j=1}^{N}\delta_{ij}p_{r+1,\,j} - \sum_{j=1}^{N}\delta_{ij}n_{r+1,\,j} + n_d - n_a\right) \quad (48)$$

$$G + \gamma\sum_{k=1}^{N}\delta_{ik}n_{r,\,k}\sum_{j=1}^{N}\delta_{ij}p_{r,\,j} - (k_{diss} + k_{rec})\sum_{j=1}^{N}\delta_{ij}X_j = \sum_{j=1}^{N}\overline{\mathcal{R}}_{ij}^{(1)} X_j \quad (49)$$

4. Study Results

The implemented numerical methods exhibit convergence and efficiency in analyzing photocurrent transients within organic polymer solar cells. This analysis aims to optimize power efficiency. Each scheme's computational characteristics are tailored to achieve high accuracy, ensuring an error margin on the order of 10^{-8} or less. The error analysis draws upon the methodology presented in [55,56]:

$$L_\infty = \left\|u_{exact} - u_{computed}\right\|_\infty = max_j\left|u_j^{exact} - u_j^{computed}\right| \quad (50)$$

The following section presents the results obtained for each proposed method. A subsequent comparative analysis will be conducted to evaluate their relative performance.

The PDQM approach tackles this problem by employing a non-uniform grid. This grid is constructed using a Gauss–Chebyshev–Lobatto (GCL) discretization technique, as described in detail within Equations (36) and (37). The size of the grid (N) is systematically varied, encompassing a range of 5 to 30 points within a single block ($\mathcal{H}$). Table 1 showcases the L_∞ error norms obtained using this non-uniform PDQM method for various temporal grid sizes (δt). The computations are conducted on a domain of [0, 1] with a fixed spatial step size ($\Delta x = 0.01$) and a specified fractional order ($\beta = 2$). The table also includes additional parameters (μ_n, μ_p, k_{rec}, and G) for reference. An important observation from Table 1 is that the L_∞ error norms exhibit a decrease as the temporal discretization (δt) is refined for both $\alpha = 1$ and $\alpha = 0.8$. This behavior confirms the convergence of the non-uniform PDQM method. Furthermore, the CPU times associated with the non-uniform PDQM method are generally lower than those reported in prior studies [19,44] for both $\alpha = 1$ and $\alpha = 0.8$. This finding suggests that the non-uniform PDQM method might be more computationally efficient compared to the methods employed in previous research [19,44]. Table 1 also reveals that the L_∞ error norms are slightly lower for $\alpha = 0.8$ compared to $\alpha = 1$. This implies that the non-uniform PDQM method might achieve higher accuracy for $\alpha = 0.8$. However, it is crucial to note that this enhanced accuracy comes at the cost of increased CPU times, as observed previously. Therefore, selecting the appropriate fractional order necessitates a careful consideration of the trade-off between accuracy and computational efficiency.

Table 1. L_∞ Error norms computed using non-uniform PDQM at various temporal discretizations (δt) with fixed spatial discretization $\Delta x = 0.01$ and fractional order $\beta = 2$ ($\mu_n = \mu_p = 2 \times 10^{-4}$ cm^{2}V^{-1}S^{-1}, $k_{rec} = 10^7$ s^{-1}, and $G = 4.3 \times 10^{26}$ m^{-3}s^{-1}).

δt	$\alpha = 1$		δt	$\alpha = 1$		δt	$\alpha = 0.8$		δt	$\alpha = 0.8$	
	Non-Uniform PDQM	CPU Time		Previous Studies [19,44]	CPU Time		Non-Uniform PDQM	CPU Time		Previous Studies [19,44]	CPU Time
1/5	0.0006	1.15	1/100	1.118×10^{-4}	15.8	1/5	0.0003	1.18	1/100	4.443×10^{-5}	16.1
1/10	3.6325×10^{-5}	1.17	1/200	5.416×10^{-5}	26.4	1/10	1.0445×10^{-5}	1.205	1/200	1.277×10^{-5}	27.3
1/15	2.2635×10^{-5}	1.2	1/400	2.300×10^{-5}	49.0	1/15	8.2147×10^{-6}	1.22	1/400	3.033×10^{-6}	49.6
1/20	7.5990×10^{-5}	1.23	1/800	6.886×10^{-6}	89.5	1/20	5.1110×10^{-6}	1.25	1/800	1.103×10^{-6}	91.4
1/25	4.0251×10^{-6}	1.3	1/1600	2.005×10^{-6}	156.8	1/25	1.3281×10^{-6}	1.33	1/1600	3.946×10^{-7}	162.8
1/30	3.9523×10^{-6}	1.35	---	---	---	1/30	9.0147×10^{-7}	1.4	---	---	---

Table 2 presents the L_∞ error norms computed using a non-uniform PDQM method for various discretizations of the problem. The discretizations include:

- Number of blocks ($\mathcal{H}$): This controls the overall number of subintervals in the time domain. The L_∞ error norms generally decrease as the number of blocks ($\mathcal{H}$) increases for a fixed number of time levels (L) and temporal discretization (δt). This suggests that using more blocks can improve the accuracy of the non-uniform PDQM method. However, the CPU time also increases with the number of blocks, as there are more subintervals to compute over.
- Time levels associated with each block (L): This determines the number of grid points within each block. The L_∞ error norms generally decrease as the number of time levels (L) increases for a fixed number of blocks ($\mathcal{H}$) and temporal discretization (δt). This indicates that using more time levels within each block refines the grid and leads to higher accuracy. As with block numbers, this improvement in accuracy comes at the cost of increased CPU time.
- Temporal discretization (δt): This represents the size of the time steps used in the computations. The L_∞ error norms decrease as the temporal discretization (δt) gets smaller (finer grid) for all values of $\mathcal{H}$ and L shown in the table. This confirms that the non-uniform PDQM method is convergent for the given conditions. There is a trade-off here as well, with a finer grid size leading to more accurate results but requiring more computational resources.

Table 2. L_∞ Error norms computed using non-uniform PDQM at various numbers of blocks ($\mathcal{H}$), time levels associated with each block (L), and temporal discretizations (δt) with fixed spatial discretization $\Delta x = 0.01$ and fractional orders $\alpha = 0.9$ and $\beta = 2$ ($\mu_n = \mu_p = 2 \times 10^{-4}$ cm^{2}V^{-1}S^{-1}, $k_{rec} = 10^7$ s^{-1}, and $G = 4.3 \times 10^{26}$ m^{-3}s^{-1}).

L	δt	$\mathcal{H}$=1		$\mathcal{H}$=3		$\mathcal{H}$=5		$\mathcal{H}$=7		δt	Previous Studies [19,44]	CPU Time
		Non-Uniform PDQM	CPU Time	Non-Uniform PDQM	CPU Time	Non-Uniform PDQM	CPU Time	Non-Uniform PDQM	CPU Time			
$L = 4$	1/5	0.005	0.90	0.00099	1.20	0.0003	1.23	1.9717×10^{-5}	1.26	1/100	7.443×10^{-5}	15.6
	1/10	9.8250×10^{-4}	1.05	5.3124×10^{-5}	1.25	1.0616×10^{-5}	1.27	8.5178×10^{-6}	130	1/200	3.085×10^{-5}	26.2
	1/15	5.8749×10^{-4}	1.10	4.0198×10^{-5}	1.30	8.2288×10^{-6}	1.33	5.8777×10^{-6}	1.37	1/400	8.391×10^{-6}	48.9
	1/20	9.0230×10^{-5}	1.15	6.3132×10^{-6}	1.35	5.2317×10^{-6}	1.38	1.9466×10^{-6}	1.41	1/800	3.141×10^{-6}	88.7
	1/25	6.8764×10^{-5}	1.20	4.8327×10^{-6}	1.42	1.3660×10^{-6}	1.46	9.9989×10^{-7}	1.49	1/1600	9.358×10^{-7}	155.2
	1/30	4.0005×10^{-5}	1.25	2.2222×10^{-6}	1.47	9.1489×10^{-7}	1.51	6.7713×10^{-7}	1.54	---	---	---
$L = 8$	1/5	0.00099	1.15	0.00007	1.28	8.9470×10^{-5}	1.32	9.1397×10^{-6}	1.35	1/100	7.443×10^{-5}	15.6
	1/10	4.7315×10^{-5}	1.17	1.7146×10^{-5}	1.36	9.8732×10^{-6}	1.37	6.7486×10^{-6}	141	1/200	3.085×10^{-5}	26.2
	1/15	3.7195×10^{-5}	1.20	9.7412×10^{-6}	1.41	5.9702×10^{-6}	1.45	4.0877×10^{-6}	1.50	1/400	8.391×10^{-6}	48.9
	1/20	7.4700×10^{-6}	1.23	4.1415×10^{-6}	1.47	3.0017×10^{-6}	1.54	9.1486×10^{-7}	1.58	1/800	3.141×10^{-6}	88.7
	1/25	4.6233×10^{-6}	1.30	2.0337×10^{-6}	1.53	9.8200×10^{-7}	1.60	6.3144×10^{-7}	1.63	1/1600	9.358×10^{-7}	155.2
	1/30	2.9583×10^{-6}	1.35	9.8714×10^{-7}	1.60	7.1739×10^{-7}	1.66	4.0053×10^{-7}	1.72	---	---	---
$L = 12$	1/5	0.00045	1.18	3.8215×10^{-5}	1.35	1.7493×10^{-5}	1.40	7.0805×10^{-6}	1.42	1/100	7.443×10^{-5}	15.6
	1/10	2.1375×10^{-5}	1.19	8.7657×10^{-6}	1.40	7.0355×10^{-6}	1.44	4.6245×10^{-6}	147	1/200	3.085×10^{-5}	26.2
	1/15	1.0009×10^{-5}	1.20	6.0247×10^{-6}	1.48	3.6974×10^{-6}	1.53	1.9143×10^{-6}	1.55	1/400	8.391×10^{-6}	48.9
	1/20	6.1240×10^{-6}	1.24	2.0522×10^{-6}	1.56	1.8179×10^{-6}	1.63	8.8887×10^{-7}	1.70	1/800	3.141×10^{-6}	88.7
	1/25	2.9140×10^{-6}	1.31	9.3414×10^{-7}	1.61	6.8397×10^{-7}	1.67	3.4422×10^{-7}	1.75	1/1600	9.358×10^{-7}	155.2
	1/30	1.9975×10^{-6}	1.37	7.0329×10^{-7}	1.66	3.9274×10^{-7}	1.72	1.8005×10^{-7}	1.80	---	---	---

The table also includes fixed values for the spatial discretization ($\Delta x = 0.01$) and fractional orders ($\alpha = 0.9$, $\beta = 2$), along with references to previous studies [19,44] for comparison. The CPU times of the non-uniform PDQM method are generally lower than those reported in previous studies [19,44] for most cases. This suggests that the non-uniform PDQM method might be more computationally efficient for solving this particular problem.

Also, Table 3 investigates the convergence and computational efficiency of the non-uniform PDQM method for solving fractional-order differential equations. It presents the L_∞ error norms obtained using this method for various temporal discretizations (δt) with a fixed spatial discretization (Δx) and two specific fractional orders ($\beta = 1.9$ and $\beta = 1.7$). The grid size (N) is systematically varied within a single block ($\mathbb{R}$), ranging from 5 to 30 points. The table also includes CPU times associated with the non-uniform PDQM computations. The results demonstrate that the L_∞ error norms generally decrease as the temporal discretization (δt) gets smaller (finer grid) for both $\beta = 1.9$ and $\beta = 1.7$. This behavior suggests that the non-uniform PDQM method is convergent for these fractional orders. As the grid becomes finer, the numerical solution approaches the exact solution, leading to a reduction in the error norms. While a definitive conclusion regarding the impact of fractional order (β) on accuracy cannot be drawn solely from Table 3, it is possible to compare the error norms for different β values (e.g., $\beta = 1.9$ and $\beta = 1.7$) at the same temporal discretization (δt). If one β value consistently results in lower error norms, it might indicate that the non-uniform PDQM method exhibits higher accuracy for that particular fractional order.

In conclusion, Table 3 provides evidence that the non-uniform PDQM method is convergent for the given problem with different fractional orders (β). The CPU times included in the table further suggest that the method offers computational efficiency.

Table 4 shows the L_∞ error norms computed using a non-uniform PDQM method at various numbers of blocks ($\mathcal{H}$), time levels associated with each block (L), and temporal discretizations (δt) with a fixed spatial discretization ($\Delta x = 0.01$) and fractional orders ($\alpha = 1$ and $\beta = 1.8$). The table also includes references to previous studies [19,44].

Table 3. L_∞ Error norms computed using non-uniform PDQM at various temporal discretizations (δt) with fixed spatial discretization $\Delta x = 0.01$ and fractional order $\alpha = 1$ ($\mu_n = \mu_p = 2 \times 10^{-4}$ $cm^2V^{-1}S^{-1}$, $k_{rec} = 10^7$ s^{-1}, and $G = 4.3 \times 10^{26}$ $m^{-3}s^{-1}$).

	$\beta = 1.9$			$\beta = 1.9$			$\beta = 1.7$			$\beta = 1.7$	
δt	Non-Uniform PDQM	CPU Time	δt	Previous Studies [19,44]	CPU Time	δt	Non-Uniform PDQM	CPU Time	δt	Previous Studies [19,44]	CPU Time
1/5	0.0006	1.33	1/100	5.936×10^{-4}	18.2	1/5	0.0009	1.35	1/100	8.828×10^{-4}	18.7
1/10	8.7238×10^{-5}	1.40	1/200	5.639×10^{-4}	27.9	1/10	1.8471×10^{-4}	1.43	1/200	8.590×10^{-4}	31.7
1/15	8.544×10^{-5}	1.47	1/400	5.485×10^{-4}	55.8	1/15	1.8102×10^{-4}	1.50	1/400	8.472×10^{-4}	58.4
1/20	8.3050×10^{-5}	1.53	1/800	5.407×10^{-4}	111.5	1/20	1.7887×10^{-4}	1.56	1/800	8.413×10^{-4}	109.1
1/25	8.1201×10^{-5}	1.60	1/1600	5.368×10^{-4}	181.4	1/25	1.7524×10^{-4}	1.64	1/1600	8.384×10^{-4}	201.5
1/30	7.9003×10^{-5}	1.65	---	---	---	1/30	1.7093×10^{-4}	1.70	---	---	---

Table 4. L_∞ Error norms computed using non-uniform PDQM at various numbers of blocks ($\mathcal{H}$), time levels associated with each block (L), and temporal discretizations (δt) with fixed spatial discretization $\Delta x = 0.01$ and fractional orders $\alpha = 1$ and $\beta = 1.8$ ($\mu_n = \mu_p = 2 \times 10^{-4}$ $cm^2V^{-1}S^{-1}$, $k_{rec} = 10^7$ s^{-1}, and $G = 4.3 \times 10^{26}$ $m^{-3}s^{-1}$).

		$\mathcal{H} = 1$		$\mathcal{H} = 3$		$\mathcal{H} = 5$		$\mathcal{H} = 7$				
l	δt	Non-Uniform PDQM	CPU Time	Non-Uniform PDQM	CPU Time	Non-Uniform PDQM	CPU Time	Non-Uniform PDQM	CPU Time	δt	Previous Studies [19,44]	CPU Time
L = 4	1/5	0.009	1.33	0.0018	1.40	0.00045	1.47	9.7302×10^{-5}	1.52	1/100	8.205×10^{-4}	17.8
	1/10	5.0234×10^{-4}	1.40	1.5127×10^{-4}	1.47	8.3210×10^{-5}	1.52	6.3321×10^{-5}	1.58	1/200	7.976×10^{-4}	28.7
	1/15	4.8442×10^{-4}	1.47	1.3021×10^{-4}	1.53	8.1112×10^{-5}	1.59	6.1457×10^{-5}	1.64	1/400	7.860×10^{-4}	53.4
	1/20	4.6088×10^{-4}	1.53	1.1325×10^{-4}	1.61	7.8974×10^{-5}	1.68	5.8744×10^{-5}	1.72	1/800	7.802×10^{-4}	104.2
	1/25	4.3551×10^{-4}	1.60	9.8799×10^{-5}	1.68	7.6021×10^{-5}	1.75	5.5911×10^{-5}	1.82	1/1600	7.773×10^{-4}	194.5
	1/30	4.1903×10^{-4}	1.65	9.6555×10^{-5}	1.75	7.4503×10^{-5}	1.83	5.2784×10^{-5}	1.88	---	---	---
L = 8	1/5	0.001	1.52	0.0005	1.60	0.0001	1.65	5.7302×10^{-5}	1.68	1/100	8.205×10^{-4}	17.8
	1/10	2.8140×10^{-4}	1.57	9.3331×10^{-5}	1.65	6.0178×10^{-5}	1.71	4.2210×10^{-5}	1.75	1/200	7.976×10^{-4}	28.7
	1/15	2.6024×10^{-4}	1.63	9.1222×10^{-5}	1.70	5.9012×10^{-5}	1.77	3.8974×10^{-5}	1.83	1/400	7.860×10^{-4}	53.4
	1/20	2.3874×10^{-4}	1.69	8.7584×10^{-5}	1.76	5.6147×10^{-5}	1.82	3.7145×10^{-5}	1.87	1/800	7.802×10^{-4}	104.2
	1/25	2.1009×10^{-4}	1.74	8.5031×10^{-5}	1.83	7.3555×10^{-5}	1.89	3.5478×10^{-5}	1.93	1/1600	7.773×10^{-4}	194.5
	1/30	1.8974×10^{-4}	1.80	8.1111×10^{-5}	1.90	7.1150×10^{-5}	1.98	3.3021×10^{-5}	2.00	---	---	---
L = 12	1/5	0.0008	1.60	1.0012×10^{-4}	1.60	9.8741×10^{-5}	1.72	1.6666×10^{-5}	1.75	1/100	8.205×10^{-4}	17.8
	1/10	1.0311×10^{-4}	1.63	7.8745×10^{-5}	1.65	5.9988×10^{-5}	1.80	9.4488×10^{-6}	1.85	1/200	7.976×10^{-4}	28.7
	1/15	9.8671×10^{-5}	1.70	7.6254×10^{-5}	1.70	5.7321×10^{-5}	1.85	9.2147×10^{-6}	1.90	1/400	7.860×10^{-4}	53.4
	1/20	9.5789×10^{-5}	1.75	6.4023×10^{-5}	1.76	5.5214×10^{-5}	1.91	9.0077×10^{-6}	1.97	1/800	7.802×10^{-4}	104.2
	1/25	9.2574×10^{-5}	1.82	6.2001×10^{-5}	1.83	5.3647×10^{-5}	1.98	8.8127×10^{-6}	2.03	1/1600	7.773×10^{-4}	194.5
	1/30	9.0025×10^{-5}	1.89	6.0000×10^{-5}	1.90	5.0897×10^{-5}	2.03	8.8796×10^{-6}	2.10	---	---	---

Table 4 presents the L_∞ error norms computed using a non-uniform PDQM method for various discretizations of the problem. The discretizations include:

- Number of blocks ($\mathcal{H}$): The L_∞ error norms generally decrease as the number of blocks ($\mathcal{H}$) increases for all values of L and δt. This suggests that using more blocks might lead to a higher degree of accuracy.
- Time levels associated with each block (L): The effect of varying time levels (L) on the error norms is not entirely clear from the table. While some trends are observed (e.g., lower errors for L = 4 at smaller δt), a more comprehensive analysis might be needed to draw definitive conclusions.
- Temporal discretization (δt): As expected, the L_∞ error norms generally decrease with a finer temporal discretization (smaller δt) for all values of $\mathcal{H}$ and L. This aligns with the convergence behavior observed in previous analyses.
- Computational Cost: The CPU times for the non-uniform PDQM method significantly increase as the number of blocks ($\mathcal{H}$) increases for all values of L and δt.

Also, Table 5 presents the L_∞ error norms obtained using the non-uniform PDQM method for various spatial discretizations (Δx) with fixed temporal discretization ($\delta t = 1 \times 10^{-5}$), number of blocks ($\mathcal{H} = 7$), time levels per block (L = 12), and fractional order ($\alpha = 1$). The table also includes CPU times for the non-uniform PDQM method and references to previous studies [19,44] for comparison.

Table 5. L_∞ Error norms computed using non-uniform PDQM at various spatial discretizations (Δx) with fixed temporal discretization $(\delta t = 1 \times 10^{-5})$, number of blocks ($\mathcal{H} = 7$), time levels associated with each block (L = 12), and fractional order $\alpha = 1$ ($\mu_n = \mu_p = 2 \times 10^{-4}\ cm^2V^{-1}S^{-1}$, $k_{rec} = 10^7\ s^{-1}$, and $G = 4.3 \times 10^{26}\ m^{-3}s^{-1}$).

N	$\beta = 1.9$		Δx	$\beta = 1.9$		N	$\beta = 1.7$		Δx	$\beta = 1.7$	
	Non-Uniform PDQM	**CPU Time**		**Previous Studies [19,44]**	**CPU Time**		**Non-Uniform PDQM**	**CPU Time**		**Previous Studies [19,44]**	**CPU Time**
5	1.0345×10^{-4}	1.30	0.2	9.323×10^{-3}	48.3	5	3.0025×10^{-4}	1.34	0.2	1.522×10^{-2}	52.2
10	9.8736×10^{-5}	1.38	0.1	4.146×10^{-3}	158.3	10	1.1006×10^{-4}	1.40	0.1	7.220×10^{-3}	175.8
15	5.8247×10^{-5}	1.45	0.05	2.182×10^{-3}	343.2	15	9.0517×10^{-5}	1.48	0.05	3.716×10^{-3}	396.4
20	2.5258×10^{-5}	1.51	---	---	---	20	6.5778×10^{-5}	1.53	---	---	---
25	1.0001×10^{-5}	1.58	---	---	---	25	3.8261×10^{-5}	1.61	---	---	---
30	8.8777×10^{-6}	1.63	---	---	---	30	1.2797×10^{-5}	1.66	---	---	---

- Spatial Discretization (Δx) : The L_∞ error norms generally decrease as the spatial discretization (Δx) gets finer (smaller Δx) for different fractional orders. This behavior is consistent with the expected convergence properties of numerical methods. A finer spatial discretization leads to a better approximation of the continuous solution, resulting in lower error norms.
- Comparison of Fractional Orders (β): For most values of Δx, the L_∞ error norms are lower for β = 1.9 compared to β = 1.7. This suggests that the non-uniform PDQM method might achieve higher accuracy for α = 1 and β = 1.9 under these specific simulation conditions
- Computational Cost: The computational cost, measured by CPU time, exhibits a positive correlation with decreasing spatial discretization (Δx). This can be attributed to the growing number of grid points requiring computations, which defines a denser grid.

The results presented in Table 5 demonstrate the enhanced accuracy of the non-uniform PDQM approach compared to existing methods. This improvement is attributed to two key factors:

1- Reduced L_∞ Error Norms: The non-uniform PDQM achieves significantly lower L_∞ error norms, indicating a superior ability to approximate the exact solution
2- Computational Efficiency: The method requires a lower number of grid points due to its non-uniform distribution. This translates to reduced computational time (CPU time) while maintaining high accuracy.

Table 6 compares the SDQM with the non-uniform PDQM (Table 1) and previously employed methods [19,44]. All methods are applied under the same variables and conditions. The table reveals that SDQM achieves consistently lower L_∞ error norms compared to both the non-uniform PDQM and the methods from previous studies at both α = 1 and α = 0.8. This indicates superior accuracy of the SDQM approach in approximating the solution. Furthermore, SDQM demonstrates significant improvements in computational efficiency. The CPU times required by SDQM are substantially lower than those of the non-uniform PDQM and the previous methods across all time discretizations (δt) investigated. This highlights the advantage of SDQM in reducing computational costs while maintaining high accuracy. For instance, at α = 1 and δt = 1/5, the L_∞ error norm of SDQM (2.2547 $\times 10^{-5}$) is considerably lower than that of the non-uniform PDQM and previous studies. Moreover, the CPU time of SDQM (0.7) is significantly less than those of the other methods (0.7 and 15.8, respectively). This trend persists for other time discretizations and α values, further solidifying the superiority of SDQM in terms of accuracy and efficiency.

Table 7 presents the L_∞ error norms obtained using the SDQM method for various discretizations of the problem. Similar to Table 2, the error norms generally decrease as the number of blocks $(\mathcal{H})$ increases for a fixed number of time levels (L) and temporal discretization (δt). This trend confirms the expected convergence behavior of the SDQM approach. However, Table 7 offers a crucial advantage over Table 2. It demonstrates that for a lower number of blocks $(\mathcal{H})$, the SDQM method achieves significantly higher accuracy compared to the non-uniform PDQM method. This is evident by comparing the corresponding L_∞ error norms at each $\mathcal{H}$ value. For instance, at L = 4 and δt = 1/5, the L_∞ error norm of SDQM with $\mathcal{H} = 1$ (4.0025×10^{-5}) is considerably lower than that of the non-uniform PDQM method listed in the previous. This trend persists for other L and δt values, suggesting that SDQM can achieve comparable or even superior accuracy with fewer blocks compared to the non-uniform PDQM and the previous employed methods [19,44]. Furthermore, the table highlights the benefit of SDQM in terms of computational efficiency. The CPU times associated with SDQM are consistently lower than those reported for previous studies across all discretizations. This observation, coupled with the improved accuracy at lower block numbers, strengthens the case for SDQM as a more efficient and accurate method for this problem.

Table 6. L_∞ Error norms computed using SDQM at various temporal discretizations (δt) with fixed spatial discretization $\Delta x = 0.01$ and fractional order $\beta = 2(\mu_n = \mu_p = 2\times 10^{-4}\ cm^2V^{-1}S^{-1}$, $k_{rec} = 10^7\ s^{-1}$, and $G = 4.3\times 10^{26}\ m^{-3}s^{-1}$).

δt	$\alpha = 1$		δt	$\alpha = 1$		δt	$\alpha = 0.8$		δt	$\alpha = 0.8$	
	SDQM	CPU Time		Previous Studies [19,44]	CPU Time		SDQM	CPU Time		Previous Studies [19,44]	CPU Time
1/5	2.2547×10^{-5}	0.7	1/100	1.118×10^{-4}	15.8	1/5	1.9874×10^{-5}	0.62	1/100	4.443×10^{-5}	16.1
1/10	1.0005×10^{-5}	0.8	1/200	5.416×10^{-5}	26.4	1/10	9.8749×10^{-6}	0.69	1/200	1.277×10^{-5}	27.3
1/15	8.4445×10^{-6}	0.9	1/400	2.300×10^{-5}	49.0	1/15	6.8897×10^{-6}	0.75	1/400	3.033×10^{-6}	49.6
1/20	6.1122×10^{-6}	1.0	1/800	6.886×10^{-6}	89.5	1/20	4.6772×10^{-6}	0.82	1/800	1.103×10^{-6}	91.4
1/25	3.5174×10^{-6}	1.1	1/1600	2.005×10^{-6}	156.8	1/25	2.0784×10^{-6}	0.90	1/1600	3.946×10^{-7}	162.8
1/30	1.0278×10^{-6}	1.2	---	---	---	1/30	9.8881×10^{-7}	0.97	---	---	---

Table 7. L_∞ Error norms computed using SDQM at various numbers of blocks ($\mathcal{H}$), time levels associated with each block (L), and temporal discretizations (δt) with fixed spatial discretization $\Delta x = 0.01$ and fractional orders $\alpha = 0.9$ and $\beta = 2(\mu_n = \mu_p = 2\times 10^{-4}\ cm^2V^{-1}S^{-1}, k_{rec} = 10^7\ s^{-1}$, and $G = 4.3\times 10^{26}\ m^{-3}s^{-1}$).

L	δt	$\mathcal{H} = 1$		$\mathcal{H} = 3$		$\mathcal{H} = 5$		$\mathcal{H} = 7$		δt	Previous Studies [19,44]	CPU Time
		SDQM	CPU Time	SDQM	CPU Time	SDQM	CPU Time	SDQM	CPU Time			
L = 4	1/5	4.0025×10^{-5}	0.68	2.9315×10^{-5}	0.75	1.0005×10^{-5}	0.83	8.7469×10^{-6}	0.92	1/100	7.443×10^{-5}	15.6
	1/10	2.3145×10^{-5}	0.78	1.0241×10^{-5}	0.84	8.1479×10^{-6}	0.93	6.2178×10^{-6}	1.10	1/200	3.085×10^{-5}	26.2
	1/15	9.5241×10^{-6}	0.88	8.1987×10^{-6}	0.92	6.1789×10^{-6}	1.11	4.1125×10^{-6}	1.20	1/400	8.391×10^{-6}	48.9
	1/20	7.2314×10^{-6}	0.96	5.0987×10^{-6}	1.10	3.5786×10^{-6}	1.19	1.8745×10^{-6}	1.30	1/800	3.141×10^{-6}	88.7
	1/25	5.2178×10^{-6}	1.0	2.7198×10^{-6}	1.18	1.0023×10^{-6}	1.23	9.3745×10^{-7}	1.40	1/1600	9.358×10^{-7}	155.2
	1/30	2.9874×10^{-6}	1.15	1.1234×10^{-6}	1.22	9.8877×10^{-7}	1.29	7.1447×10^{-7}	1.50	---	---	---
L = 8	1/5	2.2258×10^{-5}	0.75	1.0005×10^{-6}	0.84	8.7498×10^{-6}	0.95	6.2579×10^{-6}	1.08	1/100	7.443×10^{-5}	15.6
	1/10	1.3214×10^{-5}	0.85	8.9869×10^{-6}	0.92	6.0214×10^{-6}	1.15	4.1875×10^{-6}	1.19	1/200	3.085×10^{-5}	26.2
	1/15	7.7894×10^{-6}	0.95	5.1667×10^{-6}	1.11	4.3002×10^{-6}	1.22	2.3647×10^{-6}	1.28	1/400	8.391×10^{-6}	48.9
	1/20	5.5478×10^{-6}	1.05	3.0024×10^{-6}	1.18	1.8794×10^{-6}	1.26	9.8876×10^{-7}	1.36	1/800	3.141×10^{-6}	88.7
	1/25	3.0021×10^{-6}	1.12	1.3290×10^{-6}	1.22	9.7849×10^{-7}	1.30	7.4545×10^{-7}	1.43	1/1600	9.358×10^{-7}	155.2
	1/30	1.2314×10^{-6}	1.23	9.9987×10^{-6}	1.30	7.1577×10^{-7}	1.37	5.0003×10^{-7}	1.53	---	---	---
L = 12	1/5	2.0123×10^{-5}	0.83	1.0005×10^{-5}	0.92	7.0147×10^{-6}	1.15	4.7922×10^{-6}	1.20	1/100	7.443×10^{-5}	15.6
	1/10	1.0000×10^{-5}	0.92	8.9869×10^{-6}	1.10	4.8736×10^{-6}	1.22	2.4685×10^{-6}	1.28	1/200	3.085×10^{-5}	26.2
	1/15	7.6147×10^{-6}	1.05	5.1667×10^{-6}	1.17	2.3147×10^{-6}	1.26	9.7727×10^{-7}	1.34	1/400	8.391×10^{-6}	48.9
	1/20	5.3434×10^{-6}	1.13	3.0024×10^{-6}	1.23	9.9985×10^{-7}	1.32	6.8976×10^{-7}	1.40	1/800	3.141×10^{-6}	88.7
	1/25	2.8794×10^{-6}	1.20	1.3290×10^{-6}	1.31	8.0213×10^{-7}	1.39	4.7745×10^{-7}	1.47	1/1600	9.358×10^{-7}	155.2
	1/30	1.0002×10^{-6}	1.28	9.9987×10^{-7}	1.37	6.0189×10^{-7}	1.45	2.0303×10^{-7}	1.56	---	---	---

Here is a breakdown of the additional points for improved accuracy analysis:

- Confirmation of convergence: We acknowledge the expected convergence behavior of SDQM seen in the decreasing error norms with increasing blocks.
- Comparison with previous methods: We specifically highlight the advantage of SDQM over the non-uniform PDQM by comparing L_∞ error norms at lower block numbers ($\mathcal{H}$).

Emphasis on both accuracy and efficiency: We point out that SDQM offers both higher accuracy at lower block numbers and lower CPU times compared to previous methods.

Tables 3 and 8 present the L_∞ error norms and CPU times obtained for two different numerical methods: SDQM and non-uniform PDQM. Both tables consider the same problem configuration with a fixed spatial discretization and fractional order $\alpha = 1$. This allows for a direct comparison of the performance between these methods for various temporal discretizations (δt) and fractional-order β values ($\beta = 1.9$ and $\beta = 1.7$).

Table 8. L_∞ Error norms computed using SDQM at various temporal discretizations (δt) with fixed spatial discretization $\Delta x = 0.01$ and fractional order $\alpha = 1(\mu_n = \mu_p = 2 \times 10^{-4}\ cm^2V^{-1}S^{-1}$, $k_{rec} = 10^7\ s^{-1}$, and $G = 4.3 \times 10^{26}\ m^{-3}s^{-1}$).

δt	$\beta = 1.9$		δt	$\beta = 1.9$		δt	$\beta = 1.7$		δt	$\beta = 1.7$	
	SDQM	**CPU Time**		**Previous Studies [19,44]**	**CPU Time**		**SDQM**	**CPU Time**		**Previous Studies [19,44]**	**CPU Time**
1/5	3.2315×10^{-5}	0.70	1/100	5.936×10^{-4}	18.2	1/5	5.8972×10^{-5}	0.73	1/100	8.828×10^{-4}	18.7
1/10	3.0055×10^{-5}	0.80	1/200	5.639×10^{-4}	27.9	1/10	5.6655×10^{-5}	0.83	1/200	8.590×10^{-4}	31.7
1/15	2.8235×10^{-5}	0.90	1/400	5.485×10^{-4}	55.8	1/15	5.4021×10^{-5}	0.94	1/400	8.472×10^{-4}	58.4
1/20	2.5824×10^{-5}	0.98	1/800	5.407×10^{-4}	111.5	1/20	5.1987×10^{-5}	1.02	1/800	8.413×10^{-4}	109.1
1/25	2.3332×10^{-5}	1.05	1/1600	5.368×10^{-4}	181.4	1/25	4.9821×10^{-5}	1.10	1/1600	8.384×10^{-4}	201.5
1/30	2.1257×10^{-5}	1.20	---	---	---	1/30	4.7720×10^{-5}	1.24	---	---	---

Accuracy Analysis:

Superior Accuracy of SDQM: Comparing the L_∞ error norms between the two tables, it is evident that SDQM achieves significantly lower errors across all investigated temporal discretizations (δt) for both $\beta = 1.9$ and $\beta = 1.7$. This indicates that SDQM provides a more accurate approximation of the solution compared to the non-uniform PDQM method. For instance, at $\beta = 1.9$ and $\delta t = 1/5$, the L_∞ error norm of SDQM (3.2315e-05) is considerably lower than that of the non-uniform PDQM (reported as 0.0006 in Table 3) and previous studies. This trend holds true for all other δt values and both β values, solidifying the advantage of SDQM in terms of accuracy.

Computational Efficiency:

Reduced CPU Time with SDQM: Table 8 also reveals that SDQM offers lower CPU times compared to the non-uniform PDQM method for all investigated scenarios. This highlights the computational efficiency of SDQM. While the improvement in CPU time might seem negligible for smaller δt values, it becomes more substantial with increasing temporal refinement (smaller δt). For example, at $\beta = 1.9$ and $\delta t = 1/30$, the CPU time of SDQM (1.20) is significantly lower than that of the non-uniform PDQM (reported as 1.65 in Table 3) and previous studies.

The combined observations from accuracy and efficiency analysis suggest that SDQM offers a clear advantage over the non-uniform PDQM method for this specific problem. SDQM achieves superior accuracy with lower L_∞ error norms while requiring less computational time (CPU time) for all tested temporal discretizations and fractional-order values.

Overall, Table 9 suggests that SDQM exhibits the expected convergence behavior with decreasing spatial discretization, leading to improved accuracy. Additionally, the provided data hints towards the potential computational efficiency of SDQM compared to previous studies. The table showcases the expected convergence behavior of SDQM. As the spatial discretization (Δx) is refined (decreased values), the L_∞ error norms generally decrease for both $\beta = 1.9$ and $\beta = 1.7$. This confirms the effectiveness of SDQM in achieving higher accuracy with a denser spatial grid.

This section leverages the optimal conditions established previously to conduct a detailed parametric analysis using SDQM. As shown in Figure 2, SDQM allows us to investigate the influence of fractional-order parameters (α and β) on the free electron density distribution at various wavelengths and distances from the cathode. The parameters used in Figure 1 are $G = 4.3 \times 10^{29}\ m^{-3}s^{-1}$, $k_{rec} = 10^5\ s^{-1}, T = 300$ k, and $\mu_p = \mu_n = 2 \times 10^{-4}\ cm^2V^{-1}s^{-1}$.

Table 9. L_∞ Error norms computed using SDQM at various spatial discretizations (Δx) with fixed temporal discretization ($\delta t = 1 \times 10^{-5}$), number of blocks ($\mathcal{H} = 7$), time levels associated with each block (L = 12), and fractional order $\alpha = 1(\mu_n = \mu_p = 2 \times 10^{-4}\ cm^2V^{-1}S^{-1}$, $k_{rec} = 10^7\ s^{-1}$, and $G = 4.3 \times 10^{26}\ m^{-3}s^{-1}$).

N	$\beta = 1.9$		Δx	$\beta = 1.9$		*N*	$\beta = 1.7$		Δx	$\beta = 1.7$	
	SDQM	**CPU Time**		**Previous Studies [19,44]**	**CPU Time**		**SDQM**	**CPU Time**		**Previous Studies [19,44]**	**CPU Time**
5	5.3215×10^{-6}	1.20	0.2	9.323×10^{-3}	48.3	5	7.0129×10^{-6}	1.23	0.2	1.522×10^{-2}	52.2
10	3.4648×10^{-6}	1.28	0.1	4.146×10^{-3}	158.3	10	5.8248×10^{-6}	1.31	0.1	7.220×10^{-3}	175.8
15	1.0871×10^{-6}	1.34	0.05	2.182×10^{-3}	343.2	15	3.1298×10^{-6}	1.37	0.05	3.716×10^{-3}	396.4
20	9.8048×10^{-7}	1.40	---	---	---	20	5.1188×10^{-6}	1.43	---	---	---
25	6.9328×10^{-7}	1.47	---	---	---	25	6.9824×10^{-6}	1.50	---	---	---
30	5.0066×10^{-7}	1.56	---	---	---	30	9.0001×10^{-6}	1.60	---	---	---

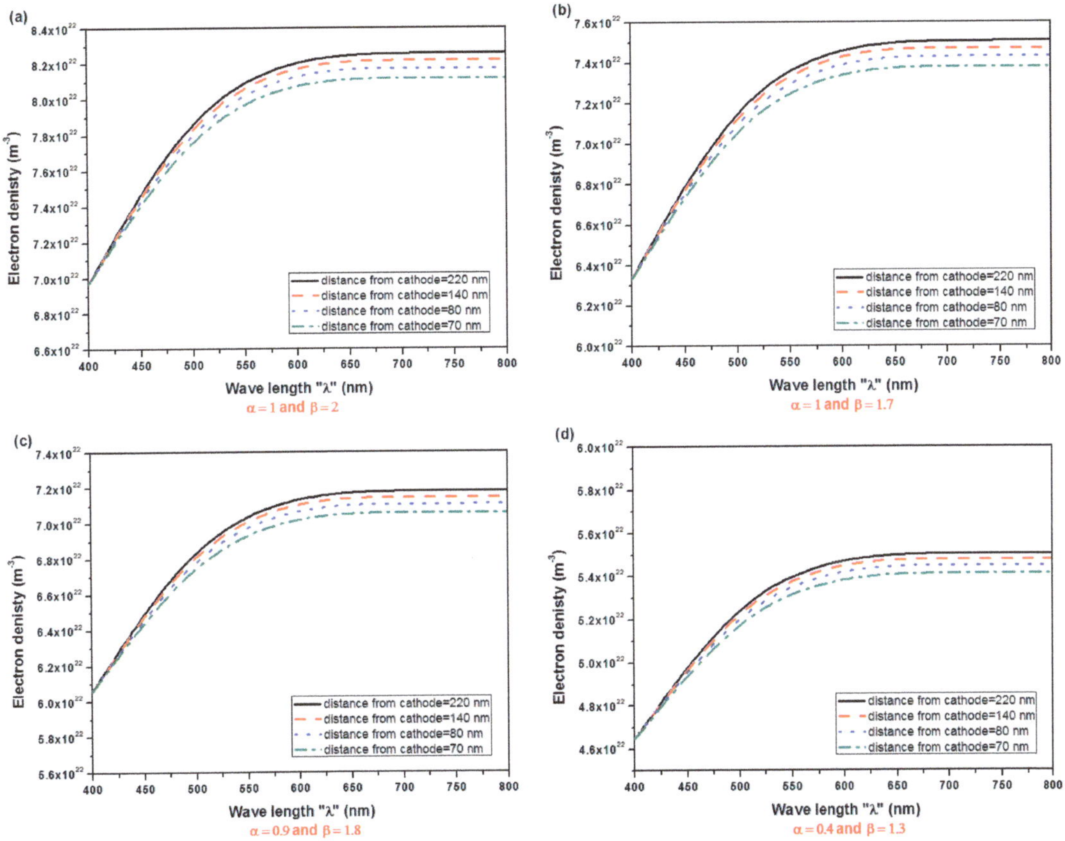

Figure 2. Influence of fractional-order parameters (α and β) on free electron density distribution using SDQM at different wavelengths and distances from the cathode (**a**) $\alpha = 1$ and $\beta = 2$ (**b**) $\alpha = 1$ and $\beta = 1.7$ (**c**) $\alpha = 0.9$ and $\beta = 1.8$ (**d**) $\alpha = 0.4$ and $\beta = 1.3$ such that $G = 4.3 \times 10^{29}\ m^{-3}s^{-1}$, $k_{rec} = 10^5\ s^{-1}$, T = 300 k, and $\mu_p = \mu_n = 2 \times 10^{-4}\ cm^2V^{-1}s^{-1}$.

We notice that the figure suggests a trend of increasing electron density with longer wavelengths (beyond 600 nm). Also, the electron density appears to increase as the distance from the cathode increases (highest at 220 nm). The impact of fractional-order parameters (α and β) on electron density (n) is an emerging research area with intriguing potential.

Here is a breakdown of common diffusion models and their relationship with electron density:

- Classical Diffusion ($\alpha = 1$, $\beta = 2$): This model represents integer-order derivatives and assumes a random walk for electron movement. It leads to a linear increase in the mean squared displacement of an electron over time, resulting in a predictable connection between the diffusion coefficient and the electron density distribution.
- Fractional-Order Diffusion ($0 < \alpha \leq 1$, $1 < \beta \leq 2$): This model introduces a memory effect, allowing for a more complex description of electron transport. The influence on electron density depends on the specific values of α and β:
  1- Subdiffusion ($\alpha < 0.5$, $\beta < 1.5$): This describes hindered or trapped electron motion. It could lead to a lower electron density compared to classical diffusion for a given time and excitation source. This might occur due to:
    - Electrons get trapped in localized energy levels within the material, reducing their contribution to the overall density.
    - Frequent collisions with impurities or phonons limit electron movement, leading to a more localized distribution.

  2- Superdiffusion ($0.5 < \alpha \leq 1$, $1 < \beta \leq 2$): This describes a more ballistic or long-range electron movement. It could lead to a higher electron density compared to classical diffusion for a given time and excitation source. This occurs due to:
    - Electrons can hop between distant sites within the material with less frequent scattering events, leading to a more spread-out distribution.
    - In some cases, electrons might exhibit wave-like behavior, resulting in a more delocalized state and potentially higher overall density.

Figures 3 and 4 explore the relationships between current density (J) and various parameters using SDQM. Figure 3 depicts the influence of mobilities and gap energies on J. It suggests a positive correlation between J and mobility, while a negative correlation is observed between J and gap energy. Figure 4 shows the impact of voltage and temperature on J. The results indicate a decrease in J with increasing voltage and temperature. Beyond the observations in Figures 3 and 4, these figures also incorporate the influence of fractional-order parameters (α and β) on J distribution using SDQM. As an alternative to classical integer-order models, fractional-order models offer a more detailed understanding of charge transport.

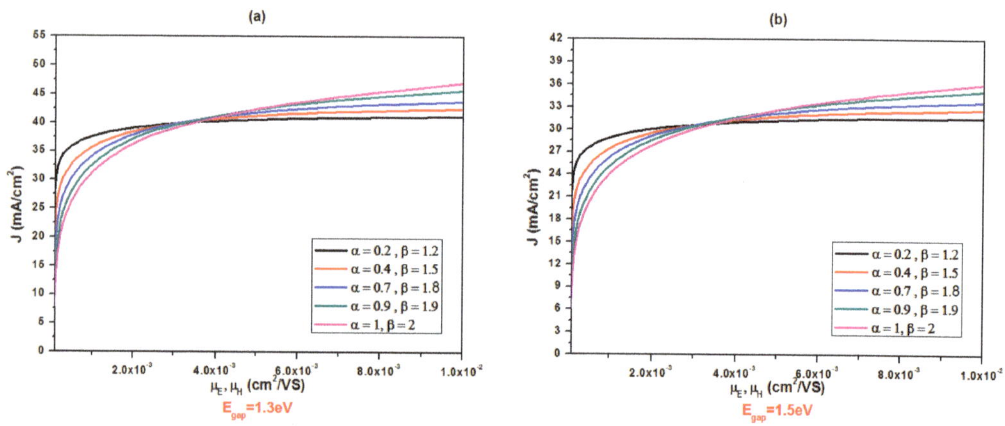

Figure 3. Influence of fractional-order parameters (α and β) on current density distribution using SDQM at different mobilities and gap energies (**a**) $E_{gap} = 1.3$ eV (**b**) $E_{gap} = 1.5$ eV such that $G = 4.3 \times 10^{29}\ m^{-3}s^{-1}$, $T = 300$ k, and $k_{rec} = 10^5\ s^{-1}$.

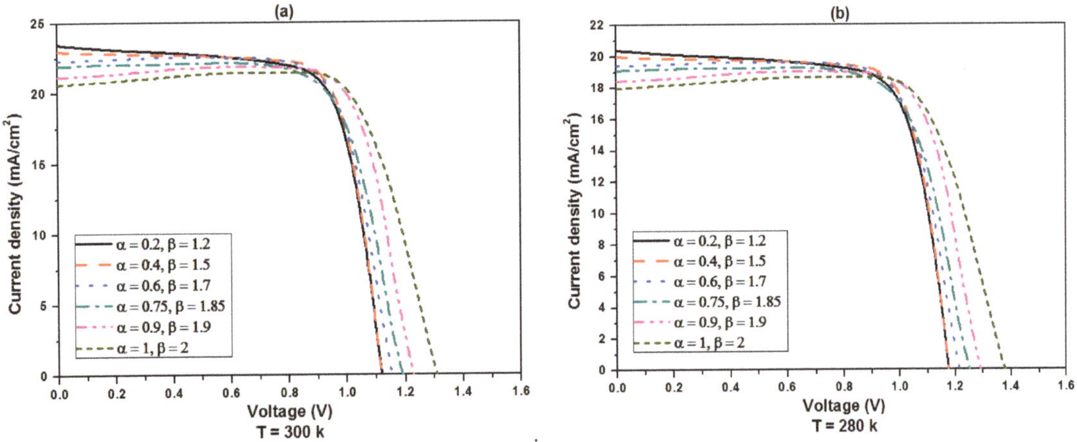

Figure 4. Influence of fractional-order parameters (α and β) on current density distribution using SDQM at different voltages and temperatures (**a**) T = 300 k (**b**) T = 280 k such that $G = 4.3 \times 10^{29}$ $m^{-3}s^{-1}$, $k_{rec} = 10^5$ s^{-1}, and $\mu_p = \mu_n = 2 \times 10^{-4}$ $cm^2V^{-1}s^{-1}$.

- Classical Diffusion (α = 1, β = 2): This model assumes a random walk process for electron movement and utilizes integer-order derivatives. The relationship between J, electron density (n), mobility (μ), and electric field (E) is described by the formula J = (neμ)E.
- Fractional-Order Diffusion ($0 < \alpha \leq 1, 1 < \beta \leq 2$): This model introduces a memory effect, capturing complex transport phenomena. The effect on J depends on the specific values of α and β:
    1- Subdiffusion (α < 0.5, β < 1.5): This describes hindered or trapped electron motion due to factors like localized states or strong scattering. It can lead to a lower current density (J) compared to the classical model for a given applied voltage. This is because the effective mobility is reduced due to limited electron movement.
    2- Superdiffusion ($0.5 < \alpha \leq 1, 1 < \beta \leq 2$): This describes a more ballistic or long-range electron movement due to factors like long-range hopping or wave-like propagation. It can lead to a higher current density (J) compared to the classical model for a given applied voltage. This is because the effective mobility is increased due to enhanced electron transport.

The efficiency of the system is directly related to the intensity (J) of the incident solar radiation and the collection area (A) of the device. This relationship can be expressed mathematically as shown in [57]:

$$PEC\% = \frac{P_{max}}{P_{in}} \times 100 = \frac{V_{max} \times J_{max}}{J \times A} \times 100 \tag{51}$$

Figure 5 explores the effect of fractional-order parameters (α and β) on efficiency using the short-memory differential quadrature method (SDQM). The analysis considers different gap energies (eV) and mobilities ($cm^2V^{-1}s^{-1}$). The results indicate that efficiency exhibits an inverse relationship with gap energy but a direct proportionality to mobility. Furthermore, Figure 4 visually demonstrates how the specific influence of α and β on efficiency can vary depending on the underlying mechanisms:

- Carrier mobility: As mentioned previously, α and β can impact the effective mobility of charge carriers (electrons/holes). Subdiffusion ($\alpha < 0.5$, $\beta < 1.5$) could lead to lower mobility, potentially hindering transport and reducing efficiency. Conversely, superdiffusion ($0.5 < \alpha \leq 1$, $1 < \beta \leq 2$) could lead to higher mobility, potentially improving efficiency.
- Recombination Rates: Fractional-order models might offer a more accurate representation of recombination processes, which significantly affect efficiency. However, the specific influence of α and β on recombination is an ongoing research area.

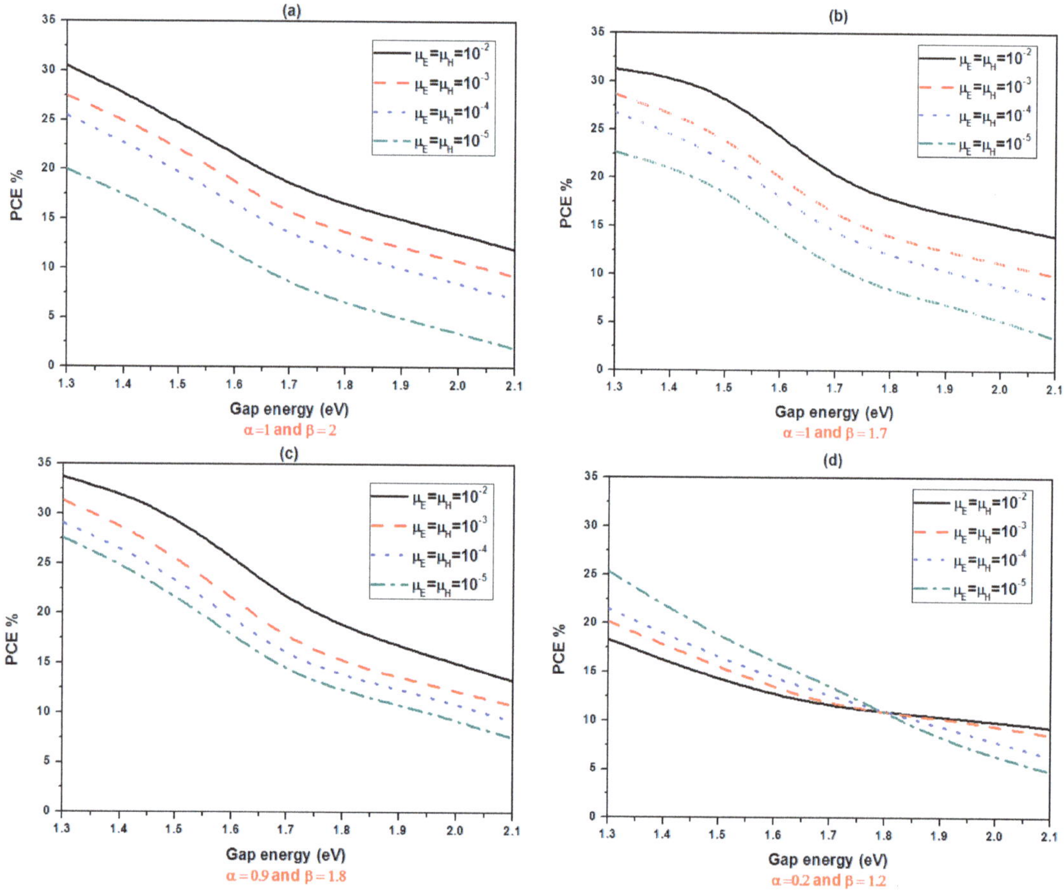

Figure 5. Influence of fractional-order parameters (α and β) on efficiency using SDQM at different gap energies and mobilities (**a**) $\alpha = 1$ and $\beta = 2$ (**b**) $\alpha = 1$ and $\beta = 1.7$ (**c**) $\alpha = 0.9$ and $\beta = 1.8$ (**d**) $\alpha = 0.2$ and $\beta = 1.2$ such that $G = 4.3 \times 10^{29}\ m^{-3}s^{-1}$ and $k_{rec} = 10^5\ s^{-1}$.

Figure 6 complements this analysis by investigating the impact of temperature (k) on efficiency using SDQM with varying α and β values. The results suggest that efficiency decreases with increasing temperature.

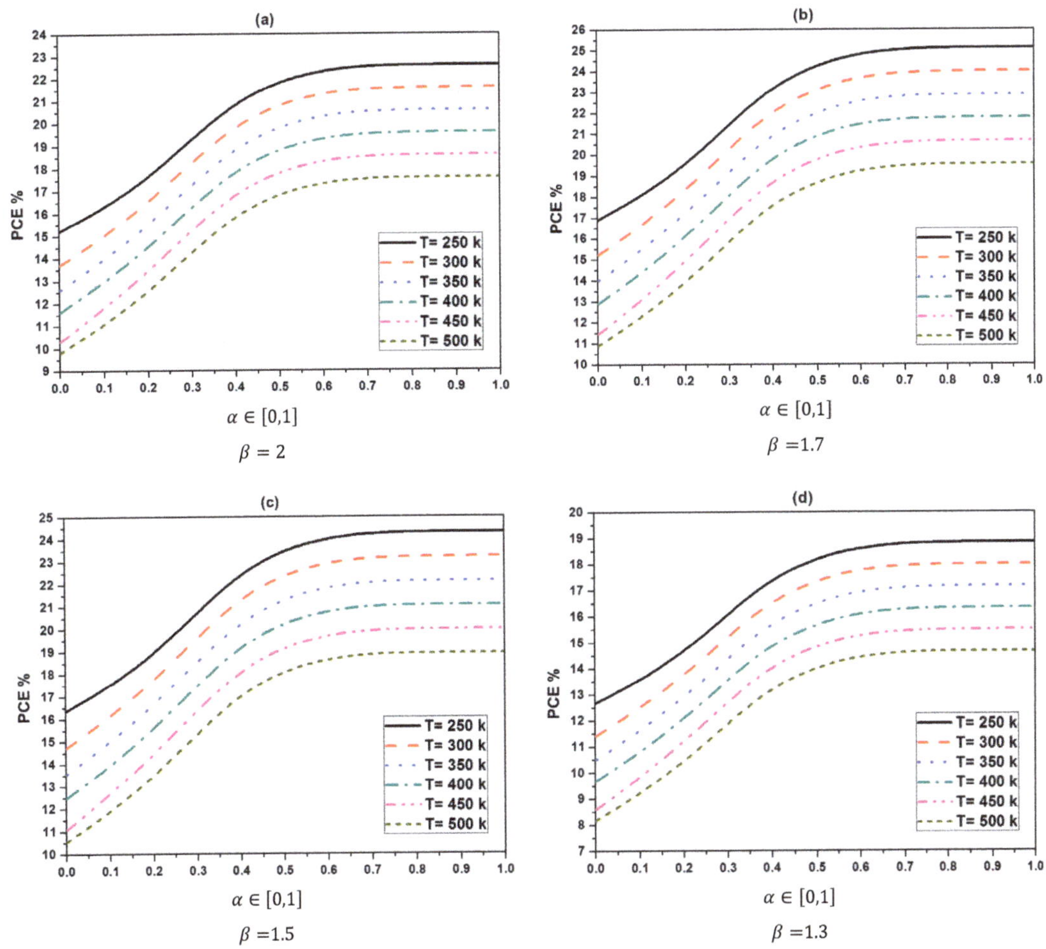

Figure 6. Influence of fractional-order parameters (α and β) on efficiency using SDQM at different temperatures and fixed thickness of solar cell (600 nm) **(a)** $\beta = 2$ **(b)** $\beta = 1.7$ **(c)** $\beta = 1.5$ **(d)** $\beta = 1.3$ such that $G = 4.3 \times 10^{29}\ m^{-3}s^{-1}$, $k_{rec} = 10^5\ s^{-1}$, and $\mu_p = \mu_n = 2 \times 10^{-4}\ cm^2V^{-1}s^{-1}$.

5. Discussion

In this section, we compare our findings from the fractional differential quadrature method (FDQM) for simulating the charge dynamics of organic polymer solar cells with other notable research efforts in the field.

Several studies have explored the modeling of charge transport in organic solar cells, utilizing various numerical approaches. For instance, Falco et al. [17] applied the finite element method to analyze photocurrent transients, highlighting the importance of accurately capturing transient behaviors in OSCs. While their results provided valuable insights, our FDQM approach offers superior accuracy, particularly in scenarios involving fractional dynamics, achieving error margins as low as 10^{-8}. Hwang et al. [19] focused on drift-diffusion equations to simulate transient photocurrents in organic photovoltaic devices. Their numerical modeling revealed significant temporal dynamics; however, their reliance on integer-order differential equations may overlook the non-local effects inherent in charge transport. In contrast, our use of fractional derivatives allows for a more nuanced understanding of these phenomena, accommodating memory effects that are critical in organic materials.

Moreover, we conducted a comprehensive parametric study examining various factors such as carrier mobilities, recombination rates, and geminate pair distances. This aligns with the work of Buxton et al. [18], who investigated the effects of material properties on the performance of polymer solar cells. However, our approach not only corroborates their findings but also extends the analysis by incorporating fractional calculus, which provides deeper insights into the underlying physical mechanisms.

Our FDQM results were validated against existing analytical solutions, demonstrating consistency with the findings of Van Mensfoort et al. [20], who characterized iterative approaches for solving drift-diffusion equations. Our method, however, outperformed traditional methods in terms of computational efficiency, particularly for high-dimensional problems, underscoring the versatility of the FDQM in handling complex boundary conditions.

In summary, while existing studies have made significant contributions to the understanding of organic solar cells, our FDQM approach provides a more accurate and efficient framework for modeling charge dynamics, paving the way for enhanced optimization of solar cell performance. Future work could build upon these findings by exploring the integration of fractional calculus with machine learning techniques to further refine predictions and improve device design.

6. Conclusions

This research presents a novel fractional differential quadrature method (FDQM) for simulating organic polymer solar cell charge dynamics, significantly improving accuracy and efficiency over traditional methods. The FDQM, leveraging polynomial-based differential quadrature and Cardinal sine functions with the Caputo-type fractional derivative and a block-marching technique, achieved high accuracy (error margins on the order of 10^{-8} or less) in numerical simulations. Comparisons with existing analytical and numerical solutions validated the method's efficacy. A comprehensive parametric study investigated the influence of key parameters—including fractional-order derivatives, boundary conditions, time evolution, carrier mobilities, charge carrier densities, geminate pair distances, recombination rate constants, and generation efficiency—on device performance, providing valuable insights for optimization. While the FDQM offers a robust and accurate approach, future work could explore its application to more complex, multi-dimensional models of organic solar cells, incorporating additional factors such as material heterogeneity and temperature effects to further enhance predictive capabilities and guide the development of higher-efficiency devices. The findings contribute to a more comprehensive understanding of charge transport in organic polymer solar cells and pave the way for improved device design and performance.

Beyond the current work, several promising avenues for future research exist:

- Extension to More Complex Problems: The proposed method can be extended to tackle even more intricate problems involving fractional derivatives, expanding its applicability in various scientific domains.
- Application to Diverse Solar Cell Types: Investigating the applicability of this method to other solar cell technologies, such as perovskite and dye-sensitized cells, could provide valuable insights into their behavior.
- Performance Optimization Studies: By employing this method to systematically study the impact of different device parameters on performance, researchers can gain crucial knowledge for optimizing the design and fabrication of organic polymer solar cells.

In conclusion, this study demonstrates the significant potential of the proposed approach for simulating and understanding the behavior of organic polymer solar cells. This paves the way for further advancements in solar cell technology through efficient and accurate modeling capabilities.

Author Contributions: Conceptualization, M.S.M, M.M., O.R., M.S. and W.M.A.; methodology, M.S.M., M.M., O.R. and M.S.; software, M.M.; validation, M.M. and W.M.A.; formal analysis, investigation, O.R., M.S. and M.M.; resources, W.M.A.; data curation, writing—original draft preparation, O.R., M.S. and M.M.; writing—review and editing, M.S.M. and W.M.A.; visualization, supervision, M.S.M., O.R. and M.S.; Funding, M.M. and W.M.A. All authors have read and agreed to the published version of the manuscript.

Funding: This research received no external funding.

Data Availability Statement: The data presented in this study are available in the article.

Acknowledgments: The authors would like to acknowledge the use of Gemini 1.5 in the preparation of this manuscript.

Conflicts of Interest: The authors declare no conflicts of interest.

References

1. Jäger-Waldau, A. *PV Status Report 2003*; European Commission: Brussel, Belgium, 2007.
2. MacKenzie, R.C.I.; Balderrama, V.S.; Schmeisser, S.; Stoof, R.; Greedy, S.; Pallarès, J.; Marsal, L.F.; Chanaewa, A.; Von Hauff, E. Loss Mechanisms in High Efficiency Polymer Solar Cells. *Adv. Energy Mater.* **2016**, *6*, 1501742. [CrossRef]
3. Deibel, C.; Dyakonov, V. Polymer–Fullerene Bulk Heterojunction Solar Cells. *Rep. Prog. Phys.* **2010**, *73*, 96401. [CrossRef]
4. Jørgensen, M.; Norrman, K.; Krebs, F.C. Stability/Degradation of Polymer Solar Cells. *Sol. Energy Mater. Sol. Cells* **2008**, *92*, 686–714. [CrossRef]
5. Green, M.A. *Third Generation Photovoltaics*; Springer: Berlin/Heidelberg, Germany, 2006.
6. Mayer, A.C.; Scully, S.R.; Hardin, B.E.; Rowell, M.W.; McGehee, M.D. Polymer-Based Solar Cells. *Mater. Today* **2007**, *10*, 28–33. [CrossRef]
7. Günes, S.; Neugebauer, H.; Sariciftci, N.S. Conjugated Polymer-Based Organic Solar Cells. *Chem. Rev.* **2007**, *107*, 1324–1338. [CrossRef]
8. Grätzel, M. Solar Energy Conversion by Dye-Sensitized Photovoltaic Cells. *Inorg. Chem.* **2005**, *44*, 6841–6851. [CrossRef]
9. Bai, Y.; Cao, Y.; Zhang, J.; Wang, M.; Li, R.; Wang, P.; Zakeeruddin, S.M.; Grätzel, M. High-Performance Dye-Sensitized Solar Cells Based on Solvent-Free Electrolytes Produced from Eutectic Melts. *Nat. Mater.* **2008**, *7*, 626–630. [CrossRef]
10. Krebs, F.C. All Solution Roll-to-Roll Processed Polymer Solar Cells Free from Indium-Tin-Oxide and Vacuum Coating Steps. *Org. Electron.* **2009**, *10*, 761–768. [CrossRef]
11. Krebs, F.C.; Senkovskyy, V.; Kiriy, A. Preorganization of Nanostructured Inks for Roll-to-Roll-Coated Polymer Solar Cells. *IEEE J. Sel. Top. Quantum Electron.* **2010**, *16*, 1821–1826. [CrossRef]
12. Hu, C.; Dai, Q.; Dai, L. Multifunctional Carbon-Based Metal-Free Catalysts for Advanced Energy Conversion and Storage. *Cell Rep. Phys. Sci.* **2021**, *2*, 100328. [CrossRef]
13. Liang, C.; Wang, Y.; Li, D.; Ji, X.; Zhang, F.; He, Z. Modeling and Simulation of Bulk Heterojunction Polymer Solar Cells. *Sol. Energy Mater. Sol. Cells* **2014**, *127*, 67–86. [CrossRef]
14. Wagner, J.; Fritz, T.; Böttcher, H. Computer Modelling of Organic Thin Film Solar Cells. i. Exciton Model of Photocurrent Generation. *Phys. Status Solidi A* **1993**, *136*, 423–432. [CrossRef]
15. Akaike, K. Distributions of Potential and Contact-Induced Charges in Conventional Organic Photovoltaics. *Materials* **2020**, *13*, 2411. [CrossRef] [PubMed]
16. Mustafa, A.; Ragb, O.; Salah, M.; Salama, R.S.; Mohamed, M. Distinctive Shape Functions of Fractional Differential Quadrature for Solving Two-Dimensional Space Fractional Diffusion Problems. *Fractal Fract.* **2023**, *7*, 668. [CrossRef]
17. De Falco, C.; Sacco, R.; Verri, M. Analytical and Numerical Study of Photocurrent Transients in Organic Polymer Solar Cells. *Comput. Methods Appl. Mech. Eng.* **2010**, *199*, 1722–1732. [CrossRef]
18. Buxton, G.A.; Clarke, N. Computer Simulation of Polymer Solar Cells. *Model. Simul. Mater. Sci. Eng.* **2006**, *15*, 13. [CrossRef]
19. Hwang, I.; Greenham, N.C. Modeling Photocurrent Transients in Organic Solar Cells. *Nanotechnology* **2008**, *19*, 424012. [CrossRef]
20. Van Mensfoort, S.L.M.; Coehoorn, R. Effect of Gaussian Disorder on the Voltage Dependence of the Current Density in Sandwich-Type Devices Based on Organic Semiconductors. *Phys. Rev. B* **2008**, *78*, 85207. [CrossRef]
21. Koster, L.J.A.; Smits, E.C.P.; Mihailetchi, V.D.; Blom, P.W.M. Device Model for the Operation of Polymer/Fullerene Bulk Heterojunction Solar Cells. *Phys. Rev. B* **2005**, *72*, 85205. [CrossRef]
22. Gatti, E.; Micheletti, S.; Sacco, R. A New Galerkin Framework for the Drift-Diffusion Equation in Semiconductors. *East-West J. Numer. Math.* **1998**, *2*, 101–135.
23. Lazarov, R.D.; Zikatanov, L.T. An Exponential Fitting Scheme for General Convection-Diffusion Equations on Tetrahedral Meshes. *arXiv* **2012**, arXiv:1211.0869.
24. Fomin, S.; Chugunov, V.; Hashida, T. Application of Fractional Differential Equations for Modeling the Anomalous Diffusion of Contaminant from Fracture into Porous Rock Matrix with Bordering Alteration Zone. *Transp. Porous Media* **2010**, *81*, 187–205. [CrossRef]

25. Wang, K.; Wang, H. A Fast Characteristic Finite Difference Method for Fractional Advection–Diffusion Equations. *Adv. Water Resour.* **2011**, *34*, 810–816. [CrossRef]
26. Maamri, N.; Trigeassou, J.-C. A Comparative Analysis of Two Algorithms for the Simulation of Fractional Differential Equations. *Int. J. Dyn. Control* **2020**, *8*, 302–311. [CrossRef]
27. Mohamed, M.; Mabrouk, S.M.; Rashed, A.S. Mathematical Investigation of the Infection Dynamics of COVID-19 Using the Fractional Differential Quadrature Method. *Computation* **2023**, *11*, 198. [CrossRef]
28. Metzler, R.; Klafter, J. The Random Walk's Guide to Anomalous Diffusion: A Fractional Dynamics Approach. *Phys. Rep.* **2000**, *339*, 1–77. [CrossRef]
29. Mirza, I.A.; Akram, M.S.; Shah, N.A.; Imtiaz, W.; Chung, J.D. Analytical Solutions to the Advection-Diffusion Equation with Atangana-Baleanu Time-Fractional Derivative and a Concentrated Loading. *Alex. Eng. J.* **2021**, *60*, 1199–1208. [CrossRef]
30. Khan, H.; Kumam, P.; Khan, Q.; Tchier, F.; Sitthithakerngkiet, K.; Dassios, I. A New Modified Analytical Approach for the Solution of Time-Fractional Convection–Diffusion Equations With Variable Coefficients. *Front. Phys.* **2022**, *10*, 900502. [CrossRef]
31. Attar, M.A.; Roshani, M.; Hosseinzadeh, K.; Ganji, D.D. Analytical Solution of Fractional Differential Equations by Akbari–Ganji's Method. Partial Differ. *Equ. Appl. Math.* **2022**, *6*, 100450.
32. Shah, R.; Khan, H.; Mustafa, S.; Kumam, P.; Arif, M. Analytical Solutions of Fractional-Order Diffusion Equations by Natural Transform Decomposition Method. *Entropy* **2019**, *21*, 557. [CrossRef]
33. Maldon, B.; Thamwattana, N. A Fractional Diffusion Model for Dye-Sensitized Solar Cells. *Molecules* **2020**, *25*, 2966. [CrossRef]
34. Aboelenen, T. A Direct Discontinuous Galerkin Method for Fractional Convection-Diffusion and Schrödinger-Type Equations. *Eur. Phys. J. Plus* **2018**, *133*, 316. [CrossRef]
35. Parvizi, M.; Eslahchi, M.R.; Dehghan, M. Numerical Solution of Fractional Advection-Diffusion Equation with a Nonlinear Source Term. *Numer. Algorithms* **2015**, *68*, 601–629. [CrossRef]
36. Singh, J.; Swroop, R.; Kumar, D. A Computational Approach for Fractional Convection-Diffusion Equation via Integral Transforms. *Ain Shams Eng. J.* **2018**, *9*, 1019–1028. [CrossRef]
37. Bi, Y.; Jiang, Z. The Finite Volume Element Method for the Two-Dimensional Space-Fractional Convection–Diffusion Equation. *Adv. Differ. Equ.* **2021**, *2021*, 379. [CrossRef]
38. Ding, H.; Zhang, Y. New Numerical Methods for the Riesz Space Fractional Partial Differential Equations. *Comput. Math. Appl.* **2012**, *63*, 1135–1146. [CrossRef]
39. Anley, E.F.; Zheng, Z. Finite Difference Approximation Method for a Space Fractional Convection–Diffusion Equation with Variable Coefficients. *Symmetry* **2020**, *12*, 485. [CrossRef]
40. Liu, J.; Zhang, J.; Zhang, X. Semi-Discretized Numerical Solution for Time Fractional Convection–Diffusion Equation by RBF-FD. *Appl. Math. Lett.* **2022**, *128*, 107880. [CrossRef]
41. Saadeh, R. Numerical Solutions of Fractional Convection-Diffusion Equation Using Finite-Difference and Finite-Volume Schemes. *J. Math. Comput. Sci.* **2021**, *11*, 7872–7891.
42. Ragb, O.; Mohamed, M.; Matbuly, M.S.; Civalek, O. Sinc and Discrete Singular Convolution for Analysis of Three-layer Composite of Perovskite Solar Cell. *Int. J. Energy Res.* **2022**, *4*, 4279–4300. [CrossRef]
43. Mustafa, A.; Salama, R.S.; Mohamed, M. Analysis of Generalized Nonlinear Quadrature for Novel Fractional-Order Chaotic Systems Using Sinc Shape Function. *Mathematics* **2023**, *11*, 1932. [CrossRef]
44. Yang, Y.; Nawrocki, R.A.; Voyles, R.M.; Zhang, H.H. A Fractional Drift Diffusion Model for Organic Semiconductor Devices. *Comput. Mater. Contin.* **2021**, *69*, 237–266. [CrossRef]
45. Choo, K.Y.; Muniandy, S.V.; Woon, K.L.; Gan, M.T.; Ong, D.S. Modeling Anomalous Charge Carrier Transport in Disordered Organic Semiconductors Using the Fractional Drift-Diffusion Equation. *Org. Electron.* **2017**, *41*, 157–165. [CrossRef]
46. Tress, W.; Leo, K.; Riede, M. Optimum Mobility, Contact Properties, and Open-Circuit Voltage of Organic Solar Cells: A Drift-Diffusion Simulation Study. *Phys. Rev. B* **2012**, *85*, 155201. [CrossRef]
47. Fallahpour, A.H.; Di Carlo, A.; Lugli, P. Sensitivity of the Drift-Diffusion Approach in Estimating the Power Conversion Efficiency of Bulk Heterojunction Polymer Solar Cells. *Energies* **2017**, *10*, 285. [CrossRef]
48. Caputo, M. Linear Models of Dissipation Whose Q Is Almost Frequency Independent—II. *Geophys. J. Int.* **1967**, *13*, 529–539. [CrossRef]
49. Weilbeer, M. *Efficient Numerical Methods for Fractional Differential Equations and Their Analytical Background*; Papierflieger: Clausthal-Zellerfeld, Germany, 2006.
50. Shu, C. *Differential Quadrature and Its Application in Engineering*; Springer Science & Business Media: Berlin/Heidelberg, Germany, 2012; ISBN 1447104072.
51. Ragb, O.; Mohamed, M.; Matbuly, M.S.; Civalek, O. Nonlinear Analysis of Organic Polymer Solar Cells Using Differential Quadrature Technique with Distinct and Unique Shape Function. *CMES Comput. Model. Eng. Sci* **2023**, *137*, 8992. [CrossRef]
52. Abdelfattah, W.M.; Ragb, O.; Salah, M.; Mohamed, M. A Robust and Versatile Numerical Framework for Modeling Complex Fractional Phenomena: Applications to Riccati and Lorenz Systems. *Fractal Fract.* **2024**, *8*, 647. [CrossRef]
53. Shu, C.; Yao, Q.; Yeo, K.S. Block-Marching in Time with DQ Discretization: An Efficient Method for Time-Dependent Problems. *Comput. Methods Appl. Mech. Eng.* **2002**, *191*, 4587–4597. [CrossRef]
54. Shu, C.; Richards, B.E. Application of Generalized Differential Quadrature to Solve Two-dimensional Incompressible Navier-Stokes Equations. *Int. J. Numer. Methods Fluids* **1992**, *15*, 791–798. [CrossRef]

55. Ahmad, S.W.; Sarwar, M.; Shah, K.; Ahmadian, A.; Salahshour, S. Fractional Order Mathematical Modeling of Novel Corona Virus (COVID-19). *Math. Methods Appl. Sci.* **2023**, *46*, 7847–7860. [CrossRef]
56. Anley, E.F.; Zheng, Z. Finite Difference Method for Two-Sided Two Dimensional Space Fractional Convection-Diffusion Problem with Source Term. *Mathematics* **2020**, *8*, 1878. [CrossRef]
57. Ragb, O.; Mohamed, M.; Matbuly, M.S.; Civalek, O. An Accurate Numerical Approach for Studying Perovskite Solar Cells. *Int. J. Energy Res.* **2021**, *45*, 16456–16477. [CrossRef]

fractal and fractional

MDPI

Article

Personalised Fractional-Order Autotuner for the Maintenance Phase of Anaesthesia Using Sine-Tests

Marcian D. Mihai [1], Isabela R. Birs [1,2], Nicoleta E. Badau [1], Erwin T. Hegedus [1], Amani Ynineb [2] and Cristina I. Muresan [1,*]

[1] Department of Automation, Technical University of Cluj-Napoca, Memorandumului Street No 28, 400114 Cluj-Napoca, Romania; marcian.mihai@aut.utcluj.ro (M.D.M.); isabela.birs@aut.utcluj.ro (I.R.B.); nicoleta.badau@aut.utcluj.ro (N.E.B.); erwin.hegedus@aut.utcluj.ro (E.T.H.)

[2] Research Group on Dynamical Systems and Control, Department of Electromechanics, Systems and Metal Engineering, Ghent University, Tech Lane Science Park 125, 9052 Gent, Belgium; amani.ynineb@ugent.be

* Correspondence: cristina.muresan@aut.utcluj.ro

Abstract: The research field of clinical practice has experienced a substantial increase in the integration of information technology and control engineering, which includes the management of medication administration for general anaesthesia. The invasive nature of input signals is the reason why autotuning methods are not widely used in this research field. This study proposes a non-invasive method using small-amplitude sine tests to estimate patient parameters, which allows the design of a personalised controller using an autotuning principle. The primary objective is to regulate the Bispectral Index through the administration of Propofol during the maintenance phase of anaesthesia, using a personalised fractional-order PID. This work aims to demonstrate the effectiveness of personalised control, which is facilitated by the proposed sine-based method. The closed-loop simulation results demonstrate the efficiency of the proposed approach.

Keywords: drug dosing; anaesthesia; closed-loop control of anaesthesia; fractional-order controllers; autotuners; sine test

1. Introduction

Automated drug dosage systems integrate real-time physiological data, such as blood pressure, heart rate, oxygen saturation, and levels of exhaled carbon dioxide, utilising computerised algorithms designed to control the delivery of anaesthetic agents. Sensors continuously monitor these parameters, and the system's algorithms adjust the rate of drug infusion to maintain a stable anaesthetic state that is neither too deep nor too light. Target-controlled infusion (TCI) systems are frequently implemented in general anaesthesia [1–3]. To obtain a specific target concentration of the anaesthetic agent in the blood or brain, these systems calculate the drug dose necessary.

The primary goal of research in automated systems for anaesthesia is to obtain precise control over the administration of drug dosage during all stages of a surgical procedure. This precision is crucial for ensuring the safety and well-being of patients, as severe complications can result from insufficient or excessive dosing [4]. Nevertheless, a closed-loop control system that is capable of continually adjusting drug delivery in response to the patient's evolving physiological state is necessary to achieve such precision.

Anaesthesia mainly comprises three stages: the induction phase, the maintenance phase and the emergence phase [5]. The induction phase commences with the administration of intravenous anaesthetic agents, which rapidly induce unconsciousness in the patient. The maintenance phase aims to ensure that the patient remains unconscious and pain-free throughout the procedure, provided that the desired depth of anaesthesia has been achieved. This is accomplished by closely monitoring vital signs while administering a continuous intravenous infusion of anaesthetic medications. Ultimately, the patient's consciousness is progressively restored during the emergence phase, as the administration of anaesthetic agents is reduced or ceased. Careful management during this stage provides a smooth recovery while reducing the likelihood of complications, including agitation, nausea, or pain. One of the most important aspects in anaesthesia is ensuring the depth of hypnosis, evaluated using the measured Bispectral Index (BIS) signal [6]. An adequate level of hypnosis is usually achieved by administering a certain Propofol drug dose at a certain rate. Several control strategies have been developed to handle Propofol drug dosing to achieve a specific BIS signal. Almost all control algorithms share a common requirement: the necessity of a mathematical model for the patient. Although the majority of research focuses on population-based models, a subset has shifted towards personalised control [7]. This results in tailored controller parameters based on patient demographics. The results of the closed-loop simulation indicate that the individualised controller enhances robustness to patient variability; however, it also demonstrates a reduction in bandwidth, leading to diminished disturbance rejection capabilities.

The primary objective of this research is to investigate the benefit of using personalised controllers, designed using autotuning methods. Such an approach has yet to be considered for anaesthesia regulation. The necessity of accurately predicting the patient response remains essential amid the development of autotuning mechanisms. Autotuners are dependent on feedback from the system they control, implying that if the system's behaviour is not well predicted, the tuning process may be inaccurate, resulting in suboptimal or even unsafe outcomes [8]. Performing classical autotuning tests, such as relay tests or Ziegler–Nichols, is completely unfeasible due to safety reasons [9]. These tests require finding the critical operating point of a system. For example, causing the patient's brain activity to experience a sustained oscillation regime having considerable amplitude is strongly against clinical safety standards. However, minimally invasive methods with small amplitude input signals would be acceptable. In this paper, such an approach is attempted, and it is based on a sine test that is compliant with patients' safety standards and provides sufficient data for tuning the controller. The data collected using this sine test are further used to design fractional-order autotuners. The choice of fractional-order controllers is based on their enhanced flexibility and robustness compared to the traditional integer order controllers [10].

Fractional-order PID (FO-PID) controllers present advantages compared to traditional integer-order PID controllers in the context of general anaesthesia, especially in regulating the depth of hypnosis and maintaining hemodynamic stability. Research indicates that FO-PID controllers demonstrate improved robustness to patient variability, resulting in more consistent performance across varied patient populations [11]. They offer enhanced disturbance rejection, effectively reducing the influence of surgical stimuli and other disruptions. Their expanded set of tuning parameters enhances flexibility and precision in control design, making them suitable for adaptive strategies that can adjust in real time to changing patient dynamics.

Fuzzy-type controllers are also appropriate in applications where mathematical models are difficult or unfeasible to establish. Additionally, fuzzy controllers are increasingly recognised for their effectiveness in managing general anaesthesia, particularly in addressing the nonlinearities, uncertainties, and imprecise characteristics of physiological responses during surgical interventions. Fuzzy logic controllers differ from traditional controllers by employing a rule-based approach that simulates human reasoning, rendering them especially appropriate for the complex and variable dynamics inherent in anaesthesia [12]. However, fuzzy rules and membership functions need to be carefully defined. The complexity can potentially increase in the context of patient intra- and inter-variability. Due to this, in this paper, a personalised fractional-order controller is preferred.

For the induction phase, a PID controller will be used for all patients. This PID controller is designed using a nominal patient model by using standard frequency domain tuning methods. The gain crossover frequency is imposed as a performance criterion to ensure a certain settling time during the induction phase. Once the BIS signal reaches a steady state value ranging between 47.5 and 52.5, indicative of an adequate level of hypnosis, the proposed sine test is applied using a frequency that matches the gain crossover frequency utilised for the induction phase. The sine test is further used to estimate the gain, phase, and derivative of the phase for each patient. This information is later employed in the autotuning of a fractional-order controller to be used during the maintenance phase. The safety range of BIS values is between 40 and 60 [13], with a steady-state value ideally equal to 50. Surgical stimuli occurring during the maintenance phase will cause variations in the BIS signal. The proposed method attempts to limit this variation and ensure that the BIS signal remains within a $\pm 5\%$ range of the steady-state value during the maintenance phase. The proposed sine test is robust to noisy signals and provides accurate estimations of the patient's gain, phase, and derivative of the phase. As such, it enables the design of a personalised fractional-order controller.

The primary contribution and novelty of this research are the introduction of a sine-test-based autotuning approach for the design of personalised fractional-order controllers that are intended to regulate the depth of hypnosis in anaesthesia. This strategy eliminates the necessity for invasive procedures or time-consuming modelling efforts by directly estimating patient-specific dynamics from data using the sine test, in contrast to traditional methods that rely on constructing detailed patient models. The proposed autotuning method is entirely non-invasive, carries no risk to the patient, and offers a considerable improvement in efficiency and adaptability. This is the first application of such a method in the context of closed-loop anaesthesia control. This work represents an advance in the development of automated and personalised anaesthetic systems by offering a computationally efficient, safe, robust to noise, and practicable alternative for customising anaesthesia delivery.

To mimic the dynamics of a patient, a novel patient simulator [14] will be used. To model the patient's BIS signal as a function of the administered Propofol, pharmacokinetic (PK) and pharmacodynamic (PD) models are most frequently used [15–17], with parameters depending on the patient's age, weight, height, and gender. These models depict the manner in which a drug interacts with the body. In general, a three-compartment PK model delineates the fast-acting compartment (blood) and two additional compartments that represent the slower-acting tissue volumes of muscle and fat. The effect site concentration is represented by the addition of a hypothetical compartment that represents the transport/mixing dynamics of the substance to the effect location. PD modelling is fundamentally based on the dose–response relationship, which seeks to explain the mechanism by which variations in drug dosage result in changes in the intensity of the drug's effect. The relationship between drug concentration and effect is frequently nonlinear, as the effects of a drug become more potent as the concentration increases. Several PK-PD models exist. In this case, the Schnider PK model [18] is employed along with a Hill function that models the PD compartment.

Closed-loop simulation results are performed. Comparative results are presented utilising both the population-based controller and the personalised controller for each patient during the maintenance phase. This demonstrates the effectiveness of personalised control.

The paper is structured as follows. Section 2 presents the mathematical foundation, while Section 3 details the procedures and methods utilised. Simulation results are included in Section 4, while the last section contains the conclusions and proposes prospective routes for further study in the field.

2. Materials and Methods

2.1. Sine Test Method

As stated in the introduction, once the BIS signal has reached steady state, a sine test is performed based on the approach in [19]. A sinusoidal input signal of small amplitude and frequency equal to ω_{gc}, denoted $u(t)$, is applied as the Propofol drug rate. The term 'small' refers to an amplitude which is significantly smaller than the dosage used for the maintenance phase. The exact quantities will be provided in the following subchapter.

The patient's behaviour (BIS level) with respect to Propofol is denoted with $P(s)$ and assumed to be unknown. The sine test will estimate the patient frequency response denoted as $P(j\omega)$, as indicated hereafter. To tune a suitable controller, the following patient's frequency response information is required: the magnitude M, the phase ϕ and the derivative of the phase $d\phi$ at the gain-crossover frequency. Computing the magnitude and phase using sine tests measurements is straightforward:

$$M = \left|P\left(j\omega_{gc}\right)\right| = \frac{A_o}{A_i}, \tag{1}$$

$$\phi = \angle P\left(j\omega_{gc}\right) = \omega_{gc}\tau = \omega_{gc}(t_i - t_o), \tag{2}$$

where A_i and A_o represent the amplitudes of the input and the output signals, respectively, and $\tau = (t_i - t_o)$ represents the time shift between the input and the output signals.

The third parameter, $d\phi$, will be used in the controller design to ensure the iso-damping property (or the robustness to gain variations). The human body is arguably one of the most unpredictable systems and prone to variations in time; therefore, the need for robust controllers is self-explanatory [11,20]. Extracting the phase derivative from a *single sine test* is not obvious, nor trivial. Figure 1 provides the innovative method proposed by the authors of [19] to compute $d\phi$, based on the magnitudes and phases of two signals: the output y(t) and the output of the process derivative, denoted as $\bar{y}(t)$.

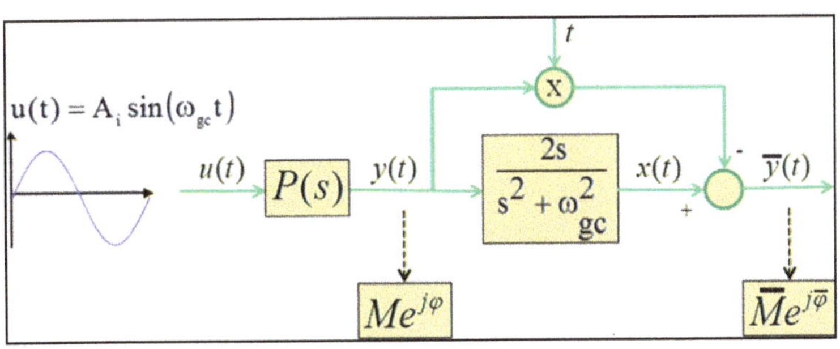

Figure 1. Proposed setup for the sine test.

The next part will demonstrate that the methodology depicted in Figure 1 effectively provides the process derivative signal. The output $\bar{y}(t)$ of the process derivative can be computed as:

$$\bar{y}(t) = x(t) - t * y(t), \tag{3}$$

where *x(t)* denotes the output of the process *P(jω)* when an input signal *t*u(t)* is applied at its input. The operator * denotes the convolution of two signals. The property of the Laplace transform regarding the derivative of a signal will be employed:

$$\frac{dF(s)}{ds} = \mathcal{L}\{-t * f(t)\}, \tag{4}$$

where $F(s) = \mathcal{L}\{f(t)\}$.

The other mathematical definition of the process derivative output, $\bar{y}(t)$, refers to the exact meaning of this signal:

$$\overline{Y}(s) = \frac{dP(s)}{ds}U(s), \tag{5}$$

where $\overline{Y}(s)$ and *U(s)* are the Laplace transforms of signals $\bar{y}(t)$ and *u(t)*, respectively.

Starting from the definition of the signal *x(t)* given in the theorem hypothesis, the following relation holds:

$$X(s) = P(s)\mathcal{L}\{t * u(t)\}, \tag{6}$$

where *X(s)* represents the Laplace transform of *x(t)*. Employing (4), (6) can be rewritten as:

$$X(s) = -P(s)\frac{dU(s)}{ds}. \tag{7}$$

The Laplace transform of the sinusoidal input signal *u(t)* is given by:

$$U(s) = \frac{A_i\omega_{gc}}{s^2 + {\omega_{gc}}^2}. \tag{8}$$

The derivative of *U(s)* is computed as follows:

$$\frac{dU(s)}{ds} = -\frac{2s}{s^2 + {\omega_{gc}}^2}U(s). \tag{9}$$

Utilising (9) in (7) leads to:

$$X(s) = -P(s)\frac{dU(s)}{ds} = \frac{2s}{s^2 + {\omega_{gc}}^2}P(s)U(s) = \frac{2s}{s^2 + {\omega_{gc}}^2}Y(s). \tag{10}$$

Equation (10) demonstrates that the signal *x(t)* can be computed utilising the output signal, *y(t)*. The derivative of the output signal in Laplace domain is computed as:

$$\frac{dY(s)}{ds} = \frac{d(P(s)U(s))}{ds} = \frac{dP(s)}{ds}U(s) + \frac{dU(s)}{ds}P(s). \tag{11}$$

If one utilises (5) and (10) in (11), it leads to:

$$\frac{dY(s)}{ds} = \overline{Y}(s) - X(s). \tag{12}$$

Applying the inverse Laplace transform to (12) demonstrates that the process derivative is achievable. This indicates the feasibility of the testing procedure outlined in Figure 1. The derivative of the process is indeed accessible without any mathematical differentiation being employed.

The modulus and phase of $\bar{y}(t)$ are computed in the same manner as in (1) and (2):

$$\overline{M} = \frac{A_{\bar{y}}}{A_i}, \tag{13}$$

$$\overline{\phi} = \omega_{gc}\tau_{\overline{y}} = \omega_{gc}(t_i - t_{\overline{y}}), \tag{14}$$

where $\overline{M}$ is the amplitude of the signal $\bar{y}(t)$ and $\overline{\phi}$ is the phase shift between $\bar{y}(t)$ and $u(t)$.

The frequency domain relation of the process derivative is given by:

$$\left.\frac{dP(j\omega)}{d\omega}\right|_{\omega=\omega_{gc}} = \overline{M}e^{j\overline{\phi}}, \tag{15}$$

By expanding both the left- and right-hand sides of (15) and complex numbers mathematical refinements, the equation becomes:

$$-j\left.\frac{dM}{d\omega}\right|_{\omega=\omega_{gc}} + M\left.\frac{d\phi}{d\omega}\right|_{\omega=\omega_{gc}} = \overline{M}\cos(\overline{\phi}-\phi) + j\overline{M}\sin(\overline{\phi}-\phi). \tag{16}$$

Equating the real and imaginary parts of the two terms in (16) results in the mathematical expression of the process phase derivative:

$$d\phi = \left.\frac{d\angle P(j\omega)}{d\omega}\right|_{\omega=\omega_{gc}} = \frac{\overline{M}}{M}\cos(\overline{\phi}-\phi), \tag{17}$$

The procedure is now complete. However, the proposed approach for estimating the frequency response slope based on filtering the output signal $y(t)$ as indicated in Figure 1 is simple, but error-prone. This study utilises a patient simulator and not real clinical data. The measurement of BIS is derived from electroencephalographic (EEG) signals through spectral and bispectral analysis. BIS measurements are often affected by noise, which can compromise their reliability. Common sources of noise include electromyographic (EMG) activity, poor electrode contact, external electrical interference, and patient-specific variability in EEG responses. To mitigate these issues, another approach that is robust to noise is presented in Appendix A.

2.2. Autotuning Mathematical Background

Upon obtaining the necessary parameters, ω_{gc}, M, ϕ and $d\phi$ (using (1), (2) and (17)), one may proceed with computing the controller parameters. Two types of fractional-order controllers are presented in this paper: FO-PI and FO-PID. Their transfer functions are indicated below:

$$H_{FO-PI}(s) = k_p\left(1 + \frac{k_i}{s^{\mu}}\right), \tag{18}$$

$$H_{FO-PID}(s) = k_p\left(1 + \frac{k_i}{s^{\mu}} + k_d s^{\lambda}\right), \tag{19}$$

where μ and λ denote the fractional orders, while k_p, k_i, k_d correspond to the proportional, integrative and derivative gains.

In this manuscript, the Grunwald–Letnikov [21] definition of the fractional-order derivative is used, which is generally preferred for applications, due to the convenient relation with the Laplace transform:

$$\mathfrak{D}^{\alpha} f(t)|_{t=kh} = \lim_{h\to 0}\frac{1}{h^{\alpha}}\sum\nolimits_{j=0}^{k}(-1)^j\binom{\alpha}{j}f(kh-jh), \tag{20}$$

where $\mathfrak{D}^{\alpha}$ is the fractional derivative of order α. The mathematical formulas for the modulus, phase, and phase derivative of the controllers can be quickly deduced due to the known structure of these controllers. These equations are presented in [21].

An algorithm has been developed to compute the controller parameters. The tuning is performed according to a set of constraints. The gain crossover frequency is correlated to the settling time requirements. Higher values of ω_{gc} are associated with quicker settling times. This is mathematically represented by the equation for magnitude:

$$|H_{OL}(j\omega_{gc})| = |H_{FO-PI/D}(j\omega_{gc})||P(j\omega_{gc})| = 1, \tag{21}$$

where $H_{OL}(j\omega_{gc}) = H_{FO-PI/D}(j\omega_{gc})P(j\omega_{gc})$ is the open loop frequency response at ω_{gc}. Phase margin (PM) serves as an essential performance metric associated with the stability of closed-loop systems, directly influencing the anticipated overshoot and undershoot. A high numerical value typically signifies a reduced excess. The equation that addresses the overshoot requirement is as follows:

$$\angle H_{OL}(j\omega_{gc}) = \angle H_{FO-PI/D}(j\omega_{gc}) + \angle P(j\omega_{gc}) = -\pi + \text{PM}, \tag{22}$$

A robustness constraint has been added to address potential gain errors arising from patient variability:

$$\begin{gathered} \left.\frac{d\angle H_{OL}(j\omega)}{d\omega}\right|_{\omega=\omega_{gc}} = 0 \\ \left.\frac{d\angle P(j\omega)}{d\omega}\right|_{\omega=\omega_{gc}} + \left.\frac{d\angle H_{FO-PI/D}(j\omega)}{d\omega}\right|_{\omega=\omega_{gc}} = 0 \end{gathered} \tag{23}$$

Several other researchers [22,23] proposed supplementary performance criteria to be used in the design of fractional-order controllers, such as the sensitivity (S), and the complementary sensitivity (T) functions, to address the rejection of disturbances, among others. Nevertheless, a model of the process is necessary for all these performance criteria. No patient model is employed in this research, as the proposed control method is an autotuning algorithm. Therefore, only the performance specifications mentioned above (21)–(23) are used in the design of the controllers.

Several performance metrics are used to evaluate the efficiency of the proposed control algorithms. These correspond to the metrics usually employed in anaesthesia control and are detailed below.

Both the control signal and the output must exhibit stable behaviour with minimum oscillation. A high overshoot value presents a serious risk of taking the BIS out of the safe range. A large PM value is selected to ensure that a small overshoot is obtained:

$$\sigma \leq 5\%. \tag{24}$$

Another important performance indicator is the time-to-target (TT), which refers to the time required for the controller to adjust the BIS signal to a desired range of values while adhering to the input safety constraints. The literature presents a range between 3 and 5 min as being appropriate for TT [24]. The condition imposed by the authors is:

$$\text{TT} \leq 200 \text{ s}. \tag{25}$$

An important aspect to be considered is that this constraint refers to the fast rejection of the disturbances and not to the response of the closed-loop system to a BIS reference. The BIS signal must stay within a range of 40 to 60 at all times, as stated in [13]; however, in this research, the values were restricted to 47.5 and 52.5 in order to have more precise control. Usually, a variation of $\pm 10\%$ is commonly employed for the Bispectral Index control. This research proposes a stricter range of only $\pm 5\%$, with respect to the ideal BIS signal value of 50. This facilitates a more precise control and a safer clinical procedure.

The Propofol rate should not exceed 200 mg/kg/h [25], a value which corresponds to 3.33 mg/kg/min. The authors proposed an even stricter limitation of a maximum of 2.5 mg/kg/min. Thus, the control signal must always be positive and less than the imposed value due to safety concerns.

A third performance indicator used in this manuscript is the Integral of Absolute Error (IAE) to evaluate the efficiency of the controllers in rejecting disturbances, defined as:

$$\mathrm{IAE} = \int_0^{\infty} |\mathrm{r(t)} - \mathrm{BIS(t)}|\mathrm{dt}, \tag{26}$$

where *BIS(t)* is the simulated output and *r(t)* is the reference value.

The frequency response of the FO-PID controller is mathematically defined as:

$$\begin{aligned} \mathrm{H_{FO-PID}}(\mathrm{j}\omega) = \mathrm{k_p}\Big(1 + \mathrm{k_i}\Big((\mathrm{j}\omega)^{-\mu}\Big(\cos\frac{\mu\pi}{2} - \mathrm{j}\sin\frac{\mu\pi}{2}\Big)\Big) \\ +\mathrm{k_d}\omega^{\lambda}\Big(\cos\frac{\lambda\pi}{2} + \mathrm{j}\sin\frac{\lambda\pi}{2}\Big)\Big), \end{aligned} \tag{27}$$

Replacing (27) into (21)–(23), leads to the following system of nonlinear equations:

$$\begin{aligned} \mathrm{k_p}\sqrt{\left(1+\mathrm{k_i}\omega_{gc}{}^{-\mu}\cos\frac{\mu\pi}{2} + \mathrm{k_d}\omega_{gc}{}^{\lambda}\cos\frac{\lambda\pi}{2}\right)^2 + \left(-\mathrm{k_i}\omega_{gc}{}^{-\mu}\sin\frac{\mu\pi}{2} + \mathrm{k_d}\omega_{gc}{}^{\lambda}\sin\frac{\lambda\pi}{2}\right)^2} \\ -\frac{1}{|\mathrm{P}(\mathrm{j}\omega_{\mathrm{gc}})|} = 0, \end{aligned} \tag{28}$$

$$\frac{-\mathrm{k_i}\omega_{gc}{}^{-\mu}\sin\frac{\mu\pi}{2} + \mathrm{k_d}\omega_{gc}{}^{\lambda}\sin\frac{\lambda\pi}{2}}{1+\mathrm{k_i}\omega_{gc}{}^{-\mu}\cos\frac{\mu\pi}{2} + \mathrm{k_d}\omega_{gc}{}^{\lambda}\cos\frac{\lambda\pi}{2}} - \tan(-\pi + PM - \angle \mathrm{P}(\mathrm{j}\omega_{\mathrm{gc}})) = 0, \tag{29}$$

$$\begin{aligned} \frac{\omega_{\mathrm{gc}}{}^{\mu-1}\left(\mathrm{k_i}\mu\sin\frac{\mu\pi}{2} + \mathrm{k_d}\mathrm{k_i}\mu\omega_{\mathrm{gc}}{}^{\mu}\sin\frac{(\mu+\lambda)\pi}{2} + \mathrm{k_d}\mathrm{k_i}\lambda\omega_{\mathrm{gc}}{}^{\lambda}\sin\frac{(\mu+\lambda)\pi}{2} + \mathrm{k_d}\mu\omega_{\mathrm{gc}}{}^{\mu+\lambda}\sin\frac{\lambda\pi}{2}\right)}{\omega_{\mathrm{gc}}{}^{2\mu} + \mathrm{k_i^2} + \mathrm{k_d^2}\omega_{\mathrm{gc}}{}^{2(\mu+\lambda)} + 2\mathrm{k_i}\omega_{\mathrm{gc}}{}^{\mu}\cos\frac{\mu\pi}{2} + 2\mathrm{k_d}\omega_{\mathrm{gc}}{}^{2\mu+\lambda}\cos\frac{\lambda\pi}{2} + 2\mathrm{k_d}\mathrm{k_i}\omega_{\mathrm{gc}}{}^{\lambda+\mu}\cos\frac{(\mu+\lambda)\pi}{2}} \\ + \left.\frac{\mathrm{d}\angle \mathrm{P}(\mathrm{j}\omega)}{\mathrm{d}\omega}\right|_{\omega=\omega_{\mathrm{gc}}} = 0. \end{aligned} \tag{30}$$

2.3. Algorithm Description

The procedure to design the personalised controllers is detailed in what follows. To determine all controller parameters, an optimisation algorithm based on the Matlab R2024A "fmincon" function is used to solve the system of equations composed of (28)–(30). For the tuning of the FO-PI controller parameters, only three parameters are estimated, namely the three controller parameters, k_p, k_i and μ. The remaining two parameters, k_d and λ in (26)–(28), are set to null. For the FO-PID, all five parameters are estimated based on solving the system of equations in (28)–(30). The gain crossover frequency and the phase margin are specified a priori as design criteria, while an initial starting guess is provided for all controller parameters in the "fmincon" function. These initial values are those reported in [11].

First, an integer order PID controller will be computed for the induction phase, based on the already existing PK-PD model of the patient, with the model parameters estimated according to patient biometric data, such as height, weight, age, and sex [26]. This part will be only briefly presented since the focus of this paper is not on the induction phase. The authors studied the control of induction in [27]. The purpose of this step is to establish the cutting frequency, ω_{gc}, which is later used for the sine test.

One relevant example of a PID autotuning algorithm can be found in [28]. Our adaptation of this algorithm provided a PID controller having the form:

$$H_{PID} = 0.205\left(1 + \frac{0.00046}{s} + \frac{82.5s}{1.66s+1}\right). \quad (31)$$

The imposed cutting frequency for this PID controller is 0.0025 rad/s. This finding is consistent with the current state of knowledge in the field of anaesthesia control, which posits that patients' responses to these medications are slow [29]. The closed-loop response for one patient is presented in Figure 2.

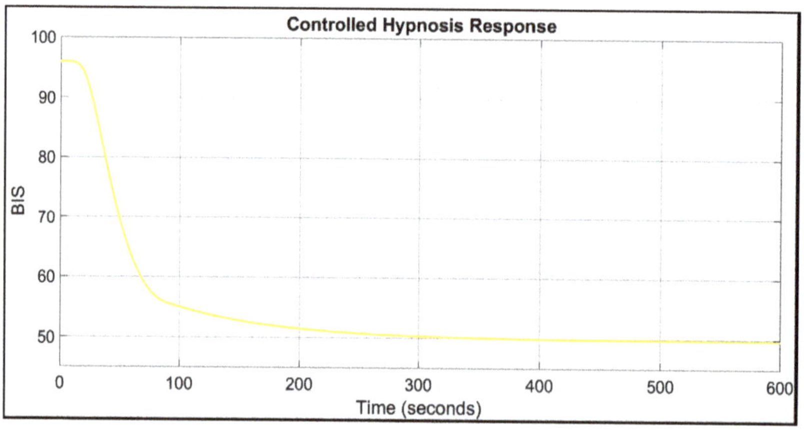

Figure 2. Closed-loop control of induction phase using PID.

As depicted in the picture above, there is a slight undershoot, and the TT is around 150 s, which is consistent with clinical protocols. This controller does not represent the main focus of this research, but merely a starting point.

The sine test will be applied to determine the patient's parameters in the next step. The sine input has a frequency equal to 0.0025 rad/s and a 0.05 amplitude of Prop. The usual dosage for maintenance is around 0.1–0.2 mg/kg/min; therefore, the sine test is minimally invasive and does not affect the sleep state of the patient. Figure 3 presents the sinusoidal signals: u, y, and $\bar{y}$. Since there is a significant difference in amplitude for these signals, a scaling operation was necessary to improve the visibility and relevancy of the picture. After computations are performed according to (1), (2) and (17), the process parameters of the studied patient are: $M = 39.47$, $\phi = -104.85°$ and $d\phi = -175.83$.

Research suggests that better control can be achieved using separate controllers for the induction and maintenance phases [30]. In fact, the controller parameters must be precisely chosen to ensure that a rapid transient response without an excessive overshoot is achieved during the induction phase, while in the maintenance phase, the BIS values are kept within the specified interval. Even though a PK-PD model can be estimated a priori, patient uncertainties are prevalent, and the control strategy is susceptible to inter- and intra-patient variability. The retuning of the controller immediately following the induction phase using the BIS signal of each patient diminishes the amount of patient uncertainties and could potentially lead to better and personalised control over the maintenance phase. Once the patient's frequency response characteristics are determined using the sine test, the FO-PI parameters will be computed using the described optimisation algorithm. Different FO-PI controllers can be obtained by imposing different ω_{gc} and PM constraints. The proposed optimisation algorithm is also used for the tuning of the FO-PID parameters. The obtained controllers and their closed-loop simulations are detailed in the next section.

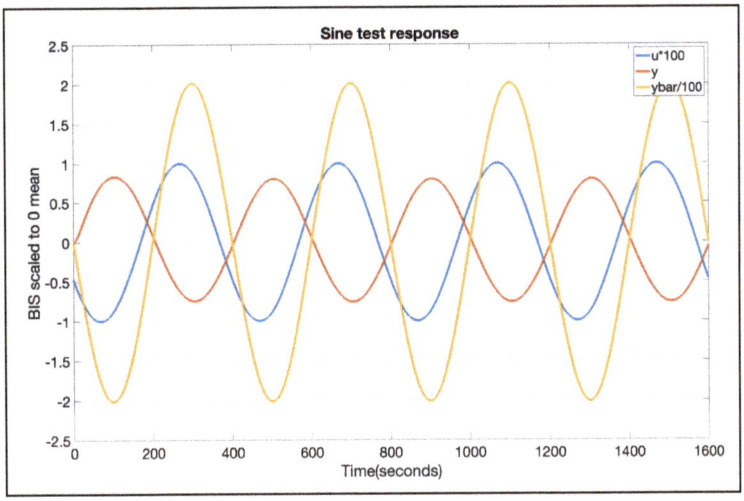

Figure 3. Sine test simulation for one patient.

Remark 1. *The primary reason for considering the sine test to extract relevant patient frequency response characteristics is the assumption that the system is linear. The proposed analysis is conducted within a stable operating point. In this regime, the PD model effectively reduces to a simple gain, thereby rendering any inherent nonlinearities negligible. While it is true that the process exhibits nonlinear behaviour in general, the chosen steady state operating point allows for a linear approximation with sufficient accuracy. Additionally, in the maintenance phase, where BIS is close to 50, the system behaviour aligns well with linear assumptions. This stability ensures that nonlinear effects do not significantly influence the proposed methodology. As a result, the system can be reliably treated as linear without compromising the validity of the proposed approach.*

3. Results

The performance of the controllers in rejecting disturbances will be analysed throughout this section. All presented results are specific to one patient, who was arbitrarily chosen to be the nominal patient. The characteristics of this patient are: age = 62 years, height = 168 cm, weight = 88 kg, sex = female. Proving the effectiveness of personalised control will be performed by using the controllers designed for the nominal case on other patients, followed by designing personalised controllers for each patient specifically. The results will prove the success of personalised control.

The parameters of the FO-PI tuned for the nominal patient are: $k_p = 0.0247$, $k_i = 0.00059$, $\mu = 1.1$, and the structure of the controller is provided in (18). The imposed constraints were: $\omega_{gc} = 0.0025$ rad/s, $PM = 50^\circ$ and the iso-damping property. Figure 4 illustrates the disturbance rejection performance of this controller. Figure 5 presents the control signal, which verifies the clinical limitations of Propofol infusion.

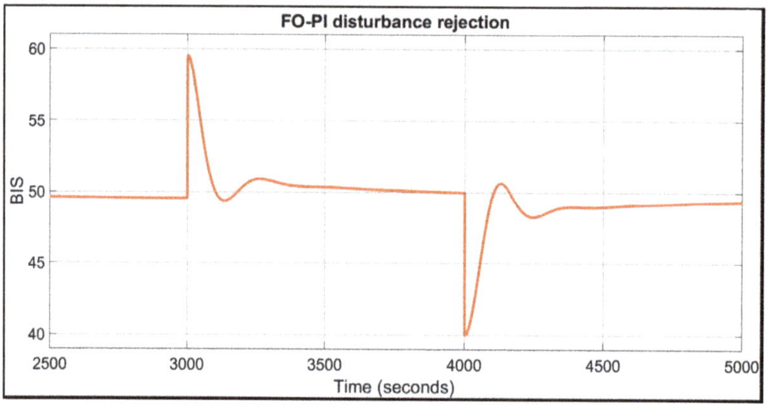

Figure 4. FO-PI disturbance rejection test for the nominal case.

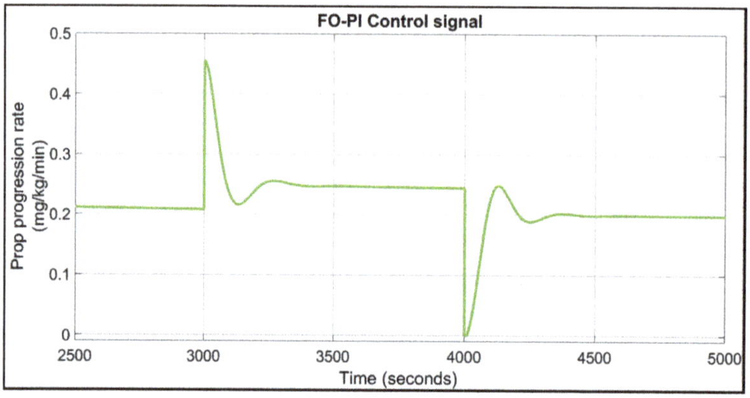

Figure 5. The control signal of the FO-PI controller for the nominal case.

The disturbance signal is composed of two step signals of amplitude 10, which occur consecutively with a 16-minute delay between them. This disturbance profile is supported by the literature [31]. This stimulus profile, or disturbance profile, simulates the patient's arousal reflexes during a surgical procedure [32]. As depicted in the figure, the first disturbance is rejected in 67 s (close to 1 min) while the second disturbance is rejected in 74 s (less than 2 min). These performances are in accordance with the clinical standards. The control signal is within the limitations for safe anaesthetic procedures since its values are positive and smaller than 2.5 mg/kg/min. The range of the control signal is between 0 and 0.5 mg/kg/min, which indicates a higher safety level for the patient. The final performance metric, the IAE, has a value of 2137. While this may initially appear high, it is important to note that the integral is computed over a duration of 2500 s.

As for the FO-PID controller, the parameters are: $k_p = 0.02$, $k_i = 0.0004$, $k_d = 53.8$, $\mu = 1.1$, $\lambda = 1.1$. Figure 6 illustrates the disturbance rejection performance, with TT values of 109 and 134 s. While these values are slightly higher than those of the FO-PI controller, the response is smoother and exhibits no overshoot. The IAE is equal to 2431, which is slightly larger than the one obtained using the FO-PI controller.

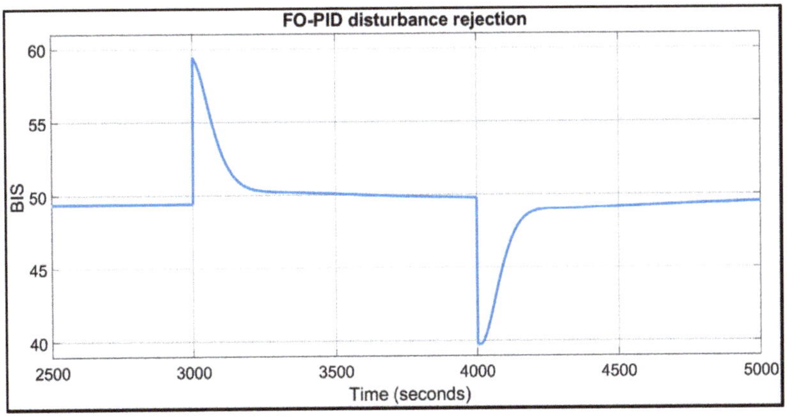

Figure 6. FO-PID disturbance rejection test for the nominal case.

The controller designed for the nominal patient is now used on different patients, and the disturbance rejection performances are analysed. One figure will be presented to illustrate the incapacity of one controller to fully compensate for inter-patient variability. Figure 7 shows that the initial FO-PI controller does not reject, according to clinical standards, the same disturbance profile when applied to another patient.

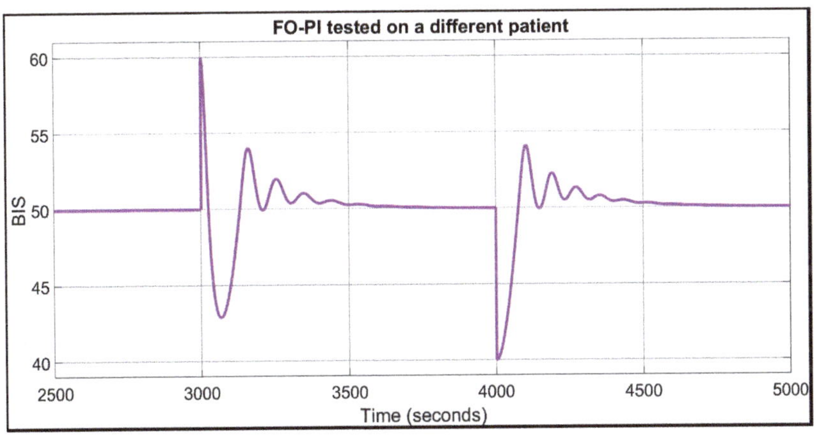

Figure 7. FO-PI disturbance rejection test for another patient.

As shown in Figure 7, the BIS signal exhibits a highly oscillatory behaviour, which could be unpleasant or even harmful for the patient. The TT performance is approximately 180 s, which is nearly three times longer than in the nominal case. The final performance indicator, the IAE, is 5542, which is more than twice the value observed in the nominal case, further emphasising the need for personalised control strategies. The patient's characteristics were: age = 50 years, height = 186 cm, weight = 96 kg, sex = male. The FO-PID response had worse performance due to the derivative component, which is more sensitive to variations in the parameters.

4. Discussion

The two initial controllers were applied to five more different patients, and the disturbance rejection performances did not comply with clinical standards. Longer TT, higher oscillations, and BIS levels not being kept within the 47.5–52.5 safe operating range were the drawbacks encountered. This finding strongly argues for the implementation of personalised control.

To design the personalised controllers, once the induction phase has been completed, a sine test similar to the one presented in Figure 3 is performed for each patient. The M, ϕ and $d\phi$ parameters are obtained for each patient, and personalised FO-PI and FO-PID controllers are designed according to the proposed approach detailed in Section 2. Closed-loop simulations were performed for seven patients. The performances of the personalised controllers are presented in Table 1. Patient 1 is the nominal patient, and it serves as a reference. The two values for TT performance correspond to the response of the system to the chosen disturbance profile. The first value corresponds to the positive disturbance rejection, while the second value refers to the rejection of the negative disturbance.

Table 1. Personalised FO-PI/PID simulations.

Patient	TTs for FO-PI (Seconds)		TTs for FO-PID (Seconds)		IAE		BIS in Safe Range of 40–60?
	Positive Dist.	Negative Dist.	Positive Dist.	Negative Dist.	FO-PI	FO-PID	
1	**67**	**74**	**109**	**134**	2138	2508	Yes
2	94	124	132	207	3002	3507	Yes
3	62	74	102	127	1977	2251	Yes
4	76	86	115	147	2304	2658	Yes
5	63	75	102	126	1987	2205	Yes
6	73	88	113	156	2285	2775	Yes
7	76	85	114	140	2238	2473	Yes

The results indicate that recovery from a positive BIS disturbance is easier for patients. The awakening of a patient, indicated by an increase in the BIS signal, can be managed more effectively than preventing a descent into dangerously deep levels of hypnosis. This finding aligns with the existing literature [33]. In control engineering, the control signal (Propofol rate) is consistently positive; therefore, an increase in the Propofol rate would reduce the BIS signal and counteract the positive disturbance. A negative control signal indicates the extraction of the anaesthetic substance from the blood, which is impractical. Consequently, this complicates the rejection of a negative disturbance, specifically a decrease in the BIS signal.

Figures 8 and 9 provide the graphical visualisation of Table 1. The results of this research are according to the clinical procedures. The nominal patient was not included in these figures for increased readability, as it has already been included in Figures 4 and 6. Both proposed structures for the fractional-order controllers proved efficient in maintaining the BIS level in the safe range and also provide fast disturbance rejection loops. The FO-PI controller proves to be faster than the FO-PID; however, the latter provides a smoother signal with no oscillations.

The findings presented in this research are compared with those documented in the literature [30,34]. These studies also proposed the use of personalised FO-PID controllers to optimise Propofol dosage during general anaesthesia. A key point to note is that none of the referenced papers utilise an autotuning method; instead, they rely on patient-specific models.

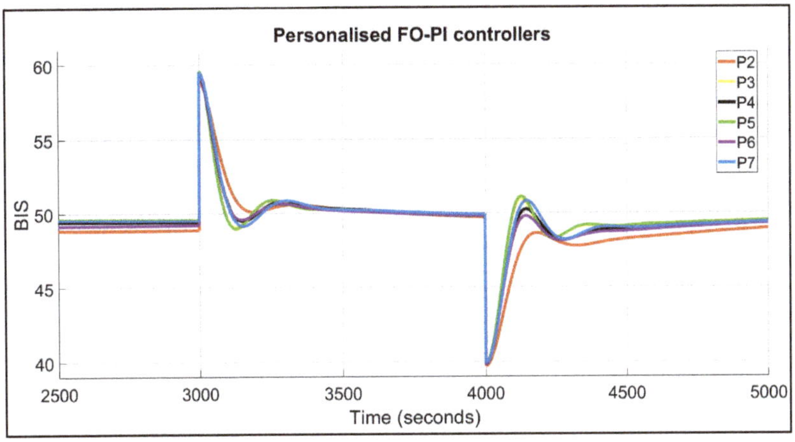

Figure 8. Personalised FO-PI controllers closed-loop simulations.

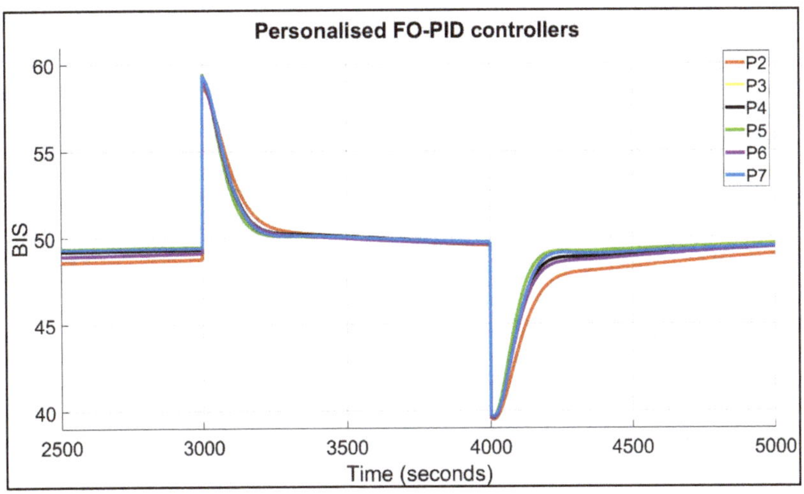

Figure 9. Personalised FO-PID controllers closed-loop simulations.

The TT performances of the FO-PI controllers average 80 s for both positive and negative disturbance steps. The FO-PID controllers present a mean value of 130 s for disturbance rejection. The same disturbance profile was utilised in [30], and the TT performances are around 120 s. Considering that the BIS range used to compute TT in this study was narrower (47.5–52.5) compared to the broader 45–55 range in prior work, the results achieved here demonstrate faster response times despite the stricter criteria. In terms of overshoot, the FO-PI controllers yield comparable performance to that reported in [30], while the FO-PID controllers provide smoother control responses. One advantage of the referenced study is its larger dataset of 13 patients, compared to 7 in the current work. Nevertheless, both studies rely on relatively small patient datasets, which underscores the continued relevance of the proposed research.

In the comparative analysis with the study presented in [34], the results are generally similar. That study introduces three versions of FO-PID controllers, each tuned based on different performance criteria. Their average TT values are 40 s for positive disturbances and 70 s for negative disturbances, which is faster than those observed in this research.

However, the overshoot values reported in [34] are higher than those achieved in the current study. The IAE values reported in [34] range from 1531 to 2354, which are comparable to those obtained in this study. Despite relying on a smaller patient dataset and a stricter BIS range, the proposed research demonstrates competitive performance in terms of TT, overshoot, and IAE when compared to existing studies. The use of personalised FO-PID controllers with an autotuning approach, in contrast to the model-dependent methods found in the literature, highlights the novelty and practical value of this work for enhancing the safety and precision of Propofol administration during general anaesthesia.

5. Conclusions

The study demonstrates the need for personalised control for the maintenance phase of anaesthesia. Two types of fractional-order controllers were developed, and both provided good performance, according to clinical practice. The TT performances are to be noted since the authors proposed a narrower range of safe operation for BIS. Instead of the classical 40–60 range found in the literature [30], the 47.5–52.5 range was used. The highest disturbance rejection time was close to 3.5 min for the FO-PID controller, whereas the FO-PI controller required no more than 2.2 min to reject disturbances. Therefore, FO-PI should be preferred when a faster response is required, while FO-PID is a suitable alternative when smoother control is prioritised. Overall, the results confirm that the FO-PI controller offers superior performance under the given constraints, while having the advantage of a decreased number of parameters to be tuned and decreased complexity compared to the FO-PID controller. This approach provides an even safer environment for the patients during clinical procedures.

The novelty of this work lies in the use of the sine-test to estimate patient information, instead of developing a model of the patient. This autotuning method is a non-invasive one, with no risks for the patient and has the considerable advantage of being faster than the modelling alternative. Introducing an autotuning method, completely novel in the literature, and providing suitable controllers may prove to be advancements in the research field of the closed-loop control of anaesthesia.

The validation of this study was performed using an existing patient simulator. Since the desired controller is an autotuner, the tests may be performed on actual patients as a future research step. However, this procedure requires substantial a priori theoretical safety guarantees. The research reported in this manuscript provides the first preliminary results in this regard. Further development ideas would be introducing more advanced control algorithms [35], which could provide even better performance.

Author Contributions: Conceptualization, C.I.M. and M.D.M.; methodology, M.D.M., E.T.H. and N.E.B.; software, M.D.M., E.T.H. and N.E.B.; validation, C.I.M. and I.R.B.; formal analysis, I.R.B.; investigation, A.Y.; resources, I.R.B. and A.Y.; data curation, M.D.M.; writing—original draft preparation, M.D.M.; writing—review and editing, C.I.M. and M.D.M.; visualization, I.R.B.; supervision, C.I.M. and I.R.B.; project administration, C.I.M.; funding acquisition, C.I.M. and I.R.B. All authors have read and agreed to the published version of the manuscript.

Funding: This work was in part supported by a grant of the Romanian Ministry of Research, Innovation and Digitization, PNRR-III-C9-2022–I8, grant number 760068/23.05.2023. I. R. Birs acknowledges the support of Flanders Research Foundation, Postdoc grant 1203224N, 2023–2026. This work was also supported by a grant of the Ministry of Research, Innovation and Digitization, CNCS -UEFISCDI, project number PN-IV-P2-2.1-TE-2023-0831, within PNCDI IV.

Data Availability Statement: The original contributions presented in this study are included in the article. Further inquiries can be directed to the corresponding author.

Conflicts of Interest: The authors declare no conflicts of interest. The funders had no role in the design of the study; in the collection, analyses, or interpretation of data; in the writing of the manuscript; or in the decision to publish the results.

Abbreviations

The following abbreviations are used in this manuscript:

TCI	Target-controlled infusion
BIS	Bispectral Index
TIVA	Total Intravenous Anaesthesia
PK	Pharmacokinetic
PD	Pharmacodynamic
FO	Fractional order
PID	Proportional-integrative-derivative
Prop	Propofol progression rate
TT	Time-to-target
EEG	Electroencephalographic
EMG	Electromyographic

Appendix A

This section presents the enhanced approach as presented in [36], robust to noises which may appear in clinical trials. The first step is to compute the amplitude A_y and phase φ_y of the output signal y(t). The procedure is based on the Transfer Function Analyzer—Discrete Fourier Transform (TFA-DFT) [37].

The steady-state response of a linear, stable system, described by a transfer function P(s), can be written as:

$$y(t) = A_y \sin\left(\overline{\omega} t + \varphi_y\right) + b + n(t), \tag{A1}$$

where *n(t)* is the stochastic disturbance with zero mean value and *b* is a non-zero bias term (in the case of an integrative process, otherwise *b* = 0). Problems of non-linear distortion and noise corruption are overcome if the measured output *y(t)* is first multiplied by the sine and cosine of the same frequency as the input $\overline{\omega}$, respectively, and then integrated over the measurement period $T_m = k\frac{2\pi}{\overline{\omega}}$:

$$\begin{gathered} y_s = \int_0^{T_m} y(t) \sin(\overline{\omega} t) dt = A_y \int_0^{T_m} (\sin(\overline{\omega} t) \cos\varphi_y + \\ \cos(\overline{\omega} t) \sin\varphi_y) \sin(\overline{\omega} t) dt + \int_0^{T_m} (b + n(t)) \sin(\overline{\omega} t) dt, \end{gathered} \tag{A2}$$

$$\begin{gathered} y_c = \int_0^{T_m} y(t) \cos(\overline{\omega} t) dt = A_y \int_0^{T_m} (\sin(\overline{\omega} t) \cos\varphi_y + \\ \cos(\overline{\omega} t) \sin\varphi_y) \cos(\overline{\omega} t) dt + \int_0^{T_m} (b + n(t)) \cos(\overline{\omega} t) dt. \end{gathered} \tag{A3}$$

With the increase in the averaging time, the contribution of the last term in the right-hand side of (A2) and (A3) can be neglected compared to the first term, which is growing with T_m. Additionally, for a long integration time, the noise will be filtered out (i.e., zero average). Since n(t) is a stochastic disturbance with zero mean value, by selecting a sufficient number of test signal periods, the desired accuracy can be reached even in the case of a low signal-to- noise ratio. In this case, (A2) reduces to:

$$y_s = A_y \cos\varphi_y \int_0^{T_m} \sin^2(\overline{\omega} t) dt + 0.5 A_y \sin\varphi_y \int_0^{T_m} 2\cos(\overline{\omega} t)\sin(\overline{\omega} t) dt. \tag{A4}$$

Rearranging (A4) leads to:

$$y_s = 0.5 T_m A_y \cos\varphi_y - 0.5 A_y \cos\varphi_y \frac{\sin(2\overline{\omega} T_m)}{2\overline{\omega}} - 0.5 A_y \sin\varphi_y \frac{(\cos(2\overline{\omega} T_m) - 1)}{2\overline{\omega}}. \tag{A5}$$

Taking the measurement (also integration) time to be an integer number of periods, as mentioned above, $T_m = k\frac{2\pi}{\overline{\omega}}$, the last two terms in (A5) will be zero, leading to:

$$y_s = 0.5T_m A_y \cos\varphi_y. \tag{A6}$$

A similar analysis can be performed for the signal in (A3), leading to:

$$y_c = 0.5T_m A_y \sin\varphi_y. \tag{A7}$$

Combining (A2) and (A3) leads to:

$$y_c - jy_s = \int_0^{T_m} y(t)(\cos(\overline{\omega}t) - j\sin(\overline{\omega}t))dt = \int_0^{T_m} y(t)e^{-j\overline{\omega}t}dt. \tag{A8}$$

The last term in (A8) can be computed via the DFT:

$$\int_0^{T_m} y(t)e^{-j\overline{\omega}t}dt = T_s \sum_0^{N-1} y(kT_s)e^{-j\overline{\omega}kT_s}, \tag{A9}$$

with a sampling period T_s adequately chosen such that $T_m = NT_s$. The left-hand side of (A9) can be written using (A6) and (A7) as:

$$y_c - jy_s = -j0.5T_m A_y(\cos\varphi_y + j\sin\varphi_y) = -j0.5T_m A_y e^{j\varphi_y}. \tag{A10}$$

Equating (A9) and (A10) leads to a robust way of computing the amplitude A_y and phase φ_y of the output signal $y(t)$:

$$A_y e^{j\varphi_y} = \frac{T_s}{-j0.5T_m} \sum_0^{N-1} y(kT_s)e^{-j\overline{\omega}kT_s} = \frac{2j}{N} \sum_0^{N-1} y(kT_s)e^{-j\overline{\omega}kT_s} \tag{A11}$$

Suppose that, apart from the pure sine of frequency $\overline{\omega}$, the output signal $y(t)$ also exhibits some other sine signals of frequencies, $\hat{\omega} \neq \overline{\omega}$, due to stochastic disturbances and noise. Then, the corresponding sine signal will be amplified by the filter with a bounded gain $\frac{2\hat{\omega}}{|\overline{\omega}^2 - \hat{\omega}^2|}$, but at the same time it will be amplified by the multiplier with the unbounded time signal, t. The effect will be an unbounded $\overline{y}(t)$ signal increasing with time, as resulting from (3). A solution to overcome this problem is based on a modification of the basic scheme in Figure 1 as indicated in Figure A1a, where $y_{TR}(t)$ and $y_{SS}(t)$ are the transient and steady-state parts of the output signal $y(t)$, with the transient component going to zero (or to a constant value for an integrating system).

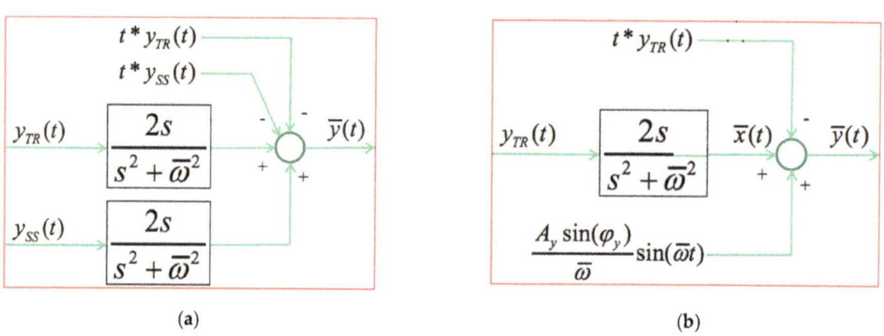

Figure A1. The robust scheme for determining the frequency response slope (**a**) intermediary solution, (**b**) final solution.

The steady-state component of the output signal is described by:

$$y_{SS}(t) = A_y \sin(\overline{\omega} t + \varphi_y) = S\sin(\overline{\omega} t) + C\cos(\overline{\omega} t), \quad \text{(A12)}$$

with the constants $S = A_y \cos(\varphi_y)$ and $C = A_y \sin(\varphi_y)$. Applying the Laplace transform to (A12) leads to:

$$Y_{SS}(s) = \frac{S\overline{\omega}}{s^2 + \overline{\omega}^2} + \frac{Cs}{s^2 + \overline{\omega}^2} = \frac{S\overline{\omega} + Cs}{s^2 + \overline{\omega}^2}, \quad \text{(A13)}$$

having the derivative equal to:

$$\frac{dY_{SS}(s)}{ds} = \frac{C(s^2 + \overline{\omega}^2) - 2s(S\overline{\omega} + Cs)}{(s^2 + \overline{\omega}^2)^2} = \frac{C}{s^2 + \overline{\omega}^2} - \frac{2s}{s^2 + \overline{\omega}^2}\frac{S\overline{\omega} + Cs}{s^2 + \overline{\omega}^2} = \frac{C}{s^2 + \overline{\omega}^2} - \frac{2s}{s^2 + \overline{\omega}^2} Y_{SS}(s). \quad \text{(A14)}$$

Applying the inverse Laplace transform to (A14) gives the following result:

$$-t * y_{SS}(t) = \frac{A_y sin(\varphi_y)}{\overline{\omega}} sin(\overline{\omega} t) - \mathcal{L}^1\left\{ \frac{2s}{s^2 + \overline{\omega}^2} Y_{SS}(s) \right\}. \quad \text{(A15)}$$

Based on the result in (A15), Figure A1a can be replaced by Figure A1b. The Laplace transform of the signal x(t) can be computed based on Figure A1b as:

$$\overline{X}(s) = \frac{2s}{s^2 + \overline{\omega}^2} Y_{TR}(s) = \frac{2s}{\overline{\omega}} Y_{TR}(s) \frac{\overline{\omega}}{s^2 + \overline{\omega}^2}, \quad \text{(A16)}$$

leading to:

$$\overline{x}(t) = \mathcal{L}^{-1}\left\{ \frac{2s}{\overline{\omega}} Y_{TR}(s) \right\} \sin(\overline{\omega} t). \quad \text{(A17)}$$

Considering the fact that the component $t^* y_{TR}(t)$ does not influence the steady-state oscillation in $\overline{y}(t)$ and the result in (A17), Figure A1b reduces to the simplified version in Figure A2.

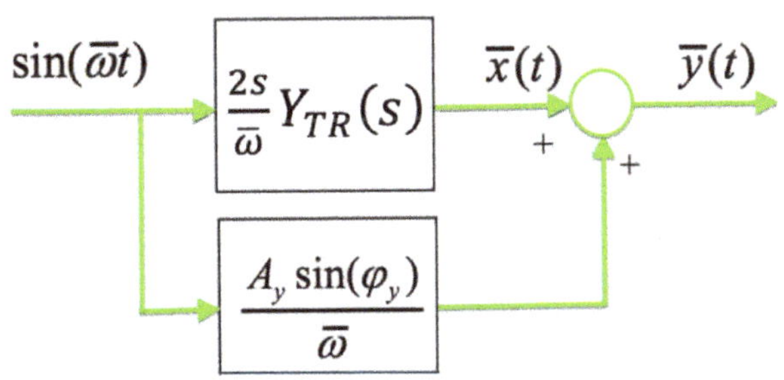

Figure A2. Simplified robust scheme for determining the frequency response slope.

Based on Figure A2, the amplitude $A_{\overline{y}}$ and phase $\varphi_{\overline{y}}$ of the signal $\overline{y}(t)$ at the specific frequency $\overline{\omega}$ can be determined as:

$$A_{\overline{y}} e^{j\varphi_{\overline{y}}} = A_{\overline{x}} e^{j\varphi_{\overline{x}}} + \frac{A_y \sin(\varphi_y)}{\overline{\omega}}. \quad \text{(A18)}$$

The corresponding amplitude $A_{\overline{x}}$ and phase $\varphi_{\overline{x}}$ at the specific frequency $\overline{\omega}$ can be obtained from the frequency response of the system $\frac{2s}{\overline{\omega}}Y_{TR}(s)$. Using the definition of the Laplace transform this results in:

$$\frac{2s}{\overline{\omega}}Y_{TR}(s) = \frac{2s}{\overline{\omega}}\int_0^\infty y_{TR}(t)e^{-st}dt, \tag{A19}$$

$$A_{\overline{x}}e^{j\varphi_{\overline{x}}} = 2j\int_0^\infty y_{TR}(t)e^{-j\overline{\omega}t}dt. \tag{A20}$$

The integral on the right-hand side of (A9) is computed based on the Discrete Fourier Transform as:

$$\int_0^\infty y_{TR}(t)e^{-j\overline{\omega}t}dt = T_s\sum_{k=0}^{N-1} y_{TR}(kT_s)e^{-j\overline{\omega}kT_s}. \tag{A21}$$

Remark A1. *The transient signal $y_{TR}(t)$ is assumed to be zero after $N.T_s$ seconds. For an integrating system, the transient signal $y_{TR}(t)$ converges to a constant value y_c. In this case, the Discrete Fourier Transform of $|y_{TR}(t) - y_c|$ is firstly calculated and afterwards corrected with the Fourier Transform of a step signal with amplitude y_c, i.e., $\frac{y_c}{j\overline{\omega}}$ should be added.*

The proposed robust method to estimate the frequency response slope of a system based on a single sine test is summarised below.

1. Perform a sine-test on the system using as the input signal a sine of the form $u(t) = A_u\sin(\overline{\omega}t)$. The sampling period for data acquisition is T_s, and the total number of measured samples is N.
2. Analyse the steady-state oscillation of y(t) to determine the amplitude A_y and phase φ_y using (42)
3. Calculate the transient part $y_{TR}(t)$ as: $y_{TR}(t) = y(t) - y_{ss}(t)$, with $y_{ss}(t) = A_y\sin(\overline{\omega}t + \varphi_y)$
4. Calculate the complex number $A_{\overline{y}}e^{j\varphi_{\overline{y}}} = 2jT_s\sum_{k=0}^{N-1} y_{TR}(kT_s)e^{-j\overline{\omega}kT_s} + \frac{A_y\sin(\varphi_y)}{\overline{\omega}}$.
5. Calculate the frequency response of the process and the frequency response slope at the frequency $\overline{\omega}$ as: $P(j\overline{\omega}) = Me^{j\varphi} = \frac{A_y}{A_u}e^{j\varphi_y}$ and $\left.\frac{dP(j\omega)}{d(j\omega)}\right|_{\omega=\overline{\omega}} = j\frac{A_{\overline{y}}}{A_u}e^{j\varphi_{\overline{y}}}$.

References

1. Casas-Arroyave, F.D.; Fernández, J.M.; Zuleta-Tobón, J.J. Evaluation of a closed-loop intravenous total anesthesia delivery system with BIS monitoring compared to an open-loop target-controlled infusion (TCI) system: Randomized controlled clinical trial. *Colomb. J. Anesthesiol.* **2019**, *47*, 84–91. [CrossRef]
2. Neckebroek, M.; Ionescu, C.M.; van Amsterdam, K.; De Smet, T.; De Baets, P.; Decruyenaere, J.; De Keyser, R.; Struys, M.M.R.F. A comparison of propofol-to-BIS post-operative intensive care sedation by means of target controlled infusion, Bayesian-based and predictive control methods: An observational, open-label pilot study. *J. Clin. Monit. Comput.* **2018**, *33*, 675–686. [CrossRef]
3. Brogi, E.; Cyr, S.; Kazan, R.; Giunta, F.; Hemmerling, T.M. Clinical performance and Safety of Closed-Loop Systems: A systematic review and meta-analysis of randomized controlled trials. *Anesth. Analg.* **2017**, *124*, 446–455. [CrossRef]
4. Carter, S.G.; Eckert, D.J. Effects of hypnotics on obstructive sleep apnea endotypes and severity: Novel insights into pathophysiology and treatment. *Sleep Med. Rev.* **2021**, *58*, 101492. [CrossRef] [PubMed]
5. Garg, N.; Kalra, Y.; Panwar, S.; Arora, M.K.; Dhingra, U. Comparison of target concentration of propofol during three phases of live donor liver transplant surgery using a target-controlled infusion of propofol total intravenous anaesthesia—A prospective, observational pilot study. *Indian J. Anaesth.* **2024**, *68*, 971–977. [PubMed]
6. Fahlenkamp, A.V.; Peters, D.; Biener, I.; Billoet, C.; Apfel, C.; Rossaint, R.; Coburn, M. Evaluation of bispectral index and auditory evoked potentials for hypnotic depth monitoring during balanced xenon anaesthesia compared with sevoflurane. *Br. J. Anaesth.* **2010**, *105*, 334–341. [CrossRef] [PubMed]
7. Schiavo, M.; Padula, F.; Latronico, N.; Paltenghi, M.; Visioli, A. Individualized PID tuning for maintenance of general anesthesia with propofol and remifentanil coadministration. *J. Process Control* **2021**, *109*, 74–82. [CrossRef]

8. Soltesz, K.; Van Heusden, K.; Dumont, G.A. In *Automated Drug Delivery in Anesthesia*; Models for control of intravenous anesthesia. Academic Press: Cambridge, MA, USA, 2020; pp. 119–166. [CrossRef]
9. West, N.; van Heusden, K.; Görges, M.; Brodie, S.; Rollinson, A.; Petersen, C.L.; Dumont, G.A.; Ansermino, J.M.; Merchant, R.N. Design and evaluation of a Closed-Loop anesthesia system with robust control and safety system. *Anesth. Analg.* **2018**, *127*, 883–894. [CrossRef]
10. Shah, P.; Agashe, S. Review of fractional PID controller. *Mechatronics* **2016**, *38*, 29–41. [CrossRef]
11. Hegedus, E.T.; Birs, I.R.; Ghita, M.; Muresan, C.I. Fractional-Order Control Strategy for Anesthesia–Hemodynamic stabilization in patients undergoing surgical procedures. *Fractal Fract.* **2022**, *6*, 614. [CrossRef]
12. Méndez, J.A.; Marrero, A.; Reboso, J.A.; León, A. Adaptive fuzzy predictive controller for anesthesia delivery. *Control Eng. Pract.* **2015**, *46*, 1–9. [CrossRef]
13. Schiavo, M.; Padula, F.; Latronico, N.; Paltenghi, M.; Visioli, A. Experimental results of an event-based PID control system for propofol and remifentanil coadministration. *Control Eng. Pract.* **2023**, *131*, 105384. [CrossRef]
14. Popescu, T.; Badau, N.; Mihai, M.; Hegedus, E.; Birs, I.; Copot, D.; Dulf, E.H.; Muresan, C.I. Advancing Anesthesia Education: Training on Modeling and Control for Enhanced Patient Care. In Proceedings of the 4th Workshop on Internet Based Control Education (IBCE), Ghent, Belgium, 18–20 September 2024.
15. Parvinian, B.; Pathmanathan, P.; Daluwatte, C.; Yaghouby, F.; Gray, R.A.; Weininger, S.; Morrison, T.M.; Scully, C.G. Credibility evidence for computational patient models used in the development of physiological Closed-Loop controlled devices for critical care medicine. *Front. Physiol.* **2019**, *10*, 220. [CrossRef]
16. Eleveld, D.J.; Colin, P.; Absalom, A.R.; Struys, M.M.R.F. Pharmacokinetic–pharmacodynamic model for propofol for broad application in anaesthesia and sedation. *Br. J. Anaesth.* **2018**, *120*, 942–959. [CrossRef] [PubMed]
17. Van Den Berg, J.P.; Vereecke, H.E.M.; Proost, J.H.; Eleveld, D.J.; Wietasch, J.K.G.; Absalom, A.R.; Struys, M.M.R.F. Pharmacokinetic and pharmacodynamic interactions in anaesthesia. A review of current knowledge and how it can be used to optimize anaesthetic drug administration. *Br. J. Anaesth.* **2017**, *118*, 44–57. [CrossRef]
18. Linassi, F.; Zanatta, P.; Spano, L.; Burelli, P.; Farnia, A.; Carron, M. Schnider and Eleveld Models for Propofol Target-Controlled Infusion Anesthesia: A Clinical comparison. *Life* **2023**, *13*, 2065. [CrossRef]
19. De Keyser, R.; Muresan, C.I.; Ionescu, C.M. A novel auto-tuning method for fractional order PI/PD controllers. *ISA Trans.* **2016**, *62*, 268–275. [CrossRef]
20. Caiado, D.V.; Lemos, J.M.; Costa, B.A.; Paz, L.A.; Mendonca, T.F. A polynomial design approach to robust control of neuromuscular blockade of patients subject to general anesthesia. In Proceedings of the 52nd IEEE Conference on Decision and Control, Firenze, Italy, 10–13 December 2013. [CrossRef]
21. Monje, C.A.; Chen, Y.; Vinagre, B.M.; Xue, D.; Feliu, V. *Fractional-Order Systems and Controls*; Springer: Berlin/Heidelberg, Germany, 2010. [CrossRef]
22. Lemos, J.; Caiado, D.V.; Costa, B.A.; Paz, L.A.; Mendonca, T.F.; Rabico, R.; Esteves, S.; Seabra, M. Robust control of Maintenance-Phase Anesthesia [Applications of control]. *IEEE Control Syst.* **2014**, *34*, 24–38. [CrossRef]
23. Pawłowski, A.; Schiavo, M.; Latronico, N.; Paltenghi, M.; Visioli, A. Event-based MPC for propofol administration in anesthesia. *Comput. Methods Programs Biomed.* **2023**, *229*, 107289. [CrossRef]
24. Ghita, M.; Ghita, M.; Copot, D. In *Automated Drug Delivery in Anesthesia*; An overview of computer-guided total intravenous anesthesia and monitoring devices—Drug infusion control strategies and analgesia assessment in clinical use and research. Academic Press: Cambridge, MA, USA, 2020; pp. 7–50. [CrossRef]
25. Bataille, A.; Guirimand, A.; Szekely, B.; Michel-Cherqui, M.; Dumans, V.; Liu, N.; Chazot, T.; Fischler, M.; Le Guen, M. Does a hypnosis session reduce the required propofol dose during closed-loop anaesthesia induction? *Eur. J. Anaesthesiol.* **2018**, *35*, 675–681. [CrossRef]
26. Schnider, T.W.; Minto, C.F.; Gambus, P.L.; Andresen, C.; Goodale, D.B.; Shafer, S.L.; Youngs, E.J. The influence of method of administration and covariates on the pharmacokinetics of propofol in adult volunteers. *Anesthesiology* **1998**, *88*, 1170–1182. [CrossRef] [PubMed]
27. Mihai, M.; Birs, I.; Erwin, H.; Copot, D.; Neckebroek, M.; De Keyser, R.; Ionescu, C.M.; Muresan, C.I. First-Hand Design of a Fractional order PID for Controlling the Depth of Hypnosis during Induction. *IFAC-Pap.* **2024**, *58*, 186–191. [CrossRef]
28. Åström, K.J.; Hägglund, T. Revisiting the Ziegler–Nichols step response method for PID control. *J. Process Control* **2004**, *14*, 635–650. [CrossRef]
29. Ghita, M.; Neckebroek, M.; Muresan, C.; Copot, D. Closed-Loop Control of Anesthesia: Survey on actual trends, challenges and perspectives. *IEEE Access* **2020**, *8*, 206264–206279. [CrossRef]
30. Padula, F.; Ionescu, C.; Latronico, N.; Paltenghi, M.; Visioli, A.; Vivacqua, G. Optimized PID control of depth of hypnosis in anesthesia. *Comput. Methods Programs Biomed.* **2017**, *144*, 21–35. [CrossRef] [PubMed]
31. Merigo, L.; Padula, F.; Latronico, N.; Paltenghi, M.; Visioli, A. Optimized PID control of propofol and remifentanil coadministration for general anesthesia. *Commun. Nonlinear Sci. Numer. Simul.* **2018**, *72*, 194–212. [CrossRef]

32. Dumont, G.A.; Martinez, A.; Ansermino, J.M. Robust control of depth of anesthesia. *Int. J. Adapt. Control Signal Process.* **2008**, *23*, 435–454. [CrossRef]
33. Thomas, E.; Martin, F.; Pollard, B. Delayed recovery of consciousness after general anaesthesia. *BJA Educ.* **2020**, *20*, 173–179. [CrossRef]
34. Paolino, N.; Schiavo, M.; Latronico, N.; Padula, F.; Paltenghi, M.; Visioli, A. On the Use of FOPID Controllers for Maintenance Phase of General Anesthesia. *Appl. Sci.* **2023**, *13*, 7381. [CrossRef]
35. De Keyser, R.; Muresan, C.I.; Ionescu, C.M. Autotuning of a robust fractional order PID controller. *IFAC-Pap.* **2018**, *51*, 466–471. [CrossRef]
36. Copot, C.; Muresan, C.; Ionescu, C.-M.; Vanlanduit, S.; De Keyser, R. Calibration of UR10 Robot Controller through Simple Auto-Tuning Approach. *Robotics* **2018**, *7*, 35. [CrossRef]
37. De Keyser, R.; Ionescu, C.M.; Festila, C. A one-step procedure for frequency response estimation based on a Switch-Mode transfer function analyzer. In Proceedings of the 50th IEEE Conference on Decision and Control and European Control Conference, Orlando, FL, USA, 12–15 December 2011. [CrossRef]

MDPI AG
Grosspeteranlage 5
4052 Basel
Switzerland
Tel.: +41 61 683 77 34

Fractal and Fractional Editorial Office
E-mail: fractalfract@mdpi.com
www.mdpi.com/journal/fractalfract

MDPI

www.ingramcontent.com/pod-product-compliance
Lightning Source LLC
Chambersburg PA
CBHW061846210926
51850CB00006B/985
9783725855117